T0093915

Clinical Care for Homeless, Runaway and Refugee Youth

Curren Warf • Grant Charles
Editors

Clinical Care for Homeless, Runaway and Refugee Youth

Intervention Approaches, Education and Research Directions

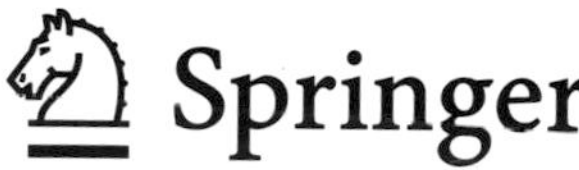

Editors
Curren Warf
Department of Pediatrics (Retired)
Division of Adolescent Health and Medicine
British Columbia Children's Hospital
University of British Columbia
Vancouver
BC
Canada

Grant Charles
School of Social Work
University of British Columbia
Vancouver
BC
Canada

ISBN 978-3-030-40677-6 ISBN 978-3-030-40675-2 (eBook)
https://doi.org/10.1007/978-3-030-40675-2

This Springer imprint is published by the registered company Springer Nature Switzerland AG
The registered company address is: Gewerbestrasse 11, 6330 Cham, Switzerland

Preface by Curren Warf

I have been working with youth for almost 30 years. I trained at Children's Hospital Los Angeles in Pediatrics and Adolescent Medicine. During that time, I became intensely interested in homeless youth and involved with the High Risk Youth Program (HRYP) led by Dr. Eric Cohen, an absolutely wonderful human being and physician, creative and fun with a natural ability to engage youth as well as students and other learners. This was in the early 1990s during the height of the HIV epidemic. HIV was a disease that had been unheard of in my own youth but was emerging as a terrifying, incurable, and infectious illness that affected many of the vulnerable young people that were on the streets. Tragically, and that word does not do justice, but tragically, my wonderful friend Eric contracted HIV. I, but in truth our entire team, witnessed Eric's decline before the first effective antiretrovirals were developed. Eric received one infusion but soon succumbed. His memory continues to inspire me. I took Eric's position as the Medical Director of the High Risk Youth Program which continued to be a pivotal learning experience for me. Always energized, always behind. Always more demands than could possibly be addressed. I worked with a wonderful interdisciplinary staff, youthful and energetic in a network of dedicated and creative community agencies. I continued as the Medical Director of the program for 15 years.

In 2009, I was recruited to the Department of Pediatrics at British Columbia Children's Hospital in Vancouver, Canada, with the goal of reinvigorating the Division of Adolescent Medicine and creating a new Subspecialty Residency Program. I had hoped to use my background with the HRYP to replicate the model. But circumstances in Vancouver were very different, and I had not come into untouched territory. There were many talented people who had developed programs targeting vulnerable youth when I arrived. The problem of literal homelessness was, frankly, much smaller than in Los Angeles, and families were much more likely to continue to be involved. The BC health-care system provides health care for all children, youth, and adults and a network of free Youth Health Clinics to address the contraceptive and sexual health needs of youth. The Ministry of Child and Family Development was deeply involved with homeless youth, and an independent advocate, the Representative for Children and Youth, was a passionate spokesperson for young people. It was a different society, a still imperfect but more equitable society, with much reduced violence and suicide, and more stably funded youth targeted programs.

For all of Canada's wonders, and there are many, there remain inequities that disproportionately affect indigenous people and youth, many of whom now live in urban environments. Refugees and immigrants are largely welcomed, though not without some barriers. I made a wonderful network of friends and colleagues in Canada and through our shared professional organizations, in particular the Society for Adolescent Health and Medicine, developed vital collaborations with others around the world in Brazil, Cuba, Mexico, Saudi Arabia, the Palestinian territories, Britain, Australia, and the United States. In conceptualizing this project, I invited many of these individuals specializing in adolescent medicine to make contributions. The results are reflected in this book.

I have now retired. I am no longer an adolescent, though somehow the youth that I had been seems as alive as ever in my heart, and I continue to reflect on the traumas and the sustaining relationships of that period of life. As I reflect upon what we have accomplished and what needs to be done, I appreciate that our goals must embrace not only our own generation, or the generation of our children or our grandchildren, but the world we will be leaving to future generations. Surrounded by the culture and natural beauty of the West Coast of North America, I continue to wonder what will be left in the face of global warming and climate change. As my wife and I drove south on our return from British Columbia through California, we were surrounded by wildfires, undoubtedly the product of global warming. It seems to me that with all the work we put into acute medical care, we may be missing the greatest public health challenge in human history, one that our descendants will have to confront.

Since returning to California, a new crisis has emerged on the US-Mexico border that has profound effects on children and youth. I worry deeply about the resurgence of white supremacy, the hateful rhetoric directed at immigrants and minorities, and the not-so-subtle threats of violence that resonate with earlier historic periods. I see children and youth growing up in this world and worry about the forces that shape their lives and conscience and sense of human decency. I remember the beautiful and idealistic youth that I have known, who survived and thrived in difficult settings, and hope that their energy, hope, and creativity will see us through.

Finally, I must express my deepest gratitude to my beloved wife and partner of over 35 years, Susan Rabinovitz, without whose support and incredible patience this book would never have been completed.

Vancouver, BC, Canada Curren Warf

Preface by Grant Charles

I have been working with young people for 50 years as a child and youth care practitioner and as a social worker. My first job was working with street-entrenched youth and adults in Central London. I was a young kid from Canada who was completely unprepared for what I experienced in England. I had no clue of the extent of homelessness in the United Kingdom or what it meant. I came up against people who had been crushed by the cruelty and apathy of their society. I was completely naive about the extent of oppression people came up against in their lives. I didn't last long at that job and ended up homeless myself for a short period of time. Again, it was eye-opening.

What has stuck with me the most all these years was the divide that was evident to me between those serving and those being served. There was an imbalance to the relationship in many cases that seemed to add to the dehumanizing aspect of being on the street. I suppose that this is to be expected on one level in that the two potentially see the "relationship" differently. To the helper, the interaction is often a one-time deal where they are simply providing a service. They are doing their job. That is not to say that the provider is trying to be detached or impersonal but rather that the nature of the circumstances almost dictates that it be structured that way. The interactions are rushed because of the context and the demand. The unfortunate result though is that the person receiving the services can feel dehumanized. This is not to say that the provider is purposely dehumanizing the other. However, to a person who is living in dehumanizing circumstances, much of their world is seen as dehumanizing. As such, it becomes important to take the time for all of us as providers to try to see our interactions through the eyes of others. It may be as a result that we become a little more "human" and a little less "clinical" in our relationships, however brief, with those receiving our services by practicing more humility and humanity we may have an impact on other people that is more influential than our intervention. From my short time on the streets, and it was only a brief period, it is the moments of humanity that stick with me the most.

In the years since that time in England, I have worked in most of the systems that provide services to young people and their families. While most of my career has been spent in the area of child and youth mental health, I have never lost my understanding that safe and secure housing needs to be at the root of all of our interventions. Without it, most of our other interventions will be ineffective or at least significantly lessened in effectiveness. The best medical or mental health interventions are diminished if the person receiving the service ends up in insecure or inadequate housing or if they end up on the streets. Regardless of where we work or the type of work we do, it is worth our while to spend at least some of our time and energy advocating for housing. It is a basic human right.

Vancouver, BC, Canada Grant Charles

Acknowledgments

This book would not have been possible without many collaborators including Abdulkarim Al Makadma, Saud Alobaida, Marvin Belzer, Meera Beharry, Diana Birch, Sara Chown, Margaret Colbourne, Bridgid Mariko Conn, Amy Dworsky, Joshua Edward, Evelyn Eisenstein, Natalie Finner, Ronald George Friesen, Kiaras Gharabaghi, Narv Gill, Ken Ginsburg, Troy Grennan, John Howard, Irene Jillson, Christine Loock, Judy Lynam, Stephanie Martin, Eva Moore, Celia Neavel, Maya Peled, Tracy Pickett, Amanda Pollicino, Nina Preto, Mari Radzik, Wingfield Rehmus, Arlene Schneir, Sara Sherer, Annie Smith, Shazeen Suleman, Gary Tennant, Jimmy Wang, Tom Warshawski, Jonathan Warus, Juliana Wu, Alice Virani, and Dzung Vo. Thank you for your contributions to this book and more importantly for your work with young people and families. This world would be much worse off without your dedicated work and daily contributions.

Finally, we would like to thank Springer Publishers, specifically Prakash Jagannathan and Miranda Finch, for their constant support, patience, organization, and flexibility that have led to the actualization of this project.

Framework for Utilizing This Book

This book is the product of the contributions of many individuals with strong backgrounds in working with homeless youth – clinically, programmatically, and in research. Each contributor has come to the table with their own special background and focus. We are fortunate and thankful to have contributors from Australia, Britain, Brazil, Canada, and the United States though the focus of most of the material is on the United States and Canada.

Youth experiencing homelessness live and survive around the world. Many live in major urban centers; others live in rural environments. Some homeless youth are members of homeless families, some couch surf from place to place, and others are unaccompanied and survive with other young people or on their own. Not all youth are affected equally by homelessness; lesbian, gay, and transgender youth are disproportionately represented and in one US study ranged from 20% to 40% of homeless youth, with the highest rates among LGBT African American youth, especially young men [1]. Despite many promises to end homelessness in the United States, we have witnessed a continuing high prevalence of youth experiencing homelessness, increasingly visible in many metropolitan areas.

Understanding and Responding to the Needs of Youth Experiencing Homelessness

In June 2010, the US Interagency Council on Homelessness released Opening Doors, the first comprehensive federal strategic plan to prevent and end homelessness, with the specific goal of ending homelessness for families, children, and youth by 2020 [2]. While that goal has clearly not been met, the plan has been useful in advancing our understanding and shaping our interventions and cogently recognized that:

> Every night, thousands of unaccompanied young people go to sleep without the safety, stability, and support of a family or a home. In contrast to common perceptions, homelessness

is not just an adult phenomenon; youth are resorting to abandoned buildings, park benches, makeshift shelters, and staying with friends and sometimes strangers. Many of these youth have experienced significant trauma before and after becoming homeless. Often they face struggles across multiple aspects of daily life that contribute to their vulnerability. At the same time, all youth have strengths, but youth experiencing homelessness often lack positive opportunities and supports to apply them. An effective strategy must account for the specific needs of adolescents and youth transitioning to adulthood and the role families can play in both the reasons for becoming homeless and the potential solutions. These considerations make an approach to ending homelessness for unaccompanied youth distinct from an approach to ending homelessness for adults…An overarching commitment to impacting core outcomes for youth experiencing homelessness – stable housing, permanent connections, education or employment, and social-emotional well-being – guides every aspect of this work…ending youth homelessness is too urgent a cause to wait for perfect solutions…

Why This Book

The goal of this book is to help provide clinicians and others with tools and resources to better understand the scope and complexity of youth homelessness, engage youth and families in care, and provide services to youth experiencing homelessness to reduce their risks and support their healthy growth and development. This book is not intended to be a complete compendium of interventions for youth experiencing homelessness, and we appreciate that we have omitted discussion of key areas of concern. We have selected content and organized chapters to help deepen the reader's understanding of the complex and overlapping social, economic, environmental, and community factors contributing to homelessness, the dominance of inequality and discriminations as key drivers, and the need for both individual interventions and structural changes to prevent and reduce homelessness among young people. We expect that interventions discussed for one type of problem – e.g., motivational interviewing for substance use – will have broad applicability and utility for other challenges confronting young people and the adults taking care of them, and we hope that we have stimulated creative ideas and innovative solutions to youth homelessness grounded in a positive youth development approach.

First things first, interviewing and communicating with adolescents requires one to recognize and value the potential of the true person. Communication with a young person experiencing homelessness requires patience, persistence, and recognition of their strengths and potentials. One of the early chapters (*Interviewing Homeless Adolescents in the Context of Clinical Care: Creating Connections, Building on Strengths, Fostering Resilience, and Improving Outcomes*) provides an authentic and valuable orientation for skill development and understanding of youth who have experienced trauma and survive in high-risk environments.

Social Pediatrics

Youth homelessness has roots in social determinants of health that have shaped the conditions in which they live, grow up, and mature including challenges of poverty, inequity of opportunity, discrimination, and lack of educational opportunities. Parents, as much as they love and want to support their children, sometimes live with an overwhelming level of stress and economic insecurity and struggle to avoid passing on to their children the legacy of the trauma that they have experienced.

Social pediatrics is an approach for children in stressed families and under-resourced communities to build expanded supports and meaningfully engage extended family and community members in building relationships and creating social and physical environments that promote stability in the face of significant challenges. It offers the potential to reduce the complex drivers of youth homelessness through community-level interventions to support youth and families. In this book, we have reviewed the history of social pediatrics and describe the development of a remarkable program in Vancouver, British Columbia, that may serve as inspiration for new programs in other localities.

Understanding the Clinical Needs of Homeless Youth

There are chapters focused on identifying and addressing the common and more difficult clinical needs of youth experiencing homelessness including evaluation and intervention for the patient at risk for suicide; access to full-spectrum contraceptive services; evaluation of the sexual assault victim; diagnosis and treatment of sexually transmitted infections; testing, prevention, and treatment for HIV; and dermatological problems. Clinical sections of the book are not intended to be comprehensive but to highlight specific areas commonly encountered in the care of youth who are experiencing homelessness and refer the reader to clinical guidelines and other resources for medical management.

Developing Skills in Motivational Interviewing for Adolescents with Substance Use Disorders

Adolescents and young adults, particularly those on the streets, commonly experiment with and may become seriously affected by substance use. This can interfere with their functioning and has long-term consequences for their education, employability, and interpersonal relationships. Motivational interviewing is a teachable, practical approach to developing clinical skills to support young people in behavior change efforts.

New Approaches for Youth in an Era of Rapid Escalation of Deaths from Opiate Overdose

With opiate overdose now the leading cause of death for adults under age 55 in both Canada and the United States and a leading and growing cause of death for adolescents, and the fact that adults addicted to opiates commonly initiate use as adolescents, we have included a chapter on assertive intervention with youth to interrupt opiate use, including certified (or mandated) hospital admission for stabilization after overdose and certified secure care to interrupt opiate use. We have engaged medical ethicists in this discussion to explore concerns related to autonomy in the treatment of adolescents. These models are not substitutes for evidence-based outpatient and inpatient treatment for substance use disorders or pharmaceutical intervention with suboxone or methadone for treatment of addiction, and they're a complement to harm reduction strategies such as safe injection sites and access to clean needles, syringes, and pharmaceuticals when these resources are available for those users who are not yet motivated to stop.

Refugees and Forced Migration as a World Driver for Homelessness of Adolescents

In recognition that youth homelessness is not unique to the United States and Canada or the developed world, we have included a brief review of international adolescent refugees that is often overlooked in discussions of youth homelessness. This chapter is necessarily abbreviated, given the historic roots, scope, and continuing rapid growth of numbers of migrants and refugees. The chapter contains four major themes: the existing international agreements to protect the rights of young refugees and migrants, the treatment of adolescent refugees and migrants in host countries, regional conditions that drive refugees to leave, and approaches to improve the conditions of refugee and migrant youth in host countries. With continued mass displacement of populations, accelerated by the climate crisis, both developing and developed countries will be faced with addressing the needs of these young people and their families.

Need for Research

Given the complexity of the challenges of addressing youth homelessness, there is a deep need for continued research both on the drivers and scope of homelessness and on the prevention and intervention strategies. We have included a section on engaging homeless youth themselves in research, a creative way to help young people find meaning in their experiences and play a significant role in guiding the development of new knowledge.

Limitations

This book represents the work of multiple collaborative teams and is intended to bring to bear the considerable expertise of many accomplished clinicians and researchers to understanding and addressing the problem of youth homelessness. Our own biases and interests are reflected in the content and the issues that have been emphasized, and we apologize if we have neglected critical concerns. Any errors and omissions are ours.

Though many of the issues that are raised in this book are distressing and the problems that young people encounter are grave, those of us who work with young people are continually refreshed by the creativity, enthusiasm, and thoughtfulness that young people demonstrate when they are genuinely engaged. Working with young people is truly a hopeful process that continually demonstrates their great resilience.

This book was completed with the hope that it will make a meaningful contribution to improving services, increasing the understanding of health professionals, and improving the lives of youth who are emerging from high-risk environments that they neither created nor deserve and who embody such great potential for our shared future.

Since the development of this book, the COVID-19 pandemic has surged into every corner of the earth at an unprecedented pace and, unfortunately, the specific challenges of the pandemic could not be directly addressed in this book. It is already abundantly clear that those who live in poverty, in crowded conditions, homeless shelters, refugee camps, migrant detention, and institutional care are most vulnerable to the infection and its complications. The infection has already demonstrated a disproportionate impact on people living in poverty, and some minority populations, in particular African Americans and Indigenous peoples. The economic slowdown has disproportionately affected people working for low wages and already confronting housing instability and food insecurity. Public health interventions including "sheltering in place," critical to reducing the spread of the coronavirus, have been implemented; however, those who do not have a "place" are faced with harsh realities. Homeless and refugee youth and their families will be profoundly affected in the coming period. At the time of this writing, we anxiously await the development of an effective vaccine, readily available, sensitive and specific tests to enable identification of those infected and contact tracing, as well as effective and readily available antiviral treatment. It is essential that all youth and their families, inclusive of migrants and refugees, be provided the necessary supports to adhere to all available public health approaches to prevention, perhaps the most fundamental of which is a place to live.

Department of Pediatrics (Retired),
Division of Adolescent Health and Medicine,
British Columbia Children's Hospital,
University of British Columbia
Vancouver, BC, Canada

Curren Warf

School of Social Work, University of British Columbia
Vancouver, BC, Canada

Grant Charles

References

1. Morton MH, Samuels GM, Dworsky A, Patel, S. Missed opportunities: LGBTQ youth homelessness in America. Chicago: Chapin Hall at the University of Chicago; 2018. http://voicesofyouthcount.org/wp-content/uploads/2018/05/VoYC-LGBTQ-Brief-Chapin-Hall-2018.pdf. Accessed 22 May 2019.
2. United States Interagency Council on Homelessness. Framework to end youth homelessness: a resource text for dialogue and action. https://www.usich.gov/resources/uploads/asset_library/USICH_Federal_Youth_Framework.pdf. Accessed 21 May 2019.

Contents

Contributors

Abdul Karim AlMakadma, MD College of Medicine, Alfaisal University, Riyadh, Saudi Arabia

Saud A. Alobaida, MBBS, FRCPC Departments of Pediatrics and Dermatology, University of British Columbia, Vancouver, BC, Canada

Meera Beharry, MD, FAAP Adolescent Medicine, McLane Children's Medical Center Specialty Clinic, Temple, TX, USA

Marvin E. Belzer, MD, FACP, FSAM Department of Pediatrics, University of Southern California, Division of Adolescent and Young Adult Medicine, Children's Hospital Los Angeles, Los Angeles, CA, USA

Diana Birch, MBBS, DCH, MSc, MD Youth Support, London, UK

Grant Charles, PhD, RSW School of Social Work, University of British Columbia, Vancouver, BC, Canada

Sarah Chown, MPH YouthCO, Vancouver, BC, Canada

Margaret Colbourne, BSc, MD FRCP Department of Paediatrics, University of British Columbia, Vancouver, BC, Canada

Bridgid Mariko Conn, PhD Division of Adolescent and Young Adult Medicine, Children's Hospital Los Angeles, Los Angeles, CA, USA

Amy Dworsky, PhD Chapin Hall at the University of Chicago, Chicago, IL, USA

Joshua Edward, PhD Dalhousie University, Halifax, NS, Canada

Evelyn Eisenstein, MD, PhD University of the State of Rio de Janeiro, Rio de Janeiro, Brazil

Ronald George Friesen, LLB, BA(PE) University of Saskatchewan, Saskatoon, SK, Canada

University of Victoria, Victoria, BC, Canada

Continuing Legal Education Society of BC, Vancouver, BC, Canada

Kiaras Gharabaghi, PhD School of Child & Youth Care, Ryerson University, Toronto, ON, Canada

Ken Ginsburg, MD, MSEd The Division of Adolescent Medicine, The Children's Hospital of Philadelphia, Philadelphia, PA, USA

Covenant House Pennsylvania, Philadelphia, PA, USA

Troy Grennan, MSc, MD BC Centre for Disease Control, Vancouver, BC, Canada

John Howard, PhD National Drug and Alcohol Research Centre, UNSW Medicine | Faculty of Medicine, University of New South Wales – Sydney, Sydney, NSW, Australia

Irene Jillson, PhD Department of Family Medicine, Georgetown University School of Medicine, Washington, DC, USA

Christine Loock, MD, FRCPC, DABP Division of Developmental Pediatrics, Department of Pediatrics, British Columbia Children's Hospital, University of British Columbia, Vancouver, BC, Canada

Judith Lynam, PhD, RN University of British Columbia, School of Nursing, Faculty of Applied Sciences, Vancouver, BC, Canada

Stephanie Martin, BA McCreary Centre Society, Vancouver, BC, Canada

Eva Moore, MD, MSPH Division of Adolescent Health and Medicine, Department of Pediatrics, University of British Columbia, Vancouver, BC, Canada

Celia Neavel, MD, FSAHM, FAAFP Center for Adolescent Health, People's Community Clinic, Austin, TX, USA

Maya Peled, PhD McCreary Centre Society, Vancouver, BC, Canada

Tracy Ann Pickett, BScHon, MD, MForensMed, FRCPC Department of Emergency Medicine, University of British Columbia, Vancouver, BC, Canada

Amanda Pollicino, MPH Vancouver, BC, Canada

Nina Preto, LL.B, MSc (Bioethics), PhD Ethics Service, Provincial Health Services Authority, Vancouver, BC, Canada

Susan Rabinovitz, RN, MPH Division of Adolescent and Young Adult Medicine (Retired), Children's Hospital Los Angeles, Los Angeles, CA, USA

Mari Radzik, PhD Department of Pediatrics, Keck School of Medicine, University of Southern California, Los Angeles, CA, USA

Division of Adolescent and Young Adult Medicine, Children's Hospital Los Angeles, Los Angeles, CA, USA

Wingfield E. Rehmus, MD, MPH, FAAD Departments of Pediatrics and Dermatology, University of British Columbia, Vancouver, BC, Canada

Arlene Schneir, MPH Division of Adolescent and Young Adult Medicine, Children's Hospital Los Angeles, Los Angeles, CA, USA

Sara Sherer, PhD Department of Pediatrics, Keck School of Medicine, University of Southern California, Los Angeles, CA, USA

Division of Adolescent and Young Adult Medicine, Children's Hospital Los Angeles, Los Angeles, CA, USA

Annie Smith, MLA, PhD McCreary Centre Society, Vancouver, BC, Canada

Shazeen Suleman, MD, MPH Department of Pediatrics, St. Michael's Hospital, Toronto, ON, Canada

Faculty of Medicine, University of Toronto, Toronto, ON, Canada

Li Ka Shing Research Institute, St. Michael's Hospital, Toronto, ON, Canada

Gary Tennant, MSW Faculty of Child, Family and Community Studies, Douglas College, Vancouver, BC, Canada

Alice Virani, MA (Oxon), MS, MPH, PhD Ethics Service, Provincial Health Services Authority, Vancouver, BC, Canada

Department of Medical Genetics, University of British Columbia, Vancouver, BC, Canada

Dzung Vo, MD, FAAP, FSAHM Division of Adolescent Health and Medicine, Department of Pediatrics, BC Children's Hospital & University of British Columbia, Vancouver, BC, Canada

Jimmy Wang, MD Department of Pediatrics, University of British Columbia, Vancouver, BC, Canada

Curren Warf, MD, MSEd Department of Pediatrics (Retired), Division of Adolescent Health and Medicine, British Columbia Children's Hospital, University of British Columbia, Vancouver, BC, Canada

Tom Warshawski, MD, FRCP(C) School of Social Work, University of British Columbia, Vancouver, BC, Canada

Child and Youth Network, Interior Health Authority, Kelowna, BC, Canada

Jonathan D. Warus, MD, FAAP Department of Pediatrics, University of Southern California, Division of Adolescent and Young Adult Medicine, Children's Hospital Los Angeles, Los Angeles, CA, USA

Chapter 1
The Prevalence of Youth Homelessness in the United States

Amy Dworsky

Prevalence of Youth Homelessness in the United States

Youth homelessness is widely recognized as a major social problem in the United States. Every night, thousands of young people find themselves without a safe and stable home in which they can sleep. Although the experiences of homeless youth vary widely, the potential adverse consequences of homelessness for young people are clear. Research indicates that young people experiencing homelessness are at high risk for a range of negative outcomes including physical and mental health problems, physical and sexual victimization, early pregnancy and parenthood, substance use, and premature death (e.g., [2, 8, 9, 12, 14, 15, 20, 25]).

Attention to homelessness among youth has grown over the past decade, and efforts to address the problem have emerged at national, state, and local levels. In fact, the US Interagency Council on Homelessness (USICH) established a goal of ending youth homelessness by 2020 as part of its federal strategic plan [23].[1] However, efforts to end homelessness among youth will only be effective if they are based on credible data on the size of the homeless youth population and the characteristics of those youth.

Unfortunately, despite decades of research on homeless youth, we still don't know how many young people experience homelessness each year. Nor do we know how the size of the population has changed over time. Without this information, it is impossible to determine whether we are making progress toward the goal of ending homelessness among youth.

---

[1] USICH is composed of several federal agencies including the three that are most closely involved in addressing the needs of homeless youth: the U.S. Department of Health and Human Services (HHS), the U.S. Department of Housing and Urban Development (HUD), and the U.S. Department of Education (ED).

A. Dworsky (✉)
Chapin Hall at the University of Chicago, Chicago, IL, USA
e-mail: adworsky@chapinhall.org

C. Warf, G. Charles (eds.), *Clinical Care for Homeless, Runaway and Refugee Youth*, https://doi.org/10.1007/978-3-030-40675-2_1

This chapter begins with an examination of how much prior estimates of the number of young people who experience homelessness have varied. Next, it explores the reasons for this variation and the challenges associated with estimating the size of the homeless youth population. This is followed by a review of recent efforts to overcome those challenges, with a focus on the first national 12-month prevalence estimate of homelessness among 13- to 25-year-olds. It concludes with a discussion of why credible data on the number of youth experiencing homelessness are important and why additional information about those youth is also needed.

How Many Youth Experience Homelessness?

Over the past two decades, efforts to estimate the number of youth who experience homelessness have produced widely varying results [19, 22], ranging from tens of thousands to over a million (see Table 1.1). Some of this variation reflects differences in the methodologies, sampling strategies, and data sources that have been used. It also reflects differences in how "homeless" and "youth" are defined and whether the estimate is for a point in time (i.e., point prevalence) or for a year (12-month prevalence).

Additionally, most of these estimates have significant limitations [17]. As described more fully below, estimates based on point-in-time counts have traditionally excluded youth experiencing more hidden forms of homelessness (i.e., couch-surfing) as well as youth who frequently move between being homeless and being housed. Likewise, estimates based on data collected by or in schools (e.g., the U.S. Department of Education's data on homeless students or the Youth Risk Behavior Survey data) systematically exclude youth who are out of school or may fail to include youth who become homeless during the school year.

Why Don't We Know How Many Young People Experience Homelessness?

Estimating the number of youth who experience homelessness is complicated for both methodological and pragmatic reasons. To begin with, there are no universally accepted definitions of either "homeless" or "youth" [17, 22]. In the United States, each of the three federal agencies that administer programs for youth experiencing homelessness—the Department of Housing and Urban Development (HUD), the Department of Health and Human Services (HHS), and the Department of Education (ED)—defines the term *unaccompanied homeless youth* in a different way according to the federal statutes that authorize their programs (see Table 1.2).

Not surprisingly, these differences across federal agencies in the term "homeless youth" result in very different estimates of the number of youth who are homeless.

Table 1.1 Estimates of the number of youth experiencing homelessness

Estimate	Citation	Data source
• 5.0% 12-month prevalence rate of homelessness among 12- to 17-year-olds	Ringwalt et al. [21]	Data collected from a nationally representative household sample of nearly 6500 12- to 17-year-olds who responded to the 1992 Youth Risk Behavior Survey, a supplement to the National Health Interview Survey
• 22,000–44,000 18- to 19-year-olds were homeless on a single day or 80,000–170,000 per year • 31,000–59,000 20- to 24-year-olds were homeless on a single day or about 124,000–236,000 per year	Burt et al. [3]	Data collected from a nationally representative sample program providing homeless assistance services as part of the National Survey of Homeless Assistance Providers and Clients
• ~1.7 million 12 to 17-year-olds experienced a runaway or throwaway episode during a 12-month period • 300,000–400,000 homeless youth on any given day	Hammer et al. [11]	Data collected in 1999 as part of the three components of the 2nd National Incidence Study of Missing, Abducted, Runaway and Thrownaway Children (NISMART-2): National Household Survey of Adult Caretakers, National Household Survey of Youth, and Juvenile Facilities Study
• 118,364 unaccompanied youth enrolled in public school during the school year	National Center for Homeless Education [18]	Aggregated data from the 2016–2017 school year
• 40,799 unaccompanied youth under age 25 on a single night – 4789 under age 18 – 36,010 ages 18–24 • 9436 homeless parents under age 25 on a single night	Henry et al. [13]	Aggregated data from the 2017 annual Department of Housing and Urban Development PIT count
• 2.2–2.9% 1-month prevalence rate for unaccompanied youth homelessness among public high school students in Connecticut, Delaware, and Philadelphia	Cutuli et al. [6]	Data from the 2011 Youth Risk Behavior Survey (YRBS) of public high school students

Large differences in estimates are also observed when data from other sources are used. For example, a number of states have added a question to measure homelessness to the Youth Risk Behavior Survey (YRBS). The YRBS is a survey developed by the Centers for Disease Control and Prevention which is administered biennially to a representative sample of high school students across the United States [4]. Prior to 2017, the "homelessness" question was not standardized, making it difficult to combine data from or compare results across different states.[2]

[2] Students were asked some version of "Where did you usually sleep at night?" but the time frame (e.g., past 12 months, past 30 days, usually) and the response options varied.

Table 1.2 Federal definitions of homeless youth

	Federal Agency		
	Department of Housing and Urban Development	Department of Health and Human Services	Department of Education
Role	Administers homeless assistance programs (i.e., emergency shelter, transitional housing, and permanent supportive housing)	Administers the Basic Center, Transitional Living, and Street Outreach programs	Administers the Education for Homeless Children and Youth Program which provides state education agencies with funding to ensure that homeless children and youth have equal access to free and appropriate public education
Federal statute	McKinney–Vento Homeless Assistance Act (reauthorized by the Homeless Emergency Assistance and Rapid Transition to Housing (HEARTH) Act of 2009)	Runaway and Homeless Youth Act (reauthorized by the Reconnecting Homeless Youth Act of 2008)	*McKinney–Vento* Homeless Assistance Act (amended by the Every *Student Succeeds Act* of 2015)
Definition	Defines a homeless individual as someone who "lacks a fixed, regular, and adequate nighttime residence" or who "will imminently lose their primary nighttime residence" Unaccompanied youth under age 25 are also defined as homeless if they meet another federal definition of homeless (e.g., Runaway and Homeless Youth Act or McKinney–Vento Homelessness Assistance Act) and additional criteria related to housing instability Couch surfing or doubled-up youth may be considered homeless under some circumstances	Defines homeless youth as individuals age 21 or under "for whom it is not possible to live in a safe environment with a relative and who have no other safe alternative living arrangement"	Subtitle B of Title VII defines youth as homeless if they "lack a fixed, regular, and adequate nighttime residence" Definition applies to unaccompanied youth who are couch surfing and to youth who are homeless or doubled up with their families

Additionally, point-in-time counts, the primary method for counting homeless individuals and families in the United States has proven to be decidedly ineffective for counting homeless youth [1]. The Department of Housing and Urban Development (HUD) requires communities that receive HUD funding to operate programs for their homeless populations to conduct a point-in-time (PIT) count of sheltered and unsheltered individuals and families experiencing homelessness on a single night in January.[3] The "sheltered" count occurs annually; the "unsheltered"

[3]Technically, the counts are organized and conducted by the local or regional Continuum of Care (CoC). The CoC promotes community-wide planning and strategic use of resources to address homelessness among individuals (including unaccompanied youth) and families.

or "street" count occurs every other year. CoCs are required to include youth in their PIT counts and, since 2013, have been required to report the number of individuals broken down by age (i.e., under age 18, 18–24, and over age 24). Nevertheless, it is widely recognized that youth are routinely underrepresented in the annual HUD PIT counts [1, 24], and in many jurisdictions, the number of youth who are counted is implausibly low [6].

Several factors make youth experiencing homelessness a difficult population to count [1, 19]. First, homeless youth tend to be more mobile than homeless adults, and homelessness among youth tends to be more transient than homelessness among adults. Second, youth often experience more hidden forms of homelessness, such as couch surfing, and couch-surfing youth are more difficult to identify than youth who are staying in a shelter or on the streets.[4]

Third, many homeless youth don't want to be found and may go to great pains to avoid being detected. They may be fleeing an abusive family situation and may fear being returned home or being placed in foster care (if they are under 18) if they seek help from service providers. They may also fear detection by the police, particularly if they are engaging in illicit activities such as drug use or survival sex. Finally, youth may be reluctant to identify themselves as homeless due to the associated stigma.

Can PIT Counts Produce Reliable Estimates of the Number of Youth Experiencing Homelessness?

In 2010, the U.S. Interagency Council on Homelessness (USICH) established a goal of ending youth homelessness by 2020 as part of its federal strategic plan [23].[5] Three years later, USICH published its *Framework to End Youth Homelessness* which outlined the steps that must be taken if the goal of ending homelessness among youth by 2020 is to be achieved [24]. One of the framework's strategies is to obtain better data on the number and characteristics of youth experiencing homelessness, and one component of that strategy is the development of better methods for counting homeless youth in conjunction of the annual HUD PIT count.

In 2012, a federal interagency youth homelessness working group launched Youth Count! to develop promising strategies for counting unaccompanied homeless youth and promote collaboration among Continuum of Care (CoC) service providers, runaway and homeless youth (RHY) providers, state and local education agencies (SEAs and LEAs), and other local stakeholders. Nine diverse communities participated in the initiative: Boston, MA; Cleveland, OH; Hennepin County, MN;

[4] In fact, couch-surfing youth are explicitly excluded from the biennial HUD PIT count which is limited to individuals and families experiencing sheltered or unsheltered homelessness.

[5] USICH is composed of several federal agencies including the three that are most closely involved in addressing the needs of homeless youth: the U.S. Department of Health and Human Services (HHS), the U.S. Department of Housing and Urban Development (HUD), and the U.S. Department of Education (ED).

Houston, TX; Los Angeles, CA; New York, NY; Seattle/King County, WA; Washington Balance of State counties; and Winston-Salem, NC.[6]

A process study conducted by researchers from the Urban Institute [5, 19] found that these nine communities used a variety of different strategies to increase the number of homeless youth who were counted, including conducting surveys, expanding their coverage areas to include places where youth congregate, involving housed and homeless youth in the counts, coordinating with schools, and holding magnet events to draw in youth who don't stay in shelters or on the street. Based on their observations, the Urban Institute researchers identified a number of strategies that have the potential to improve youth counts. These included are the following:

- Engaging youth service providers
- Engaging LGBTQ partners
- Involving youth in count outreach and design
- Hosting magnet events
- Using social media to raise awareness and conduct outreach
- Framing survey questions as being about housing status, rather than homelessness, so that youth defined as homelessness under broader definitions are counted

However, the Youth County! communities were not required to apply a standard definition of homeless youth, thereby limiting the comparability of their results.

More recently, Voices of Youth Count, a national research and policy initiative led by Chapin Hall at the University of Chicago, conducted point-in-time counts of youth experiencing homelessness in 22 diverse counties across the United States [7]. The youth counts were one of the initiative's multiple components aimed at filling critical gaps in our knowledge about homelessness among youth. Voices of Youth Count used some of the same promising strategies that the Youth Count! communities had used. However, unlike Youth Count!, Voices of Youth Count applied a consistent methodology, including a uniform definition of homeless youth, in each of the 22 counties. Among the key features of that methodology were the following:

- Targeting locations where youth experiencing homelessness are likely to be found.
- Using survey data, rather than visual cues, to determine whether youth are homeless.
- Defining homelessness broadly.
- Engaging currently and formerly homeless youth in count planning and execution.
- Engaging a broad set of service providers and other local stakeholders.

Employing these strategies may lead to more successful counts—that is, counts that capture a larger share of the local homeless youth population. They can also provide communities with important information about the characteristics of that population and their service needs. However, even the most successful point-in-time

[6] https://www.usich.gov/tools-for-action/youth-count/

counts are unlikely to yield credible prevalence estimates of homelessness among youth because it is a largely hidden and dynamic phenomenon.

How Can the Prevalence of Youth Homelessness Be Estimated?

One strategy that can be used to estimate the prevalence of youth homelessness across the United States (or any other country for that matter) is a nationally representative household survey. In fact, the *Framework to End Youth Homelessness* calls for studying the prevalence of youth homelessness by leveraging an existing nationally representative household survey and repeating that survey periodically over time to monitor progress toward the goal of ending homelessness among youth [24].

This call for a national prevalence study of youth homelessness was not new. On the contrary, the Reconnecting Homeless Youth Act of 2008 authorized funding for HHS to conduct periodic prevalence studies of homelessness among 13- to 25-year-olds. However, no prevalence studies were ever conducted. Instead, a conference report that accompanied the Consolidated Appropriations Act for Federal Fiscal Year 2016 directed HUD to spend $2 million on the national prevalence study of homeless youth that Congress had previously authorized as part of the Reconnecting Homeless Youth Act. HUD used those funds to award a Research Partnerships grant to the Chapin Hall at the University of Chicago to support its Voices of Youth Count initiative.

In addition to conducting youth counts in 22 counties, as described above, Voices of Youth Count also conducted a national prevalence study of homelessness among 13- to 25-year-olds [16].[7] Specifically, Voices of Youth Count partnered with Gallup, Inc. to add a 19-item youth homelessness module to its U.S. Politics and Economics Daily Tracking Survey (DTS) [10]. The DTS is administered by telephone (both landline and cellphone) to 500 adults.[8] During two rounds of data collection (July to September 2016 and May to July 2017), the youth homelessness module was administered to 26,161 adults whose households included at least one 13- to 25-year-old during the preceding 12 months.[9] These adults comprised 38 percent of the 68,539 DTS respondents during the two rounds of data collection.

Two types of 12-month prevalence were estimated: *household prevalence* and *population prevalence*. *Household prevalence* was estimated separately for households that included at least one 13- to 17-year old and for households that included at least one 18- to 25-year old. *Population prevalence* was estimated for 18- to 25-year-olds but not for 13- to 17-year-olds because the DTS was only administered

[7] https://www.huduser.gov/portal/pdredge/pdr-edge-frm-asst-sec-080816.html

[8] https://www.gallup.com/224855/gallup-poll-work.aspx?utm_source=link_analyticsv9&utm_campaign=item_213755&utm_medium=copy

[9] Some respondents belonged to more than one of the subsamples.

Table 1.3 Estimated household and population prevalence of youth homelessness

Sample size	12-Month prevalence rate (%)	Population estimate
13,560 households with at least one 13- to 17-year old	4.3	660,000
16,975 households with at least one 18- to 25-year-old	12.5	2.4 million
6295 18- to 25-year-olds	9.7	3.5 million

Table 1.4 Estimated 12-month prevalence rates: urban/suburban compared to rural counties

Prevalence type	Urban/suburban (%)	Rural (%)
Households with at least one 13- to 17-year old	4.4	4.2
Households with at least one 18- to 25-year-old	13.6	12.3
18- to 25-year-olds	9.2	9.6

to adults. In all cases, homelessness was defined broadly to include couch surfing. The estimated 12-month prevalence of youth homelessness was 4.3% for households that included 13- to 17-year-olds and 12.5% for households that included 18- to 25-year-olds. The estimated 12-month population prevalence for 18- to 25-year-olds was 9.7%.[10]

When the household prevalence rates were applied to household population numbers derived from the U.S. Census Bureau's 2015 American Community Survey (ACS),[11] the number of households in which at least one 13- to 17-year-old experienced homelessness during the past 12 months was estimated to be 660,000, and the number of households in which at least one 18- to 25-year-old experienced homelessness during the past 12 months was estimated to be 2.4 million. When the population prevalence rate was applied to ACS population numbers, the number of 18- to 25-year-olds who had experienced homelessness during the past 12 months was estimated to be 3.5 million (see Table 1.3). These estimates are considerably higher than the estimates that prior studies had produced.

In addition to producing the first national 12-month prevalence estimate of youth homelessness in the United States, the study also compared the prevalence of youth homelessness in urban/suburban counties to the prevalence of youth homelessness in rural counties. Although youth homelessness tends to be far more visible in urban than in rural areas, urban/suburban and rural counties had very similar prevalence rates (see Table 1.4).

[10] See Morton et al. for more details about the estimating methodology.

[11] https://www.census.gov/programs-surveys/acs/about.html

Why Is Knowing the Number of Youth Who Experience Homelessness Important?

Credible data on the number of youth who experience homelessness are critical for a number of different reasons [1, 17]. First, communities need credible data on the number of youth who experience homelessness to inform the development of their continuum of care, particularly with respect to shelter beds, transitional housing, and other services and supports specifically for youth. Second, it is difficult to advocate effectively on both local and national levels for adequate resources to address the needs of homeless youth in the absence of credible data on the number of youth who experience homelessness. And third, credible data on the number of youth who experience homeless are essential if progress toward the goal of preventing and ending youth homelessness is to be measured.

Knowing the number of youth who experience homelessness is unquestionably important. Equally important, however, is knowing who these young people are and what their experiences with homelessness have been. Homeless youth comprise a heterogeneous population with diverse needs [7]. A clearer picture of the characteristics of the homeless youth population, especially the overrepresentation of certain subpopulations (e.g., youth who identify as lesbian, gay, bisexual, or transgender, pregnant and parenting youth, youth with a history of foster care, and African-American youth), is crucial if those diverse needs are to be addressed (e.g., [7, 8, 17]).

References

1. Auerswald C, Lin J, Petry L, Hyatt S. Hidden in plain sight: an assessment of youth inclusion in point-in-time counts of California's unsheltered homeless population. Sacramento: California Homeless Youth Project; 2013.
2. Auerswald C, Lin J, Parriott A. Six-year mortality in a street-recruited cohort of homeless youth in San Francisco, California. PeerJ. 2016;4:e1909.
3. Burt M, Aron L, Lee E. Helping America's homeless: emergency shelter or affordable housing? Washington, DC: Urban Institute Press; 2001.
4. Centers for Disease Control and Prevention. Methodology of the youth risk behavior surveillance system—2013. Morbid Mortal Wkly. 2013;62:1–20.
5. Cunningham M, Pergamit M, Astone N, Luna J. Counting homeless youth: promising practices from the youth count! initiative. Washington, DC: Urban Institute; 2014.
6. Cutuli J, Steinway C, Perlman S, Herbers J, Eyrich Garg K. Youth homelessness: prevalence and associations with weight in three regions. Health Soc Work. 2015;40:316–24.
7. Dworsky A, Horwitz B. Missed opportunities: counting youth experiencing homelessness in America. Chicago: Chapin Hall at the University of Chicago; 2018.
8. Dworsky A, Morton MH, Samuels GM. Missed opportunities: pregnant and parenting youth experiencing homelessness in America. Chicago: Chapin Hall at the University of Chicago; 2018.
9. Feldmann J, Middleman A. Homeless adolescents: common clinical concerns. Semin Pediatr Infect Dis. 2003;14:6–11.
10. Gallup I. Gallup daily methodology. New York: Gallup, Inc.; 2016.

11. Hammer H, Finkelhor D, Sedlak A. Runaway/thrownaway children: national estimates and characteristics. National Incident Studies of Missing, Abducted, Runaway, and Thrownaway Children. Washington, DC: US Department of Justice, Office of Justice Programs, Office of Juvenile Justice and Delinquency Prevention; 2002.
12. Heerde J, Hemphill S, Scholes-Balog K. Fighting for survival: a systematic review of physically violent behavior perpetrated and experienced by homeless young people. Aggress Violent Behav. 2014;19:50–66.
13. Henry M, Watt R, Rosenthal L, Shivji A. The 2017 annual homeless assessment report (AHAR) to congress: part one. Washington, DC: Department of Housing and Urban Development; 2017.
14. Hodgson K, Shelton K, van den Bree M, Los F. Psychopathology in young people experiencing homelessness: a systematic review. Am J Public Health. 2013;103:24–37.
15. Medlow S, Klineberg E, Steinbeck K. The health diagnoses of homeless adolescents: a systematic review of the literature. J Adolesc. 2014;37:531–42.
16. Morton MH, Dworsky A, Samuels GM. Missed opportunities: youth homelessness in America. National estimates. Chicago: Chapin Hall at the University of Chicago; 2017.
17. Morton MH, Samuels GM, Dworsky A, Patel S. Missed opportunities: LGBTQ youth homelessness in America. Chicago: Chapin Hall at the University of Chicago; 2018.
18. National Center for Homeless Education. National overview. 2018. Retrieved on 16 Sept 2018 from http://profiles.nche.seiservices.com/ConsolidatedStateProfile.aspx
19. Pergamit M, Cunningham M, Burt M, Lee P, Howell B, Bertumen K. Counting homeless youth: promising practices from the youth count! initiative. Washington, DC: Urban Institute; 2014.
20. Perlman S, Willard J, Herbers J, Cutuli J, Eyrich Garg K. Youth homelessness: prevalence and mental health correlates. J Soc Soc Work Res. 2014;5:361–77.
21. Ringwalt C, Greene J, Robertson M, McPheeters M. The prevalence of homelessness among adolescents in the United States. Am J Public Health. 1998;88:1325–9.
22. Toro P, Dworsky A, Fowler P. Homeless youth in the United States: recent research findings and intervention approaches. In: 2007 National symposium on homelessness research. Washington, DC: U.S. Department of Housing and Urban Development and the U.S. Department of Health and Human Services; 2007.
23. U.S. Interagency Council on Homelessness. *Opening doors: federal strategic plan to prevent and end homelessness*. Washington, DC: US Interagency Council on Homelessness; 2010.
24. U.S. Interagency Council on Homelessness. *Framework to end youth homelessness: a resource text for dialogue and action*. Washington, DC: US Interagency Council on Homelessness; 2013.
25. Whitbeck L, Hoyt D, Yoder K, Cauce A, Paradise M. Deviant behavior and victimization among homeless and runaway adolescents. J Interpers Violence. 2001;16:1175–204.

Chapter 2
Youth Homelessness in Canada: An Overview

Grant Charles, Curren Warf, and Gary Tennant

Introduction

As in the United States, there are many unknowns about youth who are homeless in Canada. There is a great deal we do not know about youth who are homeless in Canada. This is in part due to the difficulty in gathering information about the young people. It is also because until fairly recently, this population has been understudied or seen simply as a younger version of the adult homeless population. A third reason has been a lack of agreement on a definition of youth homelessness. This chapter will provide an overview on what we do know, the movement toward a common definition of homelessness, as well a synopsis of a recently developed prevention and intervention strategy framework.

Estimates of Prevalence

Having a consistently applied definition is critical not only because interventions need to be geared toward specific age groups to be effective but also how homelessness is defined influences the estimates of how many people are considered homeless. A definition that suggests that youth ranges from 13 to 18 years of age would provide a lower estimate than one that defines youth as 12–25. Policy and program

G. Charles
School of Social Work, University of British Columbia, Vancouver, BC, Canada

C. Warf (✉)
Department of Pediatrics (Retired), Division of Adolescent Health and Medicine, British Columbia Children's Hospital, University of British Columbia, Vancouver, BC, Canada

G. Tennant
Faculty of Child, Family and Community Studies, Douglas College, Vancouver, BC, Canada

C. Warf, G. Charles (eds.), *Clinical Care for Homeless, Runaway and Refugee Youth*, https://doi.org/10.1007/978-3-030-40675-2_2

development are often driven by numbers, and as such variations in definitions can have a significant impact upon how seriously the problem is taken or how many resources are dedicated toward supports and services.

It is difficult to accurately estimate the number of young people experiencing homelessness. As Dworsky points out in the previous chapter, there are significant differences in how homeless is defined. There can be variations in how youth is defined or what constitutes homelessness. The sampling strategies used to collect the data are also problematic [1, 11]. A common strategy for determining prevalence is a point-in-time count. For example, the City of Vancouver conducts a count every year that involves briefly surveying people in shelters and on the streets. While this provides a good gross measure that provides a general picture of homelessness on the day the count is conducted, this methodology has been criticized for underestimating the extent of youth homelessness as young people are more likely than their adult peers to experience hidden homelessness or to move in and out of being homeless [1, 9].

It should be noted that until quite recently much of what we knew about youth who are homeless in Canada was largely drawn upon from studies conducted in the United States. Apart from local or regional studies, often with small sample sizes, we had had little information systematically gathered to date about youth homelessness in Canada. This has changed in recent years although there is still a great deal we do not know about youth homelessness.

What we do know is that young people aged 13–24 make up approximately 20% of the homeless population in Canada [13]. This translates into roughly 35,000–40,000 youth being homeless in this country during the year with somewhere between 6000 and 7000 being homeless on any given night. Approximately 58% of young homeless self-identify as male [13].

Characteristics

People who identified as being indigenous and/or racialized were overrepresented with this homeless youth population [8, 13]. Young people who identify as LGBTQ2S (lesbian, gay, bisexual, transgender, questioning or two-spirited) are also overrepresented [13], particularly those who identify as transgender and gender expansive [33]. Many of these young people find it particularly difficult to access services because of the lack of LGBTQ2S-friendly or LGBTQ2S-specific services [31].

Although a still under-identified segment of the homeless population, it would appear that young people with disabilities are also overrepresented [2, 28]. Staff in support and intervention services often do not have the training to recognize youth with disabilities and as a result cannot be able to provide the support youth with disabilities need.

This under-identification is particularly true for young people with cognitive problems [6]. Youth with cognitive issues have a number of unique characteristics compared to other young people who are homeless. They have been found to have higher levels of vulnerability, in part as a result of their difficulties with attention, working memory, and processing speed. Given these issues young people in this population are less likely to benefit from conventional services and require specialized services that take into account their specific levels of functioning.

Approximately 40% of homeless young people experienced some form of homelessness before age 16 and were more likely to have suffered significant hardship prior to becoming homeless [13]. Those who became homeless prior to age 16 were also more likely to experience greater subsequent difficulties. They were more likely than their peers to have been involved in child protective services, to have experienced bullying, and to have been tested for ADHD. Once homeless they were more likely to become victims of crime, have mental health and substance misuse issues, have attempted suicide, and to become chronically homeless.

While those who first became homeless before the age of 16 have more commonly had significant early childhood aversive experiences, the majority of homeless young people, regardless of their age of entry, came from traumatic backgrounds. Many had histories prior to becoming homeless of abuse and neglect, school difficulties and adversity, mental health issues, and interactions with the child welfare and youth justice systems [10, 20, 22, 30].

These difficulties continue after the young people become homeless, particularly among certain populations such as Indigenous youth. Young people who are homeless and self-identify as Indigenous are more likely than their peers to be incarcerated [4]. They are also more likely to be involved in child protective services, engage in survival sex, and be diagnosed with HIV [21].

Young people who are homeless tend to differ significantly from their peers in a number of ways. In a study of young people in Vancouver, they were found to be over 160 times more likely to be involved in child protective services [3]. The young people who had been in state care were most likely to be Indigenous. There were also more likely to have started consuming hard substances at an earlier age than their peers and to have a parent who misused substances. They were also more likely to have been physically abused and less likely to have finished high school.

Substance misuse is a common feature among many of the youth that are homeless [7]. There is a relationship between incarceration, homelessness, and daily stimulant use [15]. Youth who are homeless also have a significantly higher risk for suicide than their peers [16, 19].

The vast majority of the studies about youth who are homeless tend to be conducted in urban and southern Canadian centers. There have been few studies involving young people in rural and remote communities. As a result, we know little about how these young people may differ from their urban peers in terms of characteristics and needs [17, 32].

Intervention Framework

It is widely recognized that while there need to be actions taken to help young people who are homeless secure housing and the associated supports, the only way to ultimately deal with homelessness is to address the issues causing it in the first place. Gaetz and Dej [12] have developed the New Directions Framework for homelessness prevention within which to conceptually understand how to address the factors which ultimately lead to people becoming homeless. They have provided the following definition of homelessness prevention:

> Homeless prevention refers to policies, practices and interventions that reduce the likelihood that someone will experience homelessness. (p. 6)

This New Directions Framework is based upon the understanding that since the causes of homelessness are the result of a combination of individual, relational factors, broader structural factors, and institutional failures to protect people from homelessness, then the solution has to address each of these areas. Given the range of what is needed to prevent homelessness, the development of the necessary interventions requires the establishment of a systems integration model that involves not just the homelessness sector but also all those other systems that serve people who ultimately are at risk of becoming homeless. This includes the broad systems that begin to work with people at an early age such as education and healthcare as well as those that provide specific services based upon individual circumstances such as housing, child protection, and criminal justice. This means engaging government ministries, nonprofit agencies, and community organizations. Based upon a human rights perspective, the New Directions Framework integrates an acknowledgment that prevention work also requires an intersectional and anti-oppressive orientation that addresses the specific needs of people who are systematically discriminated against in Canada due to colonization, sexism, racism, ableism, ageism, homophobia, transphobia, and other forms of oppression.

The New Directions Framework is based on a public health foundation that involves primary, secondary, and tertiary prevention interventions which focus on supporting people at points of vulnerability throughout their lives. Since there is rarely a single factor that contributes to homelessness, there need to be multiple structural interventions provided throughout the life span, as well as individually specific supports provided on an as-needed basis, to assist people with their unique needs.

The framework includes five categories, each of which addresses primary, secondary, and tertiary prevention. The typology includes the following:

1. Structural prevention
2. Systems prevention
3. Early intervention
4. Eviction prevention
5. Housing stability [12]

Structural prevention focuses on addressing risk factors through universal, selected, and indicated prevention through legislation, policy, and investment. This includes a continuum of services ranging from programs to support people facing discrimination such as members of the LGBTQ2S communities to violence prevention interventions to living wage strategies to health and mental health services.

Systems prevention looks to address organizational, institutional, and systems failures that, rather than assist in addressing homelessness, contribute to putting people at risk. There are three components to systems prevention. The first component involves addressing policy and procedural barriers that work against receiving the support they need. This might include agency policies that state that a young person has to be in a shelter by a certain hour even though they have a job that goes later than the time at which the doors close. The second component includes enhancing access to appropriate services and supports. Among many, this might include problems with mobility and transportation or linguistic, cultural, or class barriers. The third component includes the provision of reintegration supports for people transitioning from public systems such as child protection, criminal justice, and health and mental health services.

Early intervention in this framework involves the provision of services and supports to young people who are at imminent risk of becoming homeless. This includes outreach, identification and engagement supports, coordinated intake and assessment services, client-centered case management, and assistance with systems navigation, place-based supports, and shelter diversion. Gaetz and Dej [12] suggest that this may include services such as family mediation and reunification, school-based, intervention and intimate partner violence victim supports.

The last two components of systems prevention are evictions prevention and support of housing stability. Evictions prevention involves a range of strategies such as strengthening landlord–tenant laws and emergency financial assistance. The housing stability component involves assuring availability and engagement with services and supports that help people access and retain housing. This may include services that range from promoting social inclusion to supports dealing with life skills training to rent supplements.

Exiting

It appears the optimal time for youth to successfully exit the street is within the first year of becoming homeless. The longer one is homeless, the harder it is to make the transition back into the community [18]. This reflects the difficulty people have leaving the streets once they start to identify as being street involved. It is important to note that success in exiting is not just a matter of finding housing. It is clear that in order to transition from the streets to a community setting, what is required is a range of supports and services geared to the individual needs of each young person [19, 24]. The use of supportive housing is showing promising results [23, 24]. Young people in supportive housing do better than their peers who live in independent settings in terms of community engagement, quality of life, and mental health [18]. It would appear that a key component of this support needs to include the development of healthy and positive relationships with the young people in order [25, 26]. It would appear that having a sense of hope for a better future is also important as a component of a successful transition [19].

While previous studies have shown significant differences between the success rates of males and females, recent findings suggest that differences between males and females of exiting the streets and successfully transitioning may not be as great as previously thought [18]. This study found no significant differences in terms of gender or sexual orientation in the areas of mental health, quality of life, self-concept, and community integration among young people leaving the streets.

A key component of supporting the young people is ensuring that they have access to supportive and youth-friendly health services [5, 29]. This need for accessible services goes beyond basic healthcare. Inaccessibility or unavailability of services is among the most significant barriers to being able to leave the streets. Availability of mental health and substance abuse services geared to the specific needs of each young person is critical especially for youth with more serious problems [5, 27, 30]. Not having the right services at the right time significantly increases the likelihood of the young people becoming street entrenched and therefore less likely to successfully transition to a community setting. Conversely, being mentally healthy significantly contributes to successful transition [18].

Conclusion

There have been some significant steps forward in addressing the issue of adolescent homelessness in Canada, not the least being an increased focus on understanding the specific characteristics and needs of youth who are homeless or at risk of becoming homeless. This movement away from depending upon the US data is critical in our understanding of the needs and characteristics of young people in Canada. Without this country-specific knowledge, it will be more difficult to develop appropriate and targeted services given the significant differences between the health and social care systems in the two countries. It is possible to intervene in ways that successfully address youth homelessness through early prevention, intervention, and stabilization. Significant steps in dealing with youth homelessness have been taken in recent years in Canada although there is still much we need to understand before we are at the point that a serious impact can be made. However, we need to move beyond the traditional way we have looked at the solutions to youth homelessness [14]. Moving to this next level though will take a political will we have not seen to date in Canada.

References

1. Auerswald C, Lin J, Petry L, Hyatt S. Hidden in plain sight: an assessment of youth inclusion in point-in-time counts of California's unsheltered homeless population. Sacramento: California Homeless Youth Project; 2013.
2. Baker Collins S, Fudge Schormans A, Watt L, Idems B, Wilson T. The invisibility of disability for homeless youth. J Soc Distress Homeless. 2018;27(2):99–109.
3. Barker B, Kerr T, Alfred G, Fortin M, Nguyen P, Wood E, DeBeck K. High prevalence of exposure to the child welfare system among street-involved youth in a Canadian setting: implications for policy and practice. BMC Public Health. 2014;14:197. https://doi.org/10.1186/1471-2458-14-197.
4. Barker B, Alfred GT, Fleming K, Nguyen P, Wood E, Kerr T, DeBeck K. Aboriginal street-involved youth experience elevated risk of incarceration. Public Health. 2015a;129:1662–8.
5. Barker B, Kerr T, Nguyen P, Wood E, DeBeck K. Barriers to health and social services for street-involved youth in a Canadian setting. J Public Health Policy. 2015b;36(3):350–63.
6. Barone C, Yamamoto A, Richardson CG, Zivanovic R, Lin D, Mathias S. Examining patterns of cognitive impairment among homeless and precariously housed urban youth. J Adolesc. 2019;72:64–9.
7. Cheng T, Wood E, Feng C, Mathias S, Montaner J, Kerr T, DeBeck K. Transitions into and out of homelessness among street-involved youth in a Canadian setting. Health Place. 2013;23:122–7.
8. Cote P-B, Blais M. Between resignation, resistance and recognition: a qualitative analysis of LGBTQ+ youth profiles of homelessness agencies utilization. Child Youth Serv Rev. 2019;100:437–43.
9. Cutuli J, Steinway C, Perlman S, Herbers J, Eyrich Garg K. Youth homelessness: prevalence and associations with weight in three regions. Health Soc Work. 2015;40:316–24.
10. Doré-Gauthier V, Cote H, Jutras-Aswada D, Ouellet-Plamondon C, Abdel-Baki A. How to help homeless youth suffering from first episode psychosis and substance use disorders? The creation of a new intensive outreach intervention team. Psychiatry Res. 2019;273:603–12.
11. Dworsky A, Horwitz B. Missed opportunities: counting youth experiencing homelessness in America. Chicago: Chaplin Hall at the University of Chicago; 2018.
12. Gaetz S, Dej E. A new direction: a framework for homelessness prevention. Toronto: Canadian Observatory on Homelessness Press; 2017.
13. Gaetz S, O'Grady B, Kidd S, Schwan K. Without a home: the national youth homelessness survey. Toronto: Canadian Observatory on Homelessness Press; 2016.
14. Gaetz S, Ward A, Kimura L. Youth homelessness and housing stability: what outcomes should we be looking for? Healthc Manage Forum. 2019;32(2):73–7.
15. Goldman-Hasbun J, Nosova E, Kerr T, Wood E, DeBeck K. Homelessness and incarceration associated with relapse into stimulant and opioid use among youth who are street-involved in Vancouver, Canada. Drug Alcohol Rev. 2019;38:428–34.
16. Hadland SE, Marshall BDL, Kerr T, Qi J, Montaner JS, Wood E. Suicide and history of childhood trauma among street youth. J Affect Disord. 2012;136:377–80.
17. Karabanow J, Naylor T, Aube C. From place to space: exploring youth homelessness in rural Nova Scotia. J Rural Community Dev. 2014;9(2):112–27.
18. Kidd SA, Karabanow J, Hughes J, Frederick T. Brief report: youth pathways out of homelessness: preliminary findings. J Adolesc. 2013;36:1035–7.
19. Kidd SA, Frederick T, Karabanow J, Hughes J, Naylor T, Barbic S. A mixed methods study of recently homeless youth efforts to sustain housing and stability. J Child Adolesc Soc Work. 2016;33:207–18.
20. Kidd SA, Gaetz S, O'Grady B. The 2015 national Canadian homeless youth survey: mental health and addiction findings. Can J Psychiatry. 2017;62(7):493–500.

21. Kidd SA, Thistle J, Beaulieu T, O'Grady B, Gaetz S. A national study of indigenous youth homelessness in Canada. Public Health. 2019a;176:163–71. https://doi.org/10.1016/j.puhe.2018.06.012.
22. Kidd SA, Vitopoulos N, Frederick T, Leon S, Karabanow J, McKenzie K. More than four walls and a roof needed a complex tertiary prevention approach for recently homeless youth. Am J Orthopsychiatry. 2019b;89(2):248–57.
23. Kisely SR, Parker JK, Campbell LA, Karabanow J, Hughes JM, Gahagan JJ. Health impacts of supportive housing for homeless youth: a pilot study. Public Health. 2008;122:1089–92.
24. Kozloff N, Adair CE, Palma Lazgare LI, Poremski D, Cheung AH, Sandu R, Stergiopoulo V. "Housing first" for homeless youth with mental illness. Pediatrics. 2016;138(4):e20161514.
25. McCay E, Quesnel S, Langley J, Beanlands H, Cooper L, Blidner R, Aiello A, Mudachi N, Howes C, Bach K. A relationship-based intervention to improve social connectedness in street-involved youth: a pilot study. J Child Adolesc Psychiatr Nurs. 2011;24:208–15.
26. McKenzie-Mohr S, Coates J, McLeod H. Responding to the needs of youth who are homeless: calling for politicized trauma-informed intervention. Child Youth Serv Rev. 2012;34:136–43.
27. Phillips M, DeBeck K, Desjarlais T, Morrison T, Feng C, Kerr T, Wood E. Inability to access addiction treatment among street-involved youth in a Canadian setting. Subst Use Misuse. 2014;49:1233–40.
28. Rodrigue S. Hidden homeless in Canada. Ottawa: Statistics Canada; 2016.
29. Rowan MS, Mason M, Robitaille A, Labrecque L, Lambert Tocchi C. An innovative medical and dental hygiene clinic for street youth: results of a process evaluation. Eval Program Plann. 2013;40:10–6.
30. Saddichha S, Linden I, Krausz MR. Physical and mental health issues among homeless youth in British Columbia, Canada: are they different from older homeless adults? J Can Acad Child Adolesc Psychiatry. 2014;23(3):200–6.
31. Shelton J, Poirier J, Wheeler C, Abramovich A. Reversing erasure of youth and young adults who are LGBTQ and access homelessness services: asking about sexual orientation, gender identity, and pronouns. Sex Orientat Gend Identity Child Welfare. 2018;96(2):1–28.
32. Skott-Myhre H, Raby R, Nikolaou J. Towards a delivery system of services for rural homeless youth: a literature review and case study. Youth Child Care Forum. 2008;37(2):87–102.
33. Wagaman MA, Shelton J, Carter R, Stewart K, Stacey Jay Cavaliere SJ. "I'm totally transarific": exploring how transgender and gender-expansive youth and young adults make sense of their challenges and successes. Child Youth Serv. 2019;40(1):43–64.

Chapter 3
Interviewing Homeless Adolescents in the Context of Clinical Care: Creating Connections, Building on Strengths, Fostering Resilience, and Improving Outcomes

Curren Warf, Kiaras Gharabaghi, Grant Charles, and Ken Ginsburg

Introduction

This chapter is to prepare clinicians to interview youth who are experiencing homelessness. Many of the principles involved can be used for interviewing any young person, but young people who are experiencing homelessness are a special, if very diverse, group of vulnerable young people. From the start, we have to set out a caution about language and terminology; while the terms "clinician" and "interview" are quite standard from a professional perspective, they are not congruent with the hopes, aspirations, and needs of homeless young people. Very few such young people are looking to meet a "clinician," and almost none wish to be "interviewed." It is therefore important to remember that professional structures and processes, including language, meet the needs of professionals and their systems, but not necessarily the needs of those appearing in front of them.

Youth experiencing homelessness commonly have medical complaints and other problems complicating their unstable housing and social challenges. Medical problems are of a wide spectrum including injuries, infections, need for contracep-

C. Warf (✉)
Department of Pediatrics (Retired), Division of Adolescent Health and Medicine, British Columbia Children's Hospital, University of British Columbia, Vancouver, BC, Canada

K. Gharabaghi
School of Child & Youth Care, Ryerson University, Toronto, ON, Canada
e-mail: k.gharabaghi@ryerson.ca

G. Charles
School of Social Work, University of British Columbia, Vancouver, BC, Canada

K. Ginsburg
The Division of Adolescent Medicine, The Children's Hospital of Philadelphia, Philadelphia, PA, USA

Covenant House Pennsylvania, Philadelphia, PA, USA

C. Warf, G. Charles (eds.), *Clinical Care for Homeless, Runaway and Refugee Youth*, https://doi.org/10.1007/978-3-030-40675-2_3

tion, vaccinations, acute illnesses, chronic conditions requiring chronic medications including insulin-dependent diabetes, and more (See Chaps. 10, 11, 12, 13, 14, 15, and 16). These problems may open opportunities to link homeless youth to services that lead to housing stabilization.

Homeless young people may be members of homeless families, on their own or with groups of young people, or seen in shelters or drop-in centers. They may be encountered in clinics that are designed for youth who are homeless or other clinical settings, including hospital emergency departments. They may be encountered on the streets during outreach or even incidentally. Youth who are experiencing homelessness may be encountered through community organizations, in schools, through recreational activities, and other settings not typically associated with homeless youth (See Chap. 4). Often, professionals encounter homeless youth without knowing that the young person is homeless. Early and middle adolescents who experience homelessness, or are at high risk for experiencing homelessness, may have received little understanding or support and have little contact with their families; a significant number emerge from the foster care system. Not all homeless youth show signs of homelessness, and many are often highly motivated to hide their homelessness. Youth experiencing homelessness are present in almost every urban setting in the United States and Canada, and in rural or small-town settings, where the issues related to homelessness are quite different.

When interviewing youth who are homeless, it is essential to listen carefully and appreciate that though the interview may need to be brief, it may set the stage for future interactions. The interviewer needs to put aside preconceptions and assumptions regarding sexual orientation and gender identity, family background, or reasons that the youth is homeless. It is essential that the identified needs of the youth are addressed meaningfully as promptly as possible, especially those related to safety and shelter. Addressing many of these needs may be beyond the scope of familiarity of the individual clinician, and it is essential that others familiar with shelter and housing services are readily available and promptly engaged. Addressing the concrete and expressed needs of youth who are homeless for shelter, meals, healthcare, safety, and in other ways is key to cementing the relationship and building trust. It is important to listen carefully and patiently, to the spoken words, the body language and the expressed emotions and to identify and value the hidden strengths of the youth.

Diverse Characteristics and Circumstances of Youth Experiencing Homelessness

Homeless youth are diverse in age, ethnicity, immigration status, socioeconomic background, educational level, risk involvement, time on the streets, connection with the family of origin, and experiences with child protective services, juvenile authority, or in the case of young adults, with the criminal justice system (See Chap. 4). It is counterproductive for a clinician entering a conversation with a youth in unstable circumstances to hold presumptions of their background, capabilities, or expectations. Though the most dramatic stories commonly stay in our minds, an individual is not the summation of their most traumatic experiences. The clinician needs to be careful not to label events as "traumatic" because they might be experienced as traumatic from one's own position. Young people can guide the clinician in assessing trauma as it pertains to them; homeless young people may not recognize their own lived experiences as traumatic; after all, as with other young people, their young life is the only one that they have known and experienced, and the impact of trauma during vulnerable and formative periods of human development is not known to them and far from their minds. In fact, as with other adolescents, youth who have had complex backgrounds commonly strive for human connection; this is not a trauma response but a developmentally healthy and appropriate response.

Developmental Context of Interviewing the Adolescent

It is critical to remember that the fundamental question every adolescent, including youth experiencing homelessness, seeks to address is their sense of identity and their sense of belonging: "Who am I?" and "How do I belong?" They experiment with clothing styles, music, language, physical posturing, behaviors, and aspirations. They model themselves after influential peers and adults they encounter in families, at school, on the streets, or during other activities. They may be influenced by figures in the media or characters in literature. Alternatively, they may intentionally seek to construct themselves as an outsider or as someone not belonging to any group, not fitting with any subculture, and not having value in any context. "Who am I?" and "How do I belong?" often feel best answered by escaping spaces and cultures that are seen as uninviting or where young people have histories of rejection.

This process of self-discovery and associated behaviors sets the stage for their future development as adults and the roles for which they will be prepared. It is important to remember that young people are capable of great growth and change and that exploratory efforts at self-discovery, as they search for clues about how others see them, are not deterministic. Appreciating that young people live up to (or down to) the expectations we convey, deliberately or not through our own language and behavior, we need to surround youth with authentic messages that we see them as good people and expect the best, especially for youth living in difficult circumstances. This may mean countering messages they have heard from others or that they have constructed for themselves.

Don't mistake the behaviors, dress, cleanliness, or the social context in which the youth is encountered for the person. Some young people have engaged in self-destructive or undermining behaviors, often as a means to deal with harsh realities they have confronted, realities not of their making. These realities would pose a serious challenge to anyone and are commonly outside the scope of life experience of the clinician. As adults who care for and about them, we must engage them in positive and hopeful ways that can shift them away from harmful choices and toward those that will enhance their well-being and lead them to a more positive future. In so doing, however, we must be careful not to label as a "problem" the specific circumstances or behaviors that the young person may not see as a problem.

One of the great challenges of being with these young people is to remain committed to honoring their voice and their story, including how they make meaning of that story, which may not always correspond to how we might make meaning of it.

When we encounter a youth who is homeless, they have invariably had a difficult path, shaped and influenced by many factors beyond their control. These factors may include poverty; migration with loss of community and family support; the experience of emotional, sexual, and/or physical abuse; loss of parents or family; placement in institutional care; intergenerational trauma; and more. All of these forces and influences have been out of the control of the young person. Many experiences are internalized as shame or self-blame. Their relationships with peers are commonly the closest relationships that they have. Sometimes peer relationships are difficult, creating risks for young people to be manipulated by adults and other youth with sinister agendas, such as human trafficking, sexual exploitation, or recruitment into criminal gangs and activities.

Our job in this context goes beyond asking a list of clinical questions and identifying complaints. It includes using our potentially unique experience with the young person as an opportunity to provide a positive understanding and respectful experience, develop a meaningful connection, and truly listen to what they say. We need to be judicious and assure that the presenting clinical or social concern of the young person is actually addressed – while keeping in mind that our clinical encounter with the young person may open a fresh door to their developing a trusting relationship with a supportive adult and enable access to further services, if not at the moment, then in the near future.

Medical history questions often probe into sensitive areas of prior experiences having to do with sexual risk; substance use; difficult family relations; engagement with child protective services; history with foster care, the juvenile authority or adult criminal justice system; experiences with racism, sexual exploitation, homophobia and transphobia; or rejection for other reasons. We must never lose sight that these are exceedingly sensitive areas for the youth, and may be for us as well, and that talking about them may take time, requires deeply respecting youth's own boundaries, cannot be rushed, and may not be covered in a single encounter.

The traditional structure of much of medical interviewing is problem based, particularly regarding behavioral or social concerns. This can inadvertently derail a relationship with a vulnerable youth who may be very sensitive to feeling judged, not understood and not appreciated. They may interpret the focus on problems as an implicit blaming or criticism. Clinicians need to be prepared to be patient, and to seek out and identify genuine strengths and positive attributes. While it may not be a long-term relationship, it is nevertheless a relationship which itself can have a positive impact upon a young person who is living in circumstances that are dehumanizing and invalidating. The potential power of the human connection in this moment is profound.

For some clinicians, it may be better to refer the youth to another provider. It is useful to work in the context of an interdisciplinary and collaborative team, particularly in clinical educational environments when rotating students, residents, or other trainees do not have the consistent availability to develop a longer-term relationship. Youth workers, social workers, counselors and others can offer continuity of empathetic engagement.

Though young people may need care for acute health problems, chronic medical conditions, preventive care and stabilization, like others they will not access care if trust is not fostered and if they do not feel understood and valued. Communication and the relationship that is developed are key components to fostering stabilization and clinical engagement.

Young people who have experienced insecure or disrupted early childhood attachment, abuse and neglect, loss of parents and loved ones, instability of their social environment, multiple home placements and the traumas that commonly occur on the streets, may respond to interviews probing sensitive areas with a level of distrust reflected by difficult behaviors and are too frequently characterized as having a "conduct disorder" or "oppositional defiant disorder" or "intermittent explosive disorder." These labels commonly become barriers themselves to making connections and can promote a tragic sense of futility on the part of caregivers and influence the care provider to develop an unjustified sense of resignation, cynicism, and disconnection from the youth, blinding them to the strengths that the young person actually has. It is important that we recognize and identify youth's strengths particularly under these circumstances.

We need to assure that all young people are welcomed and viewed positively in the clinical environment and be willing to make the necessary changes in our approach. This may entail changing how these young people are viewed and approached in the clinical environment; making a shift in our language; suspending facile but undermining diagnostic labels; and emphasizing the recognition of young people's concealed strengths that have kept them alive so far despite having to deal with trauma, loss, and discrimination. There is a risk of re-traumatization or alienation if their sensitive information is treated with little respect for its gravity. There is the potential, if not explained clearly, for young people, or their parents (and other adults), to believe that the worst things that have happened to them *become* them and determine their fate.

Respecting Continued Attachment to Absent Parents

It is essential to appreciate that many homeless youth remain deeply attached emotionally to their parents regardless of circumstance, and the parents may remain key emotional figures in their lives, even if there has been high levels of conflict or they have been absent for one reason or another. This is true for youth who had been removed from their parents for legitimate concerns about safety (despite having truly loved each other), who commonly romanticize those parents in their absence and, given an opportunity as adolescents, may seek them out. We must value these relationships and be patient as youth explore the potential, or lack of potential, for a continuing role of their parents in their lives, regardless of past circumstances.

While respecting the need of youth for confidentiality, we also need to be as inclusive as we reasonably can be of parents, kinship carers, and foster parents, and appreciate ourselves that parenting is an exceedingly difficult role and that for many, our society does very little to prepare parents to take on this new vital role and even less in providing ongoing support. While it is not useful and may even be destructive to blame a young person for their troubles, it can be equally harmful to blame their parents or caregivers [2].

Intergenerational Trauma

No one is truly born anew, and we each carry the legacy of our family and of our historic and social circumstances. For vulnerable children and youth, facets of intergenerational trauma, in addition to the complex effects of poverty and oppressive forces, may include family disruption and inconsistent or exploitative relationships with caring adults. Many adolescents today live with the legacy of intergenerational trauma such as the mass involuntary placement of Indigenous children into residential schools in Canada and the United States, the pernicious effects of Jim Crow segregation of African-Americans in the United States, and the ongoing experience of racism and exclusion. This legacy is manifested by the continuing disproportionate representation of Indigenous children and youth of Canada, and African-American and Indigenous children and youth in the United States, in poverty, housing instability, child protective care, foster care, homelessness and youth justice, as well as adult incarceration [1].

Fostering Capacity to Confront Invisible Developmental Burdens

Youth who have experienced early disruption of attachment, early childhood maltreatment or serious neglect, and other significant traumas at an early developmental age may experience difficulties in trusting others and be subject to mood disturbances. Tragically, some young people who become homeless have been told that they are impulsive and thoughtless and have been blamed as the source of the family's problems. This process of being demeaned and blamed for events or circumstances completely outside their control may go back to early childhood and early developmental stages and may be absorbed and internalized; they may feel unwanted or unloved while feeling desperate to be wanted and loved. Their true strengths remain to be discovered. When we have the opportunity to follow young people over time, we commonly witness an amazing resilience and transformation when youth have an opportunity to experience supportive and caring relationships with others.

Some young people carry an invisible burden of prenatal drug or alcohol exposure that can have pernicious effects on neurological development resulting in some level of loss of impulse control and/or cognitive impairment.[1] This background is usually not known when youth experiencing homelessness present to clinic settings. These are true challenges, but the youth, especially under these circumstances, must not be reduced to the burden of their disabilities or overly characterized by the label of a purported or assumed clinical condition.

[1] American College of Obstetrics and Gynecology, Marijuana Use During Pregnancy and Lactation, October 2017, https://www.acog.org/en/Clinical/Clinical%20Guidance/Committee%20Opinion/Articles/2017/10/Marijuana%20Use%20During%20Pregnancy%20and%20Lactation

Recognizing and Building on Strengths

It is for these reasons that it is essential to recognize clearly the strengths and potential of traumatized youth, to be authentic and thoughtful, to give multiple chances for connection and acceptance, and to not be discouraged ourselves. The process of running away, of developing new close relationships of their own on the streets and with other youth who intuitively seem to understand their feelings, may feel more like home than home itself. It may take these young people some time to accept support and to develop trust with outreach workers, youth workers, social workers, or clinicians. We can encourage this process by recognizing the underlying drives and acknowledging their positive steps, striving to sustain engagement, and expect some setbacks.

Many young people can develop the self-awareness and skills to surmount significant early childhood challenges through later experiences of love, acceptance, understanding, and attachment, with greater insight as they cognitively and emotionally mature and are given opportunities to develop skills and self-confidence in sports, arts, music, employment or education. Though experiences of early childhood were beyond the control of the youth, the resiliency that young people commonly demonstrate, as they mature in gaining insight and experience through caring and thoughtful relationships and discovery of their own skills and talents, is genuinely inspiring. Every possible contact with an adult who is caring and attentive can add to this resiliency. We need to be aware that trauma is not just a physical but also a subjective experience. People can interpret similar events in many different ways and at different stages of life. As such, we have to avoid placing our interpretation of the seriousness of a traumatic event on the young person. They may have a very different view than us.

It is our challenge to foster effective support systems for each youth to enable them to succeed, and in particular to engage schools and after-school programs when available and accessible. Wherever the young person's life unfolds, we can focus on building capacity to better support the everyday needs of the young person, always with the young person's expertise about themselves and their own needs as our guide. With youth who are homeless or in unstable situations, it is important to make a serious attempt to identify a responsible adult who can help provide support to adhere to treatment, to access shelters or drop-in centers, and to provide other supports.

Risk Taking and Resiliency in Context

Risk is not destiny. In fact, it is impossible for anyone to explore life and try new things without engaging in some level of risk behavior. Youth separate from their parents early for many reasons, sometimes escaping maltreatment or neglect, sometimes because of parental demise or incarceration, and sometimes parental capacity is compromised because of mental illness or substance abuse. Poverty plays a particularly significant role given that some families cannot afford stable housing even when working full time for low wages, which adversely impacts parenting capacity, supervision, and healthy family dynamics.

Many youth who have experienced significant trauma are capable of great resiliency. We can support this process through authentic communication encouraging young people to have a hopeful view of their future. We aim to ensure a sense of realism in such views, but optimism at this stage of a young person's life is far more important than realism. The same youth who have survived so much also have the capacity to demonstrate great love and compassion in their treatment of peers, adoption of pets, and evolving sense of justice and fairness when they are safe and not in crisis. While we strive to understand where homeless young people are at, our goal as clinicians, aside from our clinical work, is to ensure that young people feel they *matter* while they are with us through integrating principles of trauma-sensitive (or trauma-informed) practices, positive youth development, and resilience building strategies in our interactions with youth.

Trauma-Sensitive Practices

A first step for a youth, and perhaps the most challenging step, in thinking about change is to consider if change is possible. The 14-year-old who declares emphatically that "this is just the way I am, I can never change" may truly believe it, though the future is open and full of possibilities. It may be easier to deny a problem exists than to confront the threat of failure. This is particularly true for those who have experienced prior failed attempts at progress or who have had adults who reinforce the idea that they are hopeless.

The first step toward positive behavioral change may be gaining the confidence that one can change. An important component of gaining such confidence is to find evidence of one's own agency. When young people feel (and often find evidence to confirm that feeling) that nothing will change no matter what they do, they reflect the sense that they do not have agency. Our work is to enable them to find their sense of agency again and learn how to use it constructively so that it enables them to contribute to positive change in themselves and in their circumstances. A core principle of trauma-sensitive practice is to restore control back to people from whom it has been taken away.

Listening, Recognizing Strengths and Avoiding Judgment

While we each see ourselves as unique, it is important to recognize that young people may not see us as such. They are likely to see us as an accumulation of every helping professional they have previously encountered. If they have had a positive experience, they are likely to initially see us in a positive light. If it has been negative, then they will likely be mistrustful and highly cautious. We may also remind them in some way of someone who has abused or exploited them in the past. All of this will impact how they view and interact with us.

We can characterize the appropriate approach to youth experiencing homelessness or living in unstable and high-risk settings as "*nonjudgmental, positive regard.*" As strong as our feelings may be regarding youth engaged in significant risk behaviors, it is important that the clinician continue to take a stance of "nonjudgmental, positive regard" to promote the continuation of a relationship; this entails listening and hearing difficult stories with the clinician not being overly reactive or communicate that the youth is being judged as a person by their behaviors. Communicating a caring attitude to the youth, notwithstanding disclosure of self-endangering behaviors, encourages communication and the willingness of the youth to sustain contact. We can add to this "*listen deeply, identify their underlying strengths,*" and let them know you genuinely want to recognize who they truly are. This is in keeping with integrating trauma-informed practices, fostering positive youth development through identifying and building on strengths, and promoting resiliency. This approach requires patience and connecting with youth while removing stigma and appreciating the profound potential young people possess to heal emotionally in a caring and understanding context.

Youth need, and usually want, an adult with empathy, sensitivity, and maturity and not a peer; the clinician should not try to act like, dress like, or speak like an adolescent.

It is important in making a connection with youth to listen intently to the young person's story and stay focused. You may comment on those things that demonstrate their honesty, empathy and compassion, adventurousness, or capacity for love. Youth who disclose traumatic experiences, but come for help or support, deserve recognition for their courage in seeking help, their resilience, and their determination in surviving a world that has been unfair to them.

Don't be surprised, and don't be discouraging if youth express a desire to go into the helping professions at the same time that they are disclosing their own need for support. Be cautious about offering unsolicited advice. Recognize the caring that they display toward friends or a pet, despite not having received the same protection or safety that they themselves needed. A young person who feels understood and valued, who feels recognized as an individual who has something to offer, is far more likely to accept support than someone who is discussed and treated as if they were a "problem."

Particularly on a first visit, the stories we hear may bear little resemblance to what has actually transpired; more commonly, these stories reflect the current mood of the young person and give clues about the tensions in their relationships with others and in their lives more generally. Don't be surprised if the story of a particular young person changes dramatically during a second encounter. This is not because they were not truthful the first time. It is simply a reflection of the young person continuing to experience tensions in their relationships with others, a lack of clarity, and often confusion and fear of loss. It also may be because they are gauging our trustworthiness and may float just enough information to determine our reactions and assess our true commitment to privacy.

Do not offer advice prematurely, at a point when the youth does not feel understood; sometimes listening is all one can do for the moment and is sufficient. It may well take time for the youth himself or herself to come to an understanding of and be able to articulate experiences.

Remember that a young person's story always gets more complex, and features more elements, than when it is first told. Allow the young person time to retell the story, focusing on different elements, relationships, events, or experiences, and don't focus too much on contradictions that will almost always be present in that story. In fact, while the truthfulness of the story will eventually matter, it does not really matter all that much at first. Determining the need is initially more important than determining the accuracy of the circumstances of the story. It is more important to determine why a young person tells a story as they are telling it; elements that may turn out to be fictional, or not entirely accurate, or simply exaggerated, may provide clues as to how the young person thinks of themselves.

Confidentiality

It is important to advise the youth from the outset about both their rights to confidentiality, from parents and others, regarding disclosure of health information, including sexual activities, contraception and engagement of substance use, and the limits of confidentiality.

All clinicians have a legal responsibility to notify child protective services or the police in the event of a disclosure by a minor of physical or sexual abuse or maltreatment, serious emotional abuse, or serious neglect. Clinicians also have a legal obligation to keep the patient safe, through involuntary hospitalization if indicated – entailing calling emergency medical services or police – if there is an imminent threat of suicide or threat to others or incapacitating mental health disability such as psychosis (See Chap. 15).

Beyond confidentiality, the clinician needs to explain to the young person their own responsibilities with respect to what is written into a case or patient file, and requirements with respect to sharing information with others. It is helpful to ask the young person if what you said makes sense to them.

Respecting confidentiality can be a very difficult challenge in the era of electronic medical records. Though pertinent medical information does clearly need to be included in the medical record, it may be in the best interests of the youth to omit some of their comments regarding very sensitive matters. One needs to be particularly sensitive in regard to inclusion of information in the medical records that may be stigmatizing to the youth or may later damage the youth's future opportunities. Some electronic medical record systems have developed systems that provide an extra barrier to access sensitive information; unfortunately, these are more the exception than the rule.

Setting the Stage with Parents or Caregivers

In caring for adolescents when they present with their parents, it is commonly useful to set the stage by proposing that there be time to meet with the parent(s) and youth together, then each alone, and then together again; parents commonly have a better understanding of chronic medical conditions. This process may or may not take place on subsequent visits, depending on circumstance, but it does communicate in practice a respect for sustaining relationships and for the needs of each individual; the clinician may ask the youth and parents what their preference would be to handle the encounter.

There is commonly a need to meet alone with parents who may be able to provide significant background and context, which the youth may either be unaware of or unable to articulate and parents may be hesitant to discuss in their child's presence. There needs to be assurance given that the youth's rights to confidentiality and privacy will be respected. Seeing the parents together with the youth allows the clinician to develop an idea of the character of their relationship at that time, the level of closeness or conflict, and the shared anxieties and fears. Youth may come in with parents at times of crisis so that the intensity of the moment may or may not reflect the day-to-day tensions in their relationship. Clinical engagement in which the wisdom, lived experience, and expertise of the young person and their parents is valued generally leads to better and more trusting relationships down the road.

It is important, particularly during periods when parents and youth have been in conflict, to articulate and point out to both the parents and the youth the strengths of the youth and the love that parents have for their child; often conflict originates from the fear and frustration that the parent has for their child's safety and future. It is important to note that the conflict may be the result of long-term environmental stressors experienced by the family, such as chronic housing instability, literal homelessness, unemployment, loss of loved ones, or other life circumstances of the young person or family. It is useful at the end of the encounter to have a summative discussion with parents and youth both present, to address any specific questions. In a very real sense, the family may be the patient.

Independently Homeless Youth

Youth who are independently homeless usually do not have an adult in their lives that accompany them to clinic. At times, they may wish to have a youth worker, social worker, or other supportive person present. It is important early in the interview to engage a youth worker or social worker to assess availability of resources and work on developing a trusting relationship. These young people are commonly confronted with urgent survival needs of finding age appropriate shelter, reliable meals, engagement in education and supports from child protective services or other agencies.

Without stabilization and prompt access to supports these youth commonly acculurate to the streets and become increasingly difficult to engage in services.

Structure of the Youth Interview

There have been several models developed to approach the psychosocial interview of homeless youth. Perhaps the most well known is the HEADSS model (home, education, activity, drugs, sex, suicide) which is an interviewing approach that was developed to identify significant concerns of homeless youth and was adapted to be more generally used with adolescents [3]; a second frequently used model is the SSHADDESS2 model, which addresses risks while contextualizing them in strengths (strengths, school, home, activities, drugs/substance use, emotions, eating, sexuality, safety). SSHADDESS is one component of a comprehensive set of strength-based, trauma-sensitive communication strategies intended to support healthy adolescent development and build youth resilience presented in Reaching Teens published by the American Academy of Pediatrics [3].

Both of these approaches require an "active listening approach," that is, it may be counterproductive to quickly run through a series of prescribed questions. The interview does not need to follow a rigid structure, and frequently can be conducted in a less structured conversational style. If the youth becomes impatient, does not seem able to attend, or does not want to continue the interview for one reason or another it should be discontinued, and reintroduced at a subsequent time. It is important to be sensitive to the mood of the youth and conscious of time. Usually, specific issues need to be prioritized depending on the situation; highly charged emotional issues may be deferred if the youth desires, or referred for a mental health counselor.

As with other clinical interviews, it should begin with warmly greeting the youth, smiling, extending a hand, and creating a welcoming environment. If there are others present, such as parents, one might ask the youth to introduce them. An open-ended question asking what his or her concerns are and what brought them into clinic can encourage the youth to feel that they have some control and initiate discussion, frequently identifying the major concern of the youth. Though their stated immediate concern may in the end seem relatively minor relative to the compelling social or family problems, it may open the door and bring a homeless youth into a broader, stabilizing system of care, and it is essential that the stated concern be addressed.

In general, peers and romantic partners should not be present during the interview, though it is commonly a good idea to have a clinical staff person present.

Clinicians need to avoid, especially early in the interview, asking multiple highly focused questions rather than open-ended questions. Though it may initially seem more efficient to do so (and in some very urgent circumstances it is unavoidable), it is important that the young person be able to tell their own story and be heard, their concerns emerge more clearly, and the clinician can gain an appreciation of the youth's abilities to express themselves, identify mood disturbances, and build a stronger relationship.

Listening for Strengths

Youth need to have their strengths identified and recognized as they tell their story. One can demonstrate that they have been heard by reflecting back a positive interpretation of what they had said, thereby focusing on their strengths. Praising too intensely while gathering information may prevent a young person from disclosing something they fear will disappoint you, or they may feel that you are being phony and don't really understand what they have gone through.

Don't rush through the interview; take time to pause and reflect back so that they can appreciate that you are making a genuine attempt to understand and hear them. It is more important that the young person feels heard than that all the information is gathered in one sitting.

Through the process of the interview, one can communicate listening and attentiveness through asking questions, reflecting back, and sustaining focus on what the young person says. Minimizing or being dismissive of the youth's concerns will immediately create a barrier to understanding.

Body Language and Reflection

Body language is important to communicate attentiveness, though making sustained eye contact can feel intimidating or even threatening to some young people. Listening and occasionally reflecting back what was said, communicating empathy ("that must have been difficult", "I'm sorry you had to go through that..."), and asking questions for clarification all communicate attentiveness and listening and are validating for a young person.

While the clinician communicates with their own body language (formality of dress, assertiveness in presentation, guiding of the conversation, comfort in the professional environment, etc.) the young person as well communicates through their own body language, through tearfulness or eye avoidance, silence and avoidance, frustration and impatience, distrust or in many other ways. Their level of hygiene, grooming or self-care may reflect lack of resources or absence of a healthy living environment, or self-neglect, or occasionally be a statement of alternative subcultural identity or sense of adventurousness.

However, there are always limits to time, and youth have limited patience with the length of time clinical encounters take; if the youth has come to clinic with a specific agenda (for example concern of an STI, need for contraception, request for condoms, worried about pregnancy, an injury, a rash, or significant mental health problem) these concerns need to be prioritized and much of the psychosocial interview may need to be taken up at subsequent visit. Even in the case of acute medical issues, concerns of immediate access to housing and concerns for safety should be covered and addressed.

Avoid writing, reading a computer screen, or typing notes on a keyboard while interviewing the youth. This can be particularly upsetting to a young person who is feeling frightened or distrustful or disclosing emotionally sensitive personal information. Your interview and conversation, which communicates respect and understanding, may be a unique experience for the youth with an adult, and contrast with having been deliberately ignored and avoided on the streets.

Guiding the Interview

The clinician can guide the discussion by providing open-ended questions regarding specific arenas. Where have you been spending the night recently? Do you have a place to stay? Who do you hang out with, or live with? Where do you go for food? Each of these questions allows for identification of needs for accessing services and can allow the interviewer to probe more as the youth responds. Not uncommonly, for recently homeless youth, the major first step is to get them off the streets as quickly as possible, engaged with a youth worker or social worker, identify a potential shelter or a drop in center and start working toward greater stability.

As the discussion progresses, pick an issue that you may feel stands in their way for progress or one that seems realistically amenable to change. Work with the young person, and try to come to agreement on that one issue. Ask if the issue may be discussed, and ask what the youth thinks would help move forward. Listen carefully, and you may add something yourself or reinforce what the youth has said. Finally, offer some concrete support in following through.

Some youth are less ready to express themselves openly. It can be intimidating to come to a clinic, to ask for help, or to see a clinician who is older and more educated. The clinician doesn't need to fill the void by talking, but can ask modest specific questions, find positive factors to acknowledge verbally such as coming to clinic, being open to getting support, having patience, having helped a friend or caring for a pet. Acknowledge the courage it took to come in to the clinic and disclose difficult experiences is empowering for youth. One can acknowlege through saying "I am so impressed that you have had the courage to talk so openly about..." or "It is so impressive that you have been able to take such good care of yourself and your friend after all you've been through." Premature advice communicates that you don't really understand, and they have not really been heard and may actually be a manifestation of the clinician's own sense of helplessness and impatience. Frequently, rather than unsolicited advice it is wiser to provide an empathetic response that builds a sense of understanding: "That must have been incredibly difficult (or hard to bear, or painful…)."

The process of building trust through one's connections with young people who have good reason not to trust requires a very high level of transparency. Excellent work can be undone in a moment if the young person feels that what had been promised or committed to is not what was done. This affects not only the credibillity of a clinician but even the credibility of the professional context, resulting in the young person being less likely in the future to seek help from medical professionals in otherwise accessible settings such as hospitals or clinics.

Education and School Involvement

Many youth experiencing homelessness retain a strong attachment to school and awareness of its importance for their future; they often remain enrolled in school and regularly attend classes. In these circumstances school becomes an extraordinarily important stabilizing factor and a strong supportive relationship with even one teacher, counselor or other person in the school setting can play a critical stabilizing role.

These school-enrolled youth may be "couch surfing" among friends in the community, staying in shelters, or literally homeless on the street. It is essential with homeless youth that consistent engagement in school and education be a high priority and they be provided places to study, opportunities to work, and access with social workers to help with stabilization.

Many secondary schools in urban settings have social workers and/or counselors with deep experience in working with these young people who can continue to work with youth and their families to gain a more stable living environment, access social services or mental health services and in many cases help work with parents and families. In some areas, Child Protective Services have developed specific schools with flexible schedules targeting youth in unstable living environments to support completion of secondary school and prepare them to enter trade school or other post-secondary education. Some publicly supported child protection agencies operate smaller schools capable of providing individually designed educational programs for secondary school students with support in applying for post-secondary education or trade school. In many urban centers, there are public and nonprofit agencies with experienced staff and significant history working with youth in high-risk environments. Clinical programs targeting youth who are homeless need to be aware of and work collaboratively with these programs (See Chap. 4).

Of course, not all homeless young people stay involved with school. Often, young people have been out of school for considerable periods of time, perhaps feeling overly anxious to be involved in what they experience as a performance-based setting, or not infrequently because they have been suspended or otherwise encountered barriers for attending school. Youth who have frequently changed schools and/or communities commonly have no social connections to solidify attachment to school. It is important, therefore, to allow young people to explain their relationship with school from their perspective and to tread carefully and respectfully to avoid creating additional pressure to connect with school for youth who may not be ready to do so. Ultimately, school is an important resource that can offer young people a sense of stability and belonging, but the timing for reconnecting with school needs to be determined in partnership with the young person rather than by the providers or clinicians alone.

Many communities have youth-focused agencies with skilled staff that can provide areas for youth to find safe recreation, job referrals, recreational opportunities, meals, and provide meaningful alternatives to surviving on the streets (See Chaps. 4 and 7).

The clinician can ask questions such as: Are you attending school? Where do you go? What grade level are you in? Do you have a special connection with a particular teacher or staff member? Are you interested in returning to school? What stands in your way of attending school? If the young person mentions barriers to school, such as having been victimized, social isolation, fear of failure, or lack of preparation or others, it is important to acknowledge these and find ways to enable the young person to have a more successful experience. It is important to connect the youth with a youth worker or social worker to help facilitate transition to school and support the youth in overcoming barriers.

Substance Use and Abuse

The level of drug and alcohol use is commonly (though not universally) a significant factor in the lives of homeless and marginalized youth and may shape the clinical interaction. Youth who are out of school and estranged from parents or family are at extraordinarily high risk for escalation of substance use. Though it must be remembered that many youth experiment with drugs of various types and do not develop serious substance abuse disorders as adults, for youth on the streets, out of school and not employed, significant and dangerous substance abuse is not uncommon and carries grave risk. As the drug use escalates, their circle of peers becomes increasingly restricted to other young people engaged in serious drug use and it becomes increasingly difficult to intervene or work toward abstention or reduction of use (See Chap. 8).

Youth who are on the streets, out of school, disconnected from families, unemployed, and with peers engaged in serious substance abuse are at highest risk. For some youth who are homeless, sharing drug use with peers is a powerful bonding experience that is self-reinforcing, particularly for young people who feel socially isolated. This shared experience may bring the youth into relationship with older youth or adults who have more advanced drug use, but seem to the naïve young person to be more experienced and can serve as unfortunate role models or who may find ways to exploit the youth for their own gain. Serious substance abuse treatment cannot be addressed without an appreciation of the many factors that shape youths' vulnerability.

Youth who are using drugs or alcohol can be very challenging to engage, particularly when pressure is exerted to abstain altogether. The most realistic approaches for many of these youth, particularly for late adolescents and young adults, are harm reduction strategies that are educative with respect to safety issues and provide alternatives to substance use at least some of the time, such as participation in recreational facilities where they can have rewarding experiences, rest, and have meals and hopefully develop a connection with facility staff. These trusted relationships can emerge as the most significant factor in engaging youth in productive activities, developing insight about substance use and becoming willing to reduce use. Many urban centers have daytime youth facilities. They may also be connected with voluntary placement in shelters where relationships with social workers, youth workers, mental health professionals or other staff, and engagement in alternative activities in sports or arts or school may enable them to become less dependent on alcohol and drugs.

Reviewing substance use provides an opportunity to asses the youth's level of understanding of risk and the conversation is an opportunity to introduce approaches to reduce risk. For example, the use of injection drugs in circumstances where needles or syringes are shared puts the young person at very high risk for contracting Hep-C and/or HIV. Assuring that they have access to clean needles and syringes and safe injection sites, as well as ready access to naloxone, may be a life-saving intervention as well as provide them future opportunities to access support if they decide to discontinue injection drug use.[2,3]

Given that overdose of opiates, in particular synthetic opiates such as fentanyl and oxycodone, has emerged as the leading cause of death for adolescents and adults under 55 years old in the United States and Canada, and continues to rise, opiate injection and snorting are exceedingly and demonstrably dangerous for youth.[4,5] For youth who have been homeless for shorter periods, there may be a rationale to introduce more assertive intervention that includes families and loved ones to assure that they are given the best chance to be deterred from continued use of opiates or enter into effective treatment (See Chap. 9).

While working with young people involved in substance use can be frustrating for the clinician because of the acute dangers involved, the assistance, guidance, or wisdom provided to the young person will likely be shared with the youth's peers in the community. Meaningful and trauma-sensitive approaches to talking about substance use with one young person often has an impact beyond the individual. Facilitating access for one young person to a needle exchange, for example, is likely to result in that young person's peers also accessing the needle exchange.

Homeless adolescents, or adolescents in precarious living situations, may come to attention through presentation to an Emergency Department (ED) with an opiate or

[2] BC Overdose Prevention Services Guide 2019, BC CDC, Provincial Health Services Authority http://www.bccdc.ca/resource-gallery/Documents/Guidelines%20and%20Forms/Guidelines%20and%20Manuals/Epid/Other/BC%20Overdose%20Prevention%20Services%20Guide_Jan2019_Final.pdf

[3] Harm Reduction Guidelines, British Columbia CDC; http://www.bccdc.ca/health-professionals/clinical-resources/harm-reduction

[4] Drug Overdose Deaths in the United States, 1999–2017

NCHS Data Brief No. 329, November 2018; Holly Hedegaard, M.D., Arialdi M. Miniño, M.P.H., and Margaret Warner, Ph.D. https://www.cdc.gov/nchs/products/databriefs/db329.htm

[5] Fentanyl Contamination of Other Drugs is Increasing Overdose Risk; Content source: Centers for Disease Control and Prevention, National Center for Injury Prevention and Control, Division of Unintentional Injury Prevention, Dec 19, 2018, https://www.cdc.gov/drugoverdose/data/other-drugs.html

alcohol overdose, infectious complications of injection drug use, or presentation with mental health alterations including psychosis. These are generally not circumstances during which a thorough psychosocial evaluation can be conducted. Most ED's have few resources or youth specific treatment guidelines to manage these young people and after they are perceived to be "medically stable" or not at risk for immediate death (often after only an hour or two of observation) they are commonly discharged to the same environment from which they came. Given the very high risk of death from opiate overdose, in particular by repeat fentanyl overdose, for those youth who had previously presented to the ED with an overdose, clinical practices regarding mandated hospitalization for minors and development of stabilization and secure care practices and resources need to be re-evaluated and revised (See Chap. 9).

Risks of serious substance use among youth experiencing homelessness may be moderated through utilization of harm reduction strategies, which have been found to be more effective among many substance-using homeless youth than abstention based approaches, particularly if the problem of homelessness has not been effectively addressed. Harm reduction strategies including access to clean needles, safe injection sites, emergent access to naloxone, and access to safe pharmaceuticals offer reduction of rates of HIV infection and reduced rates of lethal overdose.[6] Harm reduction programs may also open a door to introducing use of methadone, buprenorphine, or other opiate agonists to reduce risks associated with illicit drugs or overdose and enable individuals to participate more fully in employment, education, and foster more positive relationships with families.

It is important that the clinician, while being honest about the risks and consistently offering options for engagement in substance abuse treatment or harm reduction, continue to take a stance of "nonjudgmental, positive regard" to promote the continuation of a relationship and willingness of the youth to sustain contact.

Youth access to drugs over the last ten to twenty years has changed significantly. US pharmaceutical companies have heavily promoted oxycontin and other opiates throughout the United States, especially in rural areas, and have conscientiously influenced physicians' perceptions of the safety of oxycontin and other narcotics and shaped physician prescribing patterns.[7] In addition, the synthetic narcotic fentanyl has been widely and rapidly introduced into the illicit drug market. Fentanyl, an extremely potent synthetic opiate, has been widely introduced into illicit marijuana, amphetamine, cocaine, and other non-narcotic drugs, so that youth may not be aware of the drugs they are actually ingesting.

Cannabis is now commercially promoted, with little or no basis in research, as treatment for a wide spectrum of health concerns. Similarly, there is little research on the long term effects of chronic cannabis use on the cognitive abilities, emotional development and school and family engagement of adolescents. Chronic cannabis use may pose yet another barrier to stabilization for youth experiencing homelessness.

[6] Harm Reduction Guidelines, British Columbia Centre for Disease Control; http://www.bccdc.ca/health-professionals/clinical-resources/harm-reduction

[7] "Damage From OxyContin Continues to Be Revealed", Austin Frakt, The New York Times, April 13, 2020

Given the above, youth who are homeless, out of school, and unemployed are at extraordinary risk of escalating substance use problems. In interviewing youth, rather than asking if a youth uses drugs, one can ask how often he or she uses specific substances, including tobacco, alcohol, and cannabis, how frequently they are used, if they use any drugs with needles, if they are aware that many of the street drugs are contaminated with fentanyl, and if they know where to get naloxone if they need it. These discussions can also be educational sessions. The British Columbia Centre for Disease Control (BCCDC) has introduced the "Take Home Naloxone" program to supply Naloxone to people at risk for overdose; there are now 1300 sites in the Province.[8]

When interviewing youth in settings where homeless youth receive care, it is important to have readily available referral resources for youth who are identified as having or developing significant substance use disorders. It is best if they can be introduced on-site at the time of the interview to an individual substance use counselor who can begin to develop a relationship and engage them in care.

Later in this book there is a chapter on brief Motivational Enhancement Approaches for young people with substance use disorders experiencing homelessness with some specific approaches to supporting youth to reduce their substance use (See Chap. 8). There are also sections focused on developing interventions for youth immediately after overdose through hospital-based "stabilization care" or community-based secure care, both with involvement of parents or family as appropriate and available (See Chap. 9).

Sexuality and Sexual Behaviors

Youth who have run away and are out of school may be surprisingly ignorant of basic sexual physiology, and girls in particular may be unaware, or in denial of, their vulnerability to pregnancy. There may be a sense of resignation or disempowerment (what will happen, will happen) that becomes a barrier to contraception use or STI prevention. Boys as well may be poorly educated, feel that contraception is "the girl's thing," and feel that sexual activity is at least one thing in their life that is pleasurable and through which they can feel a meaningful connection with another person. There remain spoken and unspoken barriers related to denial, shame, adult denial, and lack of access to resources that stand in the way of healthy youthful sexuality. It is essential that condoms, oral contraceptives, injectable contraceptives, postcoital contraception, and safe and legal pregnancy termination be readily available to these exceedingly vulnerable youth[9] (See Chap. 11). It is also essential that

[8] Naloxone Programs, British Columbia Centre for Disease Control; http://www.bccdc.ca/our-services/programs/naloxone-programs

[9] Contraceptive Technology 2019, contraceptivetechnology21st.com

access to sexually transmitted infections (STI) screening, diagnosis, and treatment be readily available[10] (See Chap. 12).

Homeless youth are diverse in their sexuality; in their orientation; in their gender identity; in their expectation of gender roles; and in their experience with sexual abuse, assault, or exploitation. It is important in our language and in our interactions with youth that we do not have a "presumption of heterosexuality" or presume gender identity, and are genuinely open and listen non-judgmentally and empathetically to the experiences of youth. Discussion of sexual orientation and behavior are usually highly sensitive topics for youth to engage in, and their desire not to discuss or disclose must be respected.

It is not important that all details of a youth's sexual experiences be explored during a clinical visit. Many adolescents experiment sexually and need protection from unintended pregnancy, sexually transmitted infections, and safety from sexual assault or exploitation.

It is important that young people have confidential access to contraception and to condoms to assure that they have the ability to avoid unintended consequences for their future. It is important to know if the young person may be pregnant, if there is a need for contraception, and if they have access to and are familiar with the use of condoms.

Questions can be framed about sexual issues by initially framing sexual activity as a normal human experience. For example, one can ask, "I know that a lot of young people have been sexually active. Have you been sexually active?"

"It's important that you have control over your own body. Have you used anything to prevent pregnancy such as condoms or birth control pills?"

"Sexually transmitted infections are very common in the community. What have you done to protect yourself?" (This provides the opportunity to introduce the use of condoms, assure that the youth has had the HPV and Hep B vaccines, screen for STIs and HIV, or have a discussion about PReP or PEP for HIV prevention (See Chaps. 10 and 13) and opens the door to introducing a Health Educator to review in more detail the maintenance of sexual health.)

A 2012 study estimated that some 40% of homeless youth served by agencies in the United States were lesbian, gay, or transgender.[11] Many (though not all) gay, lesbian, and transgender youth do not receive the acceptance or understanding at home that they need and leave home at an early age. Though many families try, and often succeed, in achieving reconciliation, others do not, and the young person is faced with the challenge of surviving, prematurely independent, in an environment where they may be subject to discrimination, prejudice and exploitation (See Chap. 4).

[10] British Columbia Treatment Guidelines, Sexually Transmitted Diseases in Adolescents andAdults, 2014, BC CDC http://www.bccdc.ca/resource-gallery/Documents/Communicable-Disease-Manual/Chapter%205%20-%20STI/CPS_BC_STI_Treatment_Guidelines_20112014.pdf

[11] Serving Our Youth: Findings of a National Survey of Service Providers Working with Lesbian,Gay and Transgender Youth Who Are Homeless or at Risk for Becoming Homeless http://williamsinstitute.law.ucla.edu/wp-content/uploads/Durso-Gates-LGBT-Homeless-Youth-Survey-July-2012.pdf

Transgender youth, in particular, are very likely to experience stigmatization, blame, and a denial of their identity across public service systems as well as in the broader community. Very few shelters, clinics, drop-in centers, or public places such as libraries, schools, or shopping malls are prepared to meet the needs and everyday routines of transgender youth. In shelters, for example, questions about whether the transgender youth should stay at a boys' shelter or a girls' shelter are common and extend to issues regarding bathroom use and other circumstances in which binary gender biases are prevalent (See Chap. 4).

Homeless Adolescent Girls with Children

Young women experiencing homelessness who are pregnant need an opportunity to explore all of their options, including continuation or confidential termination (See Chap. 11). The decision is theirs and they can involve whoever they want in the decision-making process. Pregnant teens may need a number of sessions to explore their feelings about continuation of the pregnancy. It is essential that the clinician be conscientious to not impose his or her own biases on the youth and be familiar with local resources. Pregnant young women need to be strongly advised to abstain from alcohol, marijuana, or other drug use during pregnancy because of potential negative effects on fetal brain development; this is commonly new information for them.

The reality of pregnancy or having a child may be a powerful incentive for the youth to be open to reconciliation with parents and attend school. For some teen girls who have retained custody of their children, with support and stabilization, becoming a parent may have the potential to become a motivating experience and give new and deeper meaning to their lives as they come to see themselves responsible for another vulnerable person; young fathers as well can frequently be involved and need to be welcomed. The young parents' relationship with the child may well outlast the relationship between the young parents.

Young women who remain homeless and who have the responsibility to care for their child are highly vulnerable to exploitation to meet needs. Child Protective Services generally needs to become involved to assure the safety of the infant and identify resources for the young mother. It is important that young mothers have every oppportunity to be on sustained effective contraception (See Chap. 11)

Some adolescent girls experiencing homelessness have had children themselves and have lost custody. This is a highly traumatic experience for a young mother, and many of the behaviors that she later engages in may be linked to attempts in some way to deal with the pain of loss and the despair she feels. The expression of this pain is a reflection of the depth of caring that these girls experience; families and program staff of young mothers can recognize the great capacity for love that these young people carry. It is essential that when a young woman with a child of her own is identified in clinic, that her stability and the stability of the child have the highest priority. Child Protective Services should be involved immediately to identify a supportive environment for the young mother and child to find stability.

All adolescent parents, particularly those who are homeless or without the support of their own parents or family, require that effective efforts be devoted to provide stable supervised and supportive housing, inclusive of opportunities to go to school, learn about child development, and assure consistent financial support and mentorship.

It is critical to assess the need for childcare and babysitting resources, given that one common risk factor for the children of homeless youth is being cared for by an unqualified and perhaps less stable peer of the young parent. While such peers may intend to "do the right thing" when babysitting for a friend, they frequently do not have the bond with the infant that the parent has and are not capable of being reliably responsible.

The homeless youth's parents may desire to significantly engage with their daughter and grandchild; in some circumstances the youth's grandparents (or other individuals within a kinship network) can be engaged. For both boys and girls, becoming a young parent, given meaningful adult support, can be a profound and motivating experience that drives them to grow emotionally in ways that can be deeply surprising and gratifying. Having a child for some youth can be instrumental in building bridges to heal relationships with parents. It is with adolescent mothers and fathers that the true meaning of "it takes a village to raise a child" becomes apparent.

Survival Sex

Some homeless girls, boys and transgender youth engage in sexual activity for survival needs, that is, sexual relations in exchange for a place to stay, for food, for drugs or for money (See Chap. 4). This is a very risky and, for most, a severely demeaning activity. There is a social mythology about the practice of "survival sex"; however, it is generally experienced with profound regret by youth who see no other choices and is resorted to in only the most difficult circumstances. There is usually shame associated with survival sex, and having engaged in survival sex may not be disclosed until trust has been well established and perhaps not even then. There are not many qualitative studies of adolescent survival sex, but in at least one, the major motivation for homeless girls was to obtain money to support their child [4]. Interviewing youth regarding these behaviors needs to be conducted very carefully, with empathy and without judgment, as well as searching for ways to identify and encourage them to accept stable shelter and support (See Chap. 4).

It is essential when evaluating young people who may have engaged in survival sex that the clinician maintain a stance of neutrality and non-judgmentalism. Experiences with survival sex are commonly colored by a strong sense of personal shame. Questions can be asked such as: "Have you ever been in a situation when you had sex for food, or money or a place to stay?" The interviewer needs to be self-aware enough not to communicate a sense of judgment. This is important for exploring physical risks of STIs, unintended pregnancy, exploitation or HIV infection. The physical safety of young people who have been engaged in survival sex is commonly threatened. Clinical sites engaged in the care of homeless youth, know of and utilize local resources for shelter and services for prompt stabilization.

Sexual Assault

In addition, youth on the street, in particular girls but boys as well, are at high risk for sexual assault, either through coercion, manipulation, or when intoxicated. Whether effective or not, one of the common motivations disclosed by homeless youth for hanging out in groups is for self-protection and to assure that the girls and younger boys are not preyed upon. At some level, this represents a positive sense of protectiveness of others. Their peers may be felt to understand and value them in ways that their families were not felt to have done. Tragically, some individuals that are trusted in these environments may themselves manipulate or coerce their peers to have sex. Fostering an empathetic and supportive relationship with youth and connecting them with skilled social workers and youth workers can help move them to accept shelter or safer living situations.

The interviewer can ask if the youth has ever been in a situation when he or she was made to have sexual relations against their will, involuntarily when they were intoxicated, or sexually assaulted by an adult or family member. Sexual assault of a minor by a family member requires a report to Child Protective Services and/or the local police for investigation, in particular if there remain other children or adolescents in the home facing unsafe conditions. Reporting requirements in the United States vary from state to state.

Medical genital examination of a recent victim of sexual assault should not take place in a general medical clinic as any non-forensic examination will contaminate the value of later evidence collection. Most cities have one or more sexual assault evaluation centers available through designated Emergency Departments. Examination must take place between 36 and 96 hours depending on the practices of the specific center (See Chap. 14).

Summary

It is clear that life for young people is precarious under circumstances of homelessness and the protections are very fragile. Though youth may at times seem to be highly resistant to change, given it may require leaving their peers and at some level coming to terms with their own vulnerability, critical events commonly occur such as an assault, an arrest, a falling out with peers, a realization of the dangers of substance use or any of many other possible circumstances. When a critical and destabilizing event occurs, youth may become more open to support and intervention, while they may also become more vulnerable to exploitation and manipulation by skilled individuals looking to recruit them into sex trades, the drug trade or engage them in violent or exploitative dependency relationships [5]. It is important that there be readily available alternatives.

Those who work with young people experiencing homelessness can have an opportunity to play a significant role at times of these critical events, especially if there has been a prior investment in building a relationship and in expressing and identifying how valued they are. This foundation may be incrementally built by expressly and genuinely identifying their strengths in difficult circumstances, their resilience, their empathy and compassion, their determination, and their openness to make a connection.

Young people who are homeless commonly experience an underlying despair and sense of powerlessness, and may not have had the protection of responsible adults in their lives. The clinician, youth worker, or social worker who takes their concerns seriously, assures their safety and provides meaningful support without exploiting their trust can provide a model of what a caring and loving adult can be, and perhaps leave a young person with a substantive reason to hope and struggle for a meaningful future.

The interview of the vulnerable adolescent does not need to take a prescribed form, and commonly needs to be abbreviated, or take place during multiple visits, due to time constraints and the patience of both the youth and the provider. However, the discussions that take place cover sensitive areas that are moving for both the youth and the health care provider. Youth experiencing homelessness commonly deeply appreciate the experience of respect, understanding and authentic caring that health care providers bring to the visit.

Regardless of circumstance, youth who experience homelessness have survived many challenges. This chapter has been developed to enable the clinician not only to conduct an information-gathering session but to have a substantive and meaningful interaction with youth who have experienced significant trauma and difficulty and to play a role in improving their circumstances. It is hoped that the youth develops insight into their circumstances, a greater authentic appreciation of their own strengths and potential, hope for the future and a positive relationship with the clinician.

Not least of all, this chapter is designed to support the interviewer in appreciating what have they gained from getting to know these resilient and wonderful young people for whom the future remains unwritten.

References

1. Warf C, Clark L, Herz D, Rabinovitz S. Continuity of care to nowhere: poverty, child protective services, juvenile justice, homelessness and incarceration: the disproportionate representation of African American children and youth. Int J Child Adolesc Health. ; special issue on poverty and youth. 2009;2(1):48.
2. An excellent example of family-based work with homeless youth is Winlad DN, Gaetz SA, Patton T. Family matters: homeless youth and eva's initiatives family reconnect program. Toronto: The Canadian Homelssness Research Network Press; 2011.
3. Goldenring JM, Cohen E. Getting into adolescent heads. Contemp Pediatr. 1988;5:75.
4. Warf C, Clark L, Desai M, Rabinovitz S, Calvo R, Agahi G, Hoffman J. Coming of age on the streets: survival sex among homeless adolescent females in Hollywood. J Adolesc. 2013;36:1205.
5. Auerswald CL, Eyre SL. Youth homelessness in San Francisco: a life cycle approach. Soc Sci Med. 2002;54(10):1497–512.

Resources

American Academy of Pediatrics: helping foster and adoptive families cope with trauma. https://www.aap.org/en-us/Documents/hfca_foster_trauma_guide.pdf.

British Columbia Treatment Guidelines, Sexually Transmitted Diseases in Adolescents and Adults, 2014, BC CDC http://www.bccdc.ca/resource-gallery/Documents/Communicable-Disease-Manual/Chapter%205%20-%20STI/CPS_BC_STI Treatment_Guidelines_20112014.pdf.

The American Academy of Pediatrics published a number of useful resources aimed at guiding health care providers and families caring for youth in care and traumatized youth (American Academy of Pediatrics. Healthy Foster Care America. Available at:www.aap.org/fostercare. Accessed 02/25/2019.

Contraceptive Technology 2019, contraceptivetechnology21st.com

Ginsburg KR, McClain Z, editors. Reaching teens: strength based communication strategies to build resilience and support healthy adolescent development. 2nd ed. Itasca: American Academy of Pediatrics, in Print for Spring; 2020. (A Textbook and Video Toolkit)

Voices of Youth Count, Missed Opportunities: Homelessness in America. Chicago, IL: Chapin Hall at the University of Chicago, 2017. Retrieved from http://voicesofyouthcount.org/wp-content/uploads/2017/11/VoYC-National-Estimates-Brief-Chapin-Hall-2017.pdf.

Chapter 4
Homeless Adolescents: Identification, Outreach, Engagement, Housing, and Stabilization

Susan Rabinovitz, Arlene Schneir, and Curren Warf

Introduction

Homelessness and housing instability remove youth from conventional social supports and profoundly affect their ability to attend school, participate in sports or other activities, find employment, get medical care and other health services, and maintain family and social relationships necessary for healthy development. Homelessness makes youth highly vulnerable to abuse, sexual exploitation, and physical violence. On the streets, youth are deprived of consistent relationships with caring and responsible adults and exposed to serious drug use, and they may be influenced to engage in high-risk and dangerous behaviors in order to survive. Youth who become acculturated to the streets are poorly equipped to take on responsible adult roles. If not effectively addressed, their social isolation and traumatic experiences threaten their developmental trajectory and impact their ability to lead healthy, productive lives.

It is important for providers to understand the diversity of youths' experiences and circumstances, as well as the services available for them so that they can recognize homelessness and link youth with the services and supports that they need for their safety, stability, and healthy development.

S. Rabinovitz
Division of Adolescent and Young Adult Medicine (Retired), Children's Hospital Los Angeles, Los Angeles, CA, USA

A. Schneir
Division of Adolescent and Young Adult Medicine, Children's Hospital Los Angeles, Los Angeles, CA, USA
e-mail: Aschneir@chla.usc.edu

C. Warf (✉)
Department of Pediatrics (Retired), Division of Adolescent Health and Medicine, British Columbia Children's Hospital, University of British Columbia, Vancouver, BC, Canada

C. Warf, G. Charles (eds.), *Clinical Care for Homeless, Runaway and Refugee Youth*, https://doi.org/10.1007/978-3-030-40675-2_4

Understanding Youth Homelessness

The Scope of the Problem

Estimates of the prevalence of youth experiencing homelessness vary widely based on definitions of homelessness and age ranges of youth, data source and sample, differences in methodologies for counting, and whether the estimates are point in time or annual rates (see chapters on Epidemiology of Homeless Youth and Youth Homelessness in Canada). The January 2017 point-in-time (PIT) count in communities across the USA, mandated biannually by the US Department of Housing and Urban Development (HUD), identified 41,000 unaccompanied homeless youth under age 25; 88% (36,010) were between ages 18 and 25; 61% were male, 37% were girls or young women, and 2% were transgender. More than half of the unaccompanied youth (55%) in the US point-in-time (PIT) count were unsheltered, sleeping outdoors, in cars, or in other places not meant for human habitation [1].

A recent national prevalence study of unaccompanied youth homelessness in the USA, Voices of Youth Count (VoYC), found that across a 12-month period, more than 4.1 million young people between the ages of 13 and 25 experienced some form of homelessness, including youth who were literally on the streets as well as those who were couch surfing only [2]. There were no statistically significant differences in prevalence rates of youth homelessness between urban and rural communities. In the VoYC, 1 in 10 young adults ages 18–25 (3.5 million young adults), experienced some form of homelessness unaccompanied by a parent or guardian over the course of a year, with about half reporting "explicit" homelessness and half reporting couch-surfing only. At least 1 in 30 adolescents ages 13–17 (approximately 660,000 youth) experienced some form of homelessness unaccompanied by a parent or guardian over the course of a year, with approximately 75% reporting "explicit" homelessness, which included running away or being kicked out, and about 25% reporting couch surfing only [2, 3].

Youths' homelessness and housing instability are characterized by high degrees of fluidity [2, 4]. Youth may cycle in and out of homelessness, sometimes staying with friends, sometimes returning to family, and sometimes living on the streets or other places not meant for human habitation. In the VoYC household survey, nearly two-thirds (64.7%) of youth ages 18–25 who reported explicit homelessness also reported couch surfing over the last 12 months [3]. Many youth experience relatively brief periods of homelessness, returning home or to other stable housing for long periods [2]; older youth are less likely to return home compared to youth under age 18 [1].

Causes and Characteristics of Youth Homelessness

In order to intervene with homeless young people, providers need an understanding of the drivers of youth homelessness and a recognition of subpopulations at higher risk. Homelessness disproportionately affects African-American, Latino, and Native

American (indigenous) youth; youth who are gay, lesbian, bisexual, nonbinary, transgender, or questioning (LGBTQ); young parents; and youth aging out of child welfare or exiting juvenile justice systems. Additional factors associated with youth homelessness include: living in poverty; experiencing housing instability or homelessness as a child; not completing high school or obtaining a GED; severe family conflict, maltreatment, abuse, or abandonment by parents or caregivers; and caregiver or youth substance use or mental health disorders [1, 3].

The drivers of youth homelessness are complex and interdependent. It is important to recognize the intersectionality of risk, appreciating the ways that discrimination and disadvantage interact and amplify each other to constrain opportunities for young people, challenge their healthy development, and jeopardize their transition to adulthood [5].

Disproportionate Representation of Ethnic and Racial Minority Youth

Youth of color have a significantly higher prevalence of homelessness compared to their white non-Hispanic peers. According to VoYC national survey data on youth ages 18–25 years old, the relative risk of experiencing homelessness in the last 12 months in the USA is 83% higher for African-American youth compared to others and 33% higher for Hispanic youth compared to non-Hispanic youth [2] (it is interesting to note that when the analysis controlled for education and parenthood, the increased relative risk of experiencing explicit homelessness for Hispanic youth ages 18–25 was no longer significant) [3].

A similar disproportionate representation of ethnic and racial minority youth was found in the 2017 US PIT homeless count. About one-third (33.9%) of unaccompanied homeless youth under age 25 were African-American, over twice the proportion of African-American youth (15%) in the 18–24-year-old US population [6, 7]. This higher representation of African-American youth mirrors racial disparities found in school suspensions, foster care placement, and incarceration and likely represents the multigenerational impact of poverty, discrimination, and exclusion on African-American children and their families in the USA [2, 8].

In the 2017 US PIT count, one in four unaccompanied homeless youth (25%) under age 25 identified as Hispanic; the proportion of Hispanic youth increased to 30.5% of those homeless youth who were unsheltered. In comparison, Hispanic youth are about one in five (21%) of the US population ages 15–24. Over four percent (4.2%) of homeless youth in the PIT count identified as Native American, compared to about 1% of Native American youth ages 18–24 in the US population. About half (48.6%) of homeless youth under age 25 years old in the 2017 PIT count were white, compared to 54% of 18–24-year-olds in the US population [6, 7].

Family Poverty, Parental Loss, and Instability

Homelessness among youth often reflects the economic and social inequities and historical and multigenerational forces that lead families to live in poverty. In a systematic review of causes of child and youth homelessness for youth under age

25 in developed and developing countries, poverty was identified as the most commonly reported reason for youths' street involvement [9]. In the VoYC national survey, youth from low-income households (annual household income of less than $24,000) had a significantly higher risk of experiencing homelessness (RR = 2.62) [3].

Many homeless youth have experienced early housing instability and episodes of homelessness during childhood or adolescence [2]. In in-depth interviews ($n = 215$) conducted with unaccompanied homeless youth ages 13–25 as part of the VoYC study, nearly a quarter had previously experienced family homelessness. More than one-third reported the death of a parent or primary caregiver during their childhood or adolescence, with the most common causes being (in order of frequency) murder, drug overdose, cancer or other terminal illness, heart attack or stroke, and suicide [2, 10]. Their early housing and family instability and significant personal losses were key contributors to their pathways to homelessness, causing not just a loss of housing but critical disruptions in their schooling, neighborhoods, and personal relationships [10].

Family Conflict

Youth homelessness is often rooted in family conflict [11], and youth often report severe family conflict as the primary reason for their homelessness [1]. In the systematic review of causes of child and youth homelessness referenced above, family conflict (including family issues, domestic violence, substance abuse, and alcoholism) was identified as the most commonly reported reason for street involvement of youth in developed countries [9].

Among 873 homeless youth ages 14–21 participating in focus groups and interviews as part of the US Department of Health and Human Services (HHS), Administration on Children, Youth, and Families (ACYF) Street Outreach Program Data Collection Study, the most commonly reported reason for becoming homeless the first time was being asked to leave by a parent or caregiver (51.2%); 22.6% of youth reported they became homeless for the first time due to problems in the home as a result of a parent or caretaker's drug or alcohol abuse [1, 12]. In the VoYC in-depth interviews, chronic family conflict (verbal fights, volatility, escalating threats of violence, etc.) was described by all of the youth and was the most frequently mentioned cause of their homelessness. Over a quarter of youth (26%) described parents who struggled with addictions, unaddressed mental health conditions (9%), or both [10].

LGBTQ youth often describe a gradual escalation of conflict in the home and a growing sense of rejection, often from a parent's partner, as leading to their homelessness. Their risk increases when multiple stressors are present, such as addiction, housing instability, and loss, in addition to impaired family dynamics and lack of acceptance related to their sexual orientation, emerging gender identity, or gender expression [1, 5, 13].

Maltreatment and Abuse

Many homeless youth experienced significant abuse and neglect prior to becoming homeless. In the ACYF Street Outreach Program Data Collection Study, 23.8% of youth disclosed that the primary reason for their becoming homeless the first time was having been physically abused or beaten in the home [1, 12]. In the VoYC in-depth interviews, 30% of youth attributed their homelessness to growing up in families trapped in cycles of physical abuse, neglect, and violence [10].

Child abuse and neglect have profound impacts on development and long-term consequences on physical and mental health. Early exposure to trauma and adverse experiences put youth at risk for prolonged homelessness, serious substance use, mental health disorders, and victimization on the streets [1, 14].

Foster Care and Juvenile Justice

Youth who have been in foster care or juvenile justice systems and "crossover youth" who have been in both systems are at high risk for homelessness and are particularly at risk for prolonged homelessness [1]. According to brief in-person surveys ($n = 4139$) conducted through the VoYC, nearly one-third of youth who had experienced homelessness had been involved with foster care, and nearly half had been in juvenile detention, jail, or prison [2]. Although foster care is intended to stabilize and protect youth, youth interviewed through the VoYC identified their entrance into the foster care system as the beginning of their pathway to homelessness, with out-of-home placement disrupting family relationships, school involvement, neighborhood connections, and relationships with friends [10]. According to outcome data from the US National Youth in Transition Database (NYTD), which states are mandated to provide, 19% of youth who had been in foster care at age 17 years reported 2 years later that they had been homeless at some time during that period [15, 16, p. 2] (See chapter Youth in Care: A Very High-Risk Population for Homelessness.) Those youth who had experienced multiple placements in congregate care, African-American youth, and youth who had changed schools frequently faced significantly higher risks of experiencing homelessness after aging out of foster care [1].

Young Parents

Approximately 9400 parenting youth under age 25 and their approximately 12,150 children were identified as experiencing homelessness in the 2017 US PIT homeless count; almost all (95%) were in shelters or transitional living programs [1]. Data from the VoYC national household survey show a relative risk for homelessness of 3.0 (2.37–3.76) for youth ages 18–25 who were unmarried with children of their own [3]. Among the 18- to 25-year-old youth who had experienced homelessness, 43% of young women and 29% of young men reported having at least one child (by comparison, 22% of young women and 14% of young men who had not experienced homelessness during the past year reported having at least one child) [17]. In the brief youth surveys (n = 4139) conducted with youth experiencing homelessness as part of the VoYC, prevalence of pregnancy and parenthood was lower among minor youth, with ten percent (10%) of the girls reporting being pregnant or a parent and three (3%) of the boys reporting having a pregnant partner or being a parent [17].

Lesbian, Gay, Bisexual, Nonbinary, Transgender, Questioning (LGBTQ) Youth

Youth who identify as lesbian, gay, bisexual, nonbinary, gender fluid, transgender, or questioning (LGBTQ) are overrepresented among unaccompanied youth who experience homelessness [1]. In the VoYC survey, LGBTQ youth made up about 20% of young adults ages 18–25 reporting homelessness, with over twice the risk of experiencing homelessness (relative risk = 2.20) compared to youth of the same age identifying as heterosexual and cisgender [3, 5]. The proportion of youth experiencing homelessness who identified as LGBTQ was significantly higher in larger urban communities (up to 40% in one county's youth count) compared to rural communities, in contrast to the similar prevalence of youth homelessness between urban and rural communities found in the survey [5].

The risk of homelessness among LGBTQ youth is not the same for all ethnic and racial groups. In the VoYC national survey, black and multiracial LGBTQ youth ages 18–25 had some of the highest rates of homelessness. Black LGBTQ youth, particularly young men, reported the highest rates of explicit homelessness; nearly one in four young black men ages 18–25 who identified as LGBTQ reported explicit homelessness in the previous 12 months [1, 5].

LGBTQ homeless youth face increased risk of adverse experiences compared to their heterosexual and/or cisgender homeless peers. Transgender youth, in particular, often report severe types of discrimination, victimization, and trauma [5, 12, 18]. In comparison to non-LGBTQ homeless youth, LGBTQ homeless youth report having experienced more discrimination and stigma both within the family and outside the family; more harm to themselves; more victimization on the streets including rape, being beaten up, robbed, and threatened or assaulted with a weapon; more involvement in survival sex (exchanging sex for basic needs); and more involvement in sex trafficking [1, 6, 19, 20]. Among youth experiencing homelessness, LGBTQ youth have over twice the rate of early death [5].

The disproportionate risks experienced by LGBTQ youth are not limited to young people who are homeless. LGBTQ adolescents and young adults have significantly worse health outcomes than their heterosexual and/or cisgender peers, including higher rates of mental health problems such as chronic stress and depression, as well as substance abuse and suicide [13, 21]. The health disparities for LGBTQ youth as well as their increased risk of homelessness may emerge in part from the stigma, discrimination, harassment, and other forms of victimization LGBTQ youth experience in their families, schools, and communities [13, 21]. Further jeopardizing their health status and complicating their service access is the implicit heteronormative assumptions present in many healthcare settings and service environments [22].

Acculturation to the Streets and Risks of Homelessness

The more time young people spend disconnected from families or on the streets, the more they are at risk [23]. Youth who end up on the streets commonly go through stages of acculturation beginning with an initial period characterized by fear and anxiety, being and feeling alone, and insecurity about shelter and food [24]. During their initial period of homelessness, youth are often open to involving supportive services, including child protective services, working toward reconciliation with parents and returning home, if there is a home to return to, or entering a shelter or transitional living program if one is available. The longer youth remain on the streets, the more distrustful they may become of mainstream institutions including medical clinics, shelters, and social services and the more difficult it may become to engage them and get them off the streets.

Youth who remain on the streets may become more engaged in the street culture. They often develop an increased affiliation with more experienced homeless youth who serve as a kind of "mentor," helping them learn how to survive, how to make money, and where to get food. They may become more involved in the street economy of panhandling, drug dealing, survival sex, minor theft, and odd jobs [24]. Their experiences can be both exhilarating and terrifying, further cementing their connection to the streets. Their social relationships with other youth can be quite close and very meaningful, with youth commonly referring to their "street family" [24]. This reality is in contrast to the common perception of adults outside of their environment, who may not appreciate the interdependency of these relationships and the sense of community that develops. Notwithstanding the perception of protection offered by their street family, given youths' instability, lack of resources, and dependency, they remain vulnerable to exploitation and escalating risk behaviors.

Risks of Substance Use

Drugs can play a crucial role during initiation into street life. The shared use of drugs may solidify bonding with others on the street and expose youth to those with more advanced drug use, including injection drug use, who may influence their behavior [24].

Youth experiencing homelessness use alcohol and drugs at substantially higher rates than their non-homeless peers; substance use among homeless youth has been reported as two to three times higher than rates found among non-homeless young adults [6, 25]. One study of street youth found that up to 86% of homeless youth met the DSM IV diagnostic criteria for drug dependence or abuse [26].

Substance use prevalence rates are substantially higher among those homeless youth living on the streets compared to those homeless youth who are sheltered [6]. Increased drug use is associated with length of time homeless, age of onset of homelessness (under age 25), victimization on the streets, and involvement in survival sex. Homeless individuals with drug use are less likely to achieve housing stability, even when compared with homeless individuals with other physical and other nondrug-related mental health disorders [26].

Alcohol and drug use are associated with significant morbidity and mortality. The mortality rate for homeless youth has been found to be at least ten times higher than the mortality rate for housed youth, with drug overdose being one of the leading causes of death [26, 27]. With the current fentanyl and other opioid crisis, homeless youth face an escalating threat of a serious drug overdose, including lethal overdose. (See chapters on Motivational Enhancement Therapy for Adolescents with Substance Abuse and Stabilization and Secure Care Following Opiate Overdose.)

Risk of Engagement in Survival Sex and Sex Trafficking

Homeless youth, with little means of support, may engage in survival sex to meet basic needs, trading sex for food, shelter, money, protection or drugs, or to feed their children if the youth is a parent [1, 20, 28]. Prevalence rates of survival sex by homeless youth vary based on data source and definition. In a 10-city study of 621 homeless youth ages 17–25 accessed through agency sites in the USA and Canada, nearly 1 in 5 (19%) had turned to survival sex at some point in their lives in order to meet basic needs [19]. The ACYF Street Outreach Study found that approximately one-quarter of homeless youth had traded sex with at least one person for money (24.1%), a place to spend the night (27.5%), food (18.3%), protection (12.0%), or drugs (11.2%); similar proportions of females and males were involved except for protection, with significantly more females (17.8%) than males (6.7%) reporting exchanging sex for protection [12].

Homeless youth on the streets may become vulnerable to the influence of adults who demonstrate interest in them and may subject them to sex or labor trafficking through force, fraud, or coercion [6, 12, 14, 19, 29]. In the 10-city study of homeless youth, more than 9 in 10 youth (91%) said they had been approached by strangers or acquaintances offering work opportunities that turned out to be fraudulent (e.g., credit card scams, check fraud) or turned into sex or labor trafficking or commercial sex [19].

Estimates of the prevalence of young people who are sex and labor trafficked vary based on differences in data source, methodologies, and definitions used [29], with definitional ambiguity arising from issues such as differences in inclusion or exclusion criteria, age of consent, and legal codes.[1] Both the 10-city study and a 3-city study of 270 homeless youth ages 18–25 accessed through agency sites in the USA found similar rates of sex trafficking among youth (14% in the 10-city study and 17% in the 3-city study) [19, 20]. In the 10-city study, nearly 58% (57.6%) of the youth who identified as sex trafficking victims experienced force, fraud, or coercion [19]. In the 3-city study, youth who were sex trafficked were more likely than those who were not to be female or transgender, sexual minorities, or Latino and to have dropped out of high school. Perceived vulnerability, lack of resources or financial support, and isolation increased the risk of involvement [29]. While youth may become involved in sex or labor trafficking through gangs or organized criminal groups, they may have more personal relationships with those responsible for their participation, including family members, intimate partners, and peers [19].

In both studies LGBTQ youth were disproportionately affected by sex trafficking: LGBTQ youth accounted for 36% of youth reporting sex trafficking in the 10-city study though they were only 19% of youth interviewed [19], and 39% of youth reporting sex trafficking in the three-city study, though they were only 15% of youth interviewed. Transgender youth were particularly vulnerable, with 60% reporting sex trafficking [20].

Overall, both studies found high levels of commercial sex activity (any sex act in which anything of value is given to or received by any person, including survival sex, sex work, prostitution, and sex trafficking) among homeless youth interviewed: 30% of youth in the 10-city study and 36% of youth in the 3-city study [19, 20]. These behaviors carry with them an inherent danger for sexually transmitted infections, including HIV, and correlate with escalating drug use and increased risk of assault, in addition to the stigma, negative emotional repercussions, and short- and long-term mental health issues that may result from involvement. Providers hoping to support sex-trade engaged youth need to understand the compelling survival needs that push youth into participation, while appreciating that for some youth, their involvement provides a sense of agency and control as they confront the exigencies of homelessness [19].

[1] US Trafficking Victims Protection Act (TVPA) defines sex trafficking as "a commercial sex act induced by force, fraud or coercion, or when the person induced to perform such an act has not attained the age of 18 years of age." The TVPA defines a commercial sex act as any sex act in which anything of value is given to, or received by, any person. In Canada, minors must prove force, fraud, or coercion to be considered trafficking victims. (From Murphy [19, p. 10]).

Family Support, Reunification, and Sustaining Family Connections

Support for Family Reunification

Despite chronic family conflict and disruption, many homeless youth sustain relationships with their friends and family. Efforts should be made to support homeless youth's involvement with family or other caring adults from their community. Youth should be encouraged to attend school and participate in activities that provide safe spaces and create a social safety net. Facilitating young people's positive connections with families, communities, schools, and other positive social networks can be critical in fostering youths' resilience, building their competence, promoting their stabilization and healthy development, and reducing or ending their homelessness [23].

I have been told that most of the youth that return to families don't stay (according to Eric Rice). I worry that we are saying that brief homelessness isn't dangerous for young people. Family reconciliation and reunification, in particular for youth under age 18, are achievable in many cases. According to the US federal data, around 70% of youth under age 18 who entered a Family and Youth Services Bureau–funded emergency shelter left the shelter to return to a parent or guardian [16].

The use of evidence-based and promising practices in family interventions and trauma-informed care can address and reduce family conflict, strengthen and support parents' capacities to provide stability, and help youth understand and develop skills in managing complex and difficult relationships as they try to remain connected to or reunify with family members [10, 16, p. 4]. With the disproportionate risk of homelessness among LGBTQ youth, family interventions that promote acceptance can help reduce conflict and improve family functioning. LGBTQ young people can often identify a potential ally within their household or extended family network – an aunt, older sibling, or family friend – who can buffer conflict, reduce feelings of rejection, and provide support and stability [5]. In families where children and youth have experienced significant maltreatment or there is serious parental impairment due to mental illness or addiction, maintaining contact or returning home may not be realistic or in the best interests of the young person, though living with extended family or familiar and supportive adults may still be possible.

Providers need to recognize the strong need and desire that many youth have to reconnect with their families, despite a history of turbulent relationships, estrangement, or maltreatment. It is important to assess the safety of the family environment; prepare both youth and family for reunification, helping them identify and anticipate potential areas of conflict; establish agreements for managing issues that may emerge; and help them develop plans for alternative living arrangements if reunification isn't successful or they need more time to work things out. At times, youth return to home environments that are chaotic and destructive; they will need support navigating their family relationships, managing their expectations, and dealing with their feelings of disappointment and loss [30].

Homeless Young Women with Children

Being pregnant or having a child may be a compelling reason for homeless girls and young women to seek out or accept services and reconcile with parents and family. Young women want to be good parents. Their drive to protect their children may serve to increase their receptivity to housing and stabilization services and family intervention and support. It is essential to link these young women with shelter, housing, and other supports, along with public benefits, and, when appropriate, to support efforts to engage the father of their child or their current partner, explore family reunification, and build connections with parents and other family members [17].

Engaging and Serving Homeless Youth

Homeless youth need specialized services and youth-friendly approaches to address their developmental needs and overcome the challenges and negative consequences of homelessness. It is important for providers to have a broad understanding of program models and resources for homeless youth to facilitate access to care and promote stabilization and independence.

The US Interagency Council on Homelessness (USICH) in their report "Preventing and Ending Youth Homelessness, A Coordinated Community Response" has developed a comprehensive strategy with the following components: [16, pp. 3–4; 31].

- Identify and work with families who are at risk through promoting the use of evidence-based and promising practices in family interventions that can reduce family conflict and, when safe and appropriate, ensure youth remain connected to their families.
- Identify and engage youth who are at risk for, or experiencing, homelessness, and connect them to trauma-informed, culturally appropriate, and developmentally age-appropriate interventions with the goal of preventing and diverting youth from experiencing homelessness.
- Develop partnerships with schools, child protective services, juvenile and adult justice systems, mental healthcare systems, and other youth-serving programs.
- Intervene early when youth become homeless and, when safe and appropriate, work toward family reunification.
- Strengthen community capacity to provide low-barrier emergency and crisis services for youth who are unsheltered, fleeing an unsafe situation, or experiencing a housing crisis.

- Connect youth to services and developmentally appropriate housing through short- and long-term shelters, transitional housing, and host homes and access other forms of emergency assistance.
- Access shelter or other temporary housing in the community with a range of options that are culturally and linguistically responsive and not contingent on school attendance, sobriety, minimum income requirements, absence of a criminal record, or other unnecessary conditions, with options appropriate for particularly vulnerable youth, particularly LGBT youth. It is implicit in providing voluntary placement that youth have a right to refuse placement.
- Develop coordinated entry systems for appropriate types of assistance for the most vulnerable for youth in unsafe situations, such as fleeing domestic violence, dating violence, sexual violence, trafficking, or with other significant risk factors or vulnerabilities.
- Ensure access to safe shelter and emergency services when needed.
- Ensure that assessments respond to the unique needs and circumstances of youth, and emphasize strong connections to and supported exits from mainstream systems.
- Create individualized services and housing options tailored to the needs of each youth, including education and employment.
- Assure that youth can move into permanent or non-time-limited housing with appropriate services and supports.

Outreach to and Identification of Youth Experiencing Homelessness

Life on the streets can be dangerous and frightening, and young people commonly experience and/or witness traumatic or threatening events. These incidents, difficult and dangerous as they are, can be a catalyst for change and create an opportunity to connect a young person to a shelter or other supervised environment [24].

Youth who are homeless can be encountered in youth centers, parks, libraries, abandoned buildings, bus or train stations, and on the streets in cities and towns. Specialized outreach workers trained in trauma-informed care may be the youth's first point of contact with services and can play a critical role in identifying youth, building relationships, and fostering connection with a broader system of care. In some cases, outreach workers may have been homeless youth themselves and can demonstrate an extraordinary commitment and intuitive ability to make connections [32].

Outreach workers can provide for some of the basic needs of youth while they are homeless, offering food, clothing, and items for personal hygiene while connecting youth to other resources and linking youth to healthcare, drop-in centers, shelters, transitional living programs, and other supportive services. Outreach is an assertive approach that requires collaboration with schools and youth-serving agencies to identify youth and locations where youth congregate. Outreach provides an opportunity to identify young people who are new to the street and who might be open to early diversion or family reunification.

"Street medicine" that integrates assertive outreach with provision of medical care is a developing and innovative area to improve access to care [33]. Given the opportunity, clinicians may accompany outreach workers, provide limited evaluations with problem-focused acute care, and invite the young person to an accessible walk-in clinic. Through these efforts the clinician can develop a deeper appreciation of the circumstances in which homeless young people live and survive.

Program Approaches for Youth Experiencing Homelessness

To be effective, an intervention model for ending youth homelessness requires the use of a systematic approach across multiple providers and service systems (e.g., schools, housing providers, youth programs), using the best available research to guide service delivery and a risk and protective factors perspective to understand the diverse needs of homeless young people and inform individual- and system-level interventions [23].

Trauma-Informed Care and Positive Youth Development Approaches

Trauma-informed care and positive youth development are essential practice frameworks for structuring services and delivering interventions with homeless youth to help them heal and thrive [23]. Trauma-informed approaches recognize the significant role trauma has played in the lives of youth and shifts the clinical perspective from "what's wrong with you" to "what happened to you" by recognizing and accepting difficult behaviors as strategies developed to cope with childhood trauma. A trauma-informed approach focuses on creating safe, accepting, and respectful environments to help youth heal from the effects of trauma and teaches youth skills to improve coping, manage emotions, connect with others, build relationships, and find hope, purpose, and meaning [34]. Programs for homeless youth need clear strategies for providing trauma-informed care and relational skill development training, incorporating youth's perspectives, and valuing their insights regarding their needs and service priorities [10].

Positive youth development is a strength-based framework that recognizes the potential of youth. A working group from the US Department of Health and Human Services, Office of Population Affairs, developed the following definition of positive youth development for use by federal programs:

> Positive youth development is an intentional, pro-social approach that engages youth within their communities, schools, organizations, peer groups, and families in a manner that is productive and constructive; recognizes, utilizes, and enhances young people's strengths;

and promotes positive outcomes for young people by providing opportunities, fostering positive relationships, and furnishing the support needed to build on their leadership strengths [35].

Youth programs that use a positive youth development approach have been found to positively impact academic achievement, family relationships, and mental and physical health [36].

Developing the Skills for Self-Sufficiency and Independence

There are differences among young people in their ability to live independently, and it takes time to assess capability and readiness. Some youth are able to stabilize with less oversight and support, more readily learning new skills and taking on new responsibilities such as school, working, or managing a budget. Others have more challenges and need more intensive intervention, careful monitoring, and ongoing service provision. The path to independence is not smooth; one should expect setbacks and challenges as youth struggle to master skills and consolidate new abilities.

Young people need both hard and soft skills in order to succeed. The hard skills are the technical and academic skills that are necessary for education and employment. The soft skills are the interpersonal and emotional regulation skills that help them build the connections that are key to success. For young people growing up in stable environments, these skills develop gradually through school and life experiences. Adolescents and young adults who are experiencing homelessness, either alone or within families, often have significant deficits in both of these areas. Interrupted education makes homeless youth less prepared in the hard skills areas, such as reading and math. Severe family conflict, family disruption, multiple out-of-home placements, serious mental health problems, substance use, or significant traumatic experiences may interfere with youths' interpersonal skills, their ability to read social cues, and their ability to manage their impulses and regulate their emotions.

The trauma-informed care and positive youth development approaches underlying program services and interventions can help motivate youth, build their core skills and competencies, strengthen their interpersonal skills, and foster their social connections with peers and supportive adults to help prepare them for adulthood and self-sufficiency [23, 34, 37].

Engaging Homeless Youth and Promoting Youth Leadership

Youth engagement increases self-esteem, builds social connections, and develops skills and competencies [32, p. 12]. Youth engagement and leadership are core to achieving housing stability and self-sufficiency. Youth have energy, new ideas, and a willingness to question established practices and challenge adults to be more effective and responsive. Young people bring their insights and experiences, and their voices can play a meaningful role in shaping services.

There are many approaches to youth engagement; all of them build on a respect for youth input and their lived experiences and foster youth leadership skills. Opportunities include participation on speaker panels, membership on youth advisory boards, or participation in point-in-time homeless counts. Youth engagement takes time, commitment, and planning. It requires a good fit between participants and agencies and a belief by both youth and adults in its value.

Services for Youth Experiencing Homelessness

Drop-in centers, shelter, and housing, along with medical care and mental health services, are needed to help stabilize youth. Housing and services need to be aligned with youths' distinct needs and abilities, offering them safety from the streets, and the chance to develop the skills and capacity for independent living and self-sufficiency. Age, length of time homeless, trauma history, system involvement, and family relationships determine the types of housing and services that homeless youth need [38].

A continuum of resources is required, with low-barrier programs available for youth who have acculturated to the streets and won't access services with restrictions such as sobriety or early curfews, and more comprehensive, structured services available for youth who are ready to participate. Specialized services and supports should be targeted for specific subpopulations of homeless youth such as LGBTQ youth, pregnant and parenting youth, youth with substance use and mental health problems, youth fleeing intimate partner violence or trafficking, and those leaving juvenile or criminal justice systems [16, p. 3].

Case Management and Individual Service Planning

Most shelters and housing programs provide individualized and age- and culturally - appropriate case management to help stabilize youth and connect them to the resources they need. The intensity of intervention is determined by the needs and capabilities of youth, though funding limitations may constrain the level and duration of service provision. Case managers assess youths' needs and strengths, their risk and protective factors, and individual goals and circumstances to develop an individualized service plan. Relatively brief screening and assessment are required while trust is still being established between youth and youth workers. The specific combination and sequencing of housing, treatment, school and community programming, and family supports are determined by the needs and circumstances of individual youth [23]. Case managers provide risk reduction education and supportive counseling; focus on building skills, competencies, and positive connections; and link youth to on-site or community-based education, employment, healthcare, and mental health treatment services. Many programs provide aftercare case management to support stabilization.

Case managers need to create a positive alliance with youth, respecting their experiences and involving them in the decisions that affect them. Youth's personal involvement in case planning and housing decisions creates a greater sense of ownership and acceptance [32, p. 12]. Approaching young people with respect for their insights and strengths and engaging them in thoughtful considerations of options can build positive connections and promote stability. (Refer to the chapter – Interviewing Homeless Adolescents in the Context of Clinical Care: Creating Connections, Building on Strengths, Fostering Resilience, and Improving Outcomes – in this book.)

Drop-in Centers

Drop-in centers are commonly the first point of contact for homeless youth. They provide a friendly, low-barrier environment with a minimum of rules to address basic needs such as meals, laundry, showers, lockers, and clothing and usually provide on-site or referral services for substance use and mental health counseling, shelter and housing, school, and employment. Through a relationship with a healthcare agency, a limited scope of medical services can be provided. Drop-in centers are effective environments for fostering positive youth development, involving young people in arts, music, education, or physical activities, depending on youth interests and staff capacities. Youth can be engaged in identifying program needs and in designing programs. Youths' experiences at drop-in centers and the positive relationships they form with staff and peers can be bridges to further stabilization.

Medical Care for Homeless Youth

Medical care is a key component of services for homeless youth. Young people need medical care for contraception, prevention and treatment of STIs and HIV, treatment of acute illness and injuries, and management of chronic health conditions. Care provided through street outreach programs, in nontraditional settings frequented by youth (e.g., drop-in centers), in youth-specific transitional living and permanent housing programs, and in youth-friendly clinics is critical for increasing access and utilization (see chapter Clinical Care of Homeless Youth).

Housing Models for Youth Experiencing Homelessness

Young people experiencing homelessness need a range of developmentally appropriate housing options to address their unique needs and provide appropriate types and levels of support. Transitional age youth ages 18–25 need access to youth-specific housing and should not be housed with older homeless adults.

Housing options for homeless adolescents and young adults include emergency shelters, transitional living, and permanent housing programs. Youth may enter and exit housing programs multiple times before they can commit to a program or plan, and they may need one type of housing at one point and then find they need another when their circumstances change.

Youth Shelters

Shelters for minors (up to age 18) and transition age youth (usually ages 18 through 24) offer temporary safe housing, meals, and showers and provide respite from the streets. Staff can provide referrals for counseling and other services and support youth in reconnecting with families, returning to school, or preparing for employment. Youth may prefer shelters over abandoned buildings, bus stations, or parks which can be frightening and expose them to older chronically homeless adults. While not a solution to homelessness, shelters may facilitate entry into longer-term housing and stabilization.

Host Homes

Host Homes are an innovative approach to addressing youth homelessness. Host Homes are a flexible model that can offer both voluntary emergency shelter and longer-term transitional living in the home of a trained community host. Host Homes provide a safe living environment (largely for young adults) with client-driven supportive services to help youth complete education, prepare for employment, and find permanent housing, often enabling youth to stay in their communities and retain connections with friends and family [32]. Some Host Homes programs are developed to target specific populations of youth experiencing homelessness, such as LGBTQ youth or college students.

Transitional Housing/Transitional Living

Transitional living programs of time-limited supportive housing (usually 18–24 months) serve both minor and transitional-aged youth who are not yet ready for independent living. Transitional housing models vary and include congregate housing with consistent overnight staff for youth (particularly for younger adolescents under age 18), clustered housing units with or without an on-site supervisor, and scattered site or shared apartments. Many programs utilize a housing-first approach providing low-barrier entry with minimal requirements for participation [32].

Services offered and duration of stay vary according to the funding source and youth population targeted. Transitional living programs focus on preparing youth for permanent housing and independence, offering life skills training, education planning, and employment preparation. They frequently provide supportive counseling, healthcare, and mental health and substance abuse treatment either on site or by referral.

Permanent Housing: Rapid Rehousing and Permanent Supportive Housing

Rapid rehousing is a strategy for achieving housing stability quickly, providing time-limited rental assistance (typically, for no longer than 24 months) and developmentally appropriate case management and support services to help youth experiencing homelessness obtain housing and increase self-sufficiency. Rapid rehousing has become an important new tool for communities in their efforts to address youth homelessness. The intent of the program is that by the end of the rental assistance period, young people will be able to take over the lease and responsibility for paying their rent on their own.

Permanent supportive housing is non-time-limited permanent housing with indefinite leasing or rental assistance, paired with supportive services to assist homeless youth with disabilities, usually ages 18–24 years old, achieve housing stability. Permanent supportive housing is designed for youth with the highest and most complex service needs, including youth with serious traumatic backgrounds and mental health and substance abuse disorders. Service models may be scattered site units or a single-site rental building, using tenant-based or project-based rental assistance to support costs [32]. Increasingly, research efforts are focused on developing validated tools to assess youth's needs to identify the most vulnerable and prioritize them for entry into the limited permanent housing programs that are available [39].

Both rapid rehousing and permanent supportive housing utilize

- A *Housing First* model to provide immediate low-barrier access to entry and participation, with a harm reduction and trauma-informed approach.
- *Voluntary participation.* Participation in services is not required for youth to receive housing assistance.
- *Individualized and age-appropriate case management* to provide services and resources to help stabilize youth; help them meet lease responsibilities; and connect them with on-site or community-based healthcare, treatment, educational, and employment services.

Limitations of the Current Housing Continuum for Youth

These housing resources – emergency shelters, host homes, transitional living, and permanent housing programs – are essential components of the housing continuum, but there are limitations that constrain successful outcomes for youth. Age restrictions and eligibility criteria limit accessibility, particularly for transition age youth; lengths of stay are often too limited to give youth sufficient time to stabilize and heal; rules for participation are often too rigid, posing entry barriers for some youth and not providing the flexibility youth need to make mistakes, experience setbacks, and start over; and expectations of permanency are not necessarily realistic for a population of young people who are in transition [10, 38]. There is often a lack of programs in black and multiracial communities, particularly for LGBTQ youth, which limits access for populations critically affected by homelessness [5]. Many young parents struggle to obtain shelter and longer-term transitional living – many youth-specific housing providers don't serve youth with children, and family housing programs usually don't serve minor parents [17]. The restriction in most permanent housing programs to youth with a qualifying disability limits access for other homeless youth who need long-term support to fully stabilize and transition to independence. Ultimately, to end youth homelessness, we need youth-specific, developmentally appropriate housing models that provide security of tenancy, assistance with rent and living expenses, and supportive services and independent living skills training so that homeless youth can address their experiences of trauma, complete their education, effectively prepare for employment and self-sufficiency, stabilize, and thrive.

Preventing and Reducing Youth Homelessness

The scope, causes, and consequences of youth homelessness require individual-level, family-based, and community-level prevention and intervention, as well as structural changes in practices, programs, and policies, to address the complex and overlapping social, economic, physical, environmental, and community factors that shape and constrain opportunities and outcomes for youth [40].

There is the potential to strengthen and support young people and their families through earlier interventions and therapeutic approaches, particularly those that address the trauma, stigma, and discrimination that many young people and their families have experienced [10].

Interventions are needed to address the stressors that families face such as poverty, racism, housing instability, addiction, and mental health problems [5], with resources targeted to those youth most vulnerable to homelessness: LGBTQ youth; youth of color, particularly African-American, Latino, and Indigenous youth; young parents; and youth who have not completed high school or obtained a GED [2]. Interventions that build on local, regional, and federal initiatives to strengthen and extend school dropout prevention and positive youth development programs; improve public systems, particularly child welfare and juvenile and criminal justice; expand affordable housing and employment programs; and promote healthy families and communities could have a significant impact on improving outcomes and preventing and reducing youth homelessness [5].

Creating a System of Care for Homeless Youth

In order to reduce and end youth homelessness, we urgently need to expand youth-specific services and increase the capacity of systems and service providers to respond to the needs of youth and families. We need to listen to youth, provide meaningful opportunities for their leadership, and incorporate their feedback and priorities in service planning and delivery. Coordination among service providers and collaboration across systems, utilization of evidence-based interventions, data-driven strategies, and rigorous monitoring and evaluation are required to ensure that we are providing the services and supports needed to effectively support young people, their families, and communities.

Resources
The National Center for Youth Law www.youthlaw.org

Ending Youth Homelessness: Guidebook series: Promising Program Models
https://files.hudexchange.info/resources/documents/Ending-Youth-Homelessness-Promising-Program-Models.pdf

- Primary Prevention
- Identification and Engagement: Mobile "Street" Outreach, Drop-In Centers, Family Engagement
- Emergency and Crisis Response: Youth Shelters and Emergency Services, Host Homes, Transitional Housing and Transitional Living
- Tailored Housing and Services: Rapid Re-Housing, Non-Time-Limited Supportive Housing

Voices of Youth Count Chapin Hall
https://voicesofyouthcount.org/

Chapin Hall at the University of Chicago Research-to-Impact Missed Opportunities Briefs (Morton et al. [2]).
- Missed Opportunities: Youth Homelessness in America *National Estimates*
- https://voicesofyouthcount.org/brief/national-estimates-of-youth-homelessness/
- https://voicesofyouthcount.org/wp-content/uploads/2017/11/VoYC-National-Estimates-Brief-Chapin-Hall-2017.pdf
- Missed Opportunities in Youth Pathways Through Homelessness
- https://voicesofyouthcount.org/brief/missed-opportunities-youth-pathways-through-homelessness-in-america/
- https://voicesofyouthcount.org/wp-content/uploads/2019/05/ChapinHall_VoYC_Youth-Pathways-FINAL.pdf
- Missed Opportunities: LGBTQ Youth Homelessness in America
- https://voicesofyouthcount.org/brief/lgbtq-youth-homelessness/
- https://voicesofyouthcount.org/wp-content/uploads/2018/05/VoYC-LGBTQ-Brief-Chapin-Hall-2018.pdf
- Missed Opportunities: Pathways from Foster Care to Youth Homelessness in America
- https://voicesofyouthcount.org/brief/missed-opportunities-pathways-from-foster-care-to-youth-homelessness-in-america/

- https://voicesofyouthcount.org/wp-content/uploads/2019/04/Chapin-Hall_VoYC_Child-Welfare-Brief_2019-1.pdf
- Missed Opportunities: Education Among Youth Experiencing Homelessness in America
- https://voicesofyouthcount.org/brief/missed-opportunities-education-among-youth-experiencing-homelessness-in-america/
- https://voicesofyouthcount.org/wp-content/uploads/2019/11/ChapinHall_VoYC_Education-Brief.pdf
- Missed Opportunities: Pregnant and Parenting Youth Experiencing Homelessness in America
- https://voicesofyouthcount.org/brief/pregnant-and-parenting-youth-experiencing-homelessness/
- https://voicesofyouthcount.org/wp-content/uploads/2018/05/VoYC-Pregnant-and-Parenting-Brief-Chapin-Hall-2018.pdf

National Alliance to End Homelessness; LK Pope, *Housing for Homeless Youth*

- Youth Homelessness Series Brief No. 3 https://endhomelessness.org/

United States Interagency Council on Homelessness
https://www.usich.gov

- Preventing and Ending Youth Homelessness, *A Coordinated Community Response* https://www.usich.gov/resources/uploads/asset_library/Youth_Homelessness_Coordinated_Response.pdf
- Framework to End Youth Homelessness https://www.usich.gov/tools-for-action/framework-for-ending-youth-homelessness
- Homelessness in America Focus on Youth https://www.usich.gov/tools-for-action/homelessness-in-america-focus-on-youth
- Framework to End Youth Homelessness: A Resource Text for Dialogue and Action. USICH. February 2013. https://www.usich.gov/resources/uploads/asset_library/USICH_Federal_Youth_Framework.pdf

- Rice E. The TAY Triage Tool: a tool to identify homeless transition age youth most in need of permanent supportive housing. https://www.csh.org/resources/the-tay-triage-tool-a-tool-to-identify-homeless-transition-age-youth-most-in-need-of-permanent-supportive-housing/
- Byram T, Peart S. Young and homeless: exploring the education, life experiences and aspirations of homeless youth. London: UCL Institute of Education Press; 2017.
- Karabanow J, Kidd S, Frederick T, Hughes J. Homeless youth and the search for stability. Waterloo: Wilfrid Laurier University Press; 2018.
- Winlad DN, Gaetz SA, Patton T. Family matters: homeless youth and Eva's Initiatives Family Reconnect program. Toronto: The Canadian Homelessness Research Network Press; 2011.
- Homeless Youth Handbook. https://www.bakermckenzie.com/en/newsroom/2018/10/homeless-youth-handbook-video.

References

1. US Interagency Council on Homelessness. Homelessness in America: focus on youth. 2018. https://www.usich.gov/resources/uploads/asset_library/Homelessness_in_America_Youth.pdf.
2. Morton MH, Dworsky A, Samuels GM. Missed opportunities: youth homelessness in America. National Estimates. Chicago: Chapin Hall at the University of Chicago; 2017. https://voicesofyouthcount.org/wp-content/uploads/2017/11/ChapinHall_VoYC_NationalReport_Final.pdf. Accessed 7 Oct 2019.
3. Morton MH, et al. Prevalence and correlates of youth homelessness in the United States. J Adolesc Health. 2018;62(1):14–21. https://doi.org/10.1016/j.jadohealth.2017.10.006.
4. Samuels B. No more missed opportunities on youth homelessness. The Chronicle of Social Change. 2019. https://chronicleofsocialchange.org/featured/no-more-missed-opportunities-on-youth-homelessness/36302. Accessed 7 Oct 2019.
5. Morton MH, Samuels GM, Dworsky A, Patel S. Missed opportunities: LGBTQ youth homelessness in America. Chicago: Chapin Hall at the University of Chicago; 2018.
6. United States Interagency Council on Homelessness. Homelessness in America: focus on youth. 2019. https://www.usich.gov/resources/uploads/asset_library/Homelessness_in_America_Youth.pdf. Accessed 3 Oct 2019.
7. U.S. Department of Housing and Urban Development. The 2017 Annual Homeless Assessment Report (AHAR) to congress. Part 1: point-in-time estimates of homelessness. Dec 2017. https://files.hudexchange.info/resources/documents/2017-AHAR-Part-1.pdf. Accessed 25 Oct 2019.
8. Warf C, Clark L, Herz D, Rabinovitz S. Continuity of care to nowhere: poverty, child protective services, juvenile justice, homelessness and incarceration: the disproportionate representation of African American children and youth. Int J Child Adolesc Health. 2009;2(1):48–64.
9. Embleton L, Lee H, Gunn J, Ayuku D, Braitstein P. Causes of child and youth homelessness in developed and developing countries, a systematic review and meta-analysis. JAMA Pediatr. 2016;170(5):435–44. https://doi.org/10.1001/jamapediatrics.2016.0156.
10. Samuels GM, Cerven C, Curry S, Robinson SR, Patel S. Missed opportunities in youth pathways through homelessness. Chicago: Chapin Hall at the University of Chicago; 2019.
11. National Alliance to End Homelessness. Homelessness in America/Who experiences homelessness?/Youth and young adults. 2019. https://endhomelessness.org/homelessness-in-america/who-experiences-homelessness/youth/. Accessed 7 Oct 2019.
12. U.S. Dept of Health and Human Services, Administration for Children and Families, Family and Youth Services Bureau. Final report – street outreach program data collection study. 2016. Retrieved from: https://www.acf.hhs.gov/sites/default/files/fysb/data_collection_study_final_report_street_outreach_program.pdf. Accessed 14 Oct 2019.
13. Hafeez H, Zeshan M, Tahir MA, et al. Health care disparities among lesbian, gay, bisexual, and transgender youth: a literature review. Cureus. 2017;9(4):e1184. https://doi.org/10.7759/cureus.1184. Accessed 14 Oct 2019
14. Wolfe DS, Greeson JKP, Wasch S, Treglia D. Human trafficking prevalence and child welfare risk factors among homeless youth, a multi-city study. The Field Center for Children's Policy, Practice and Research. 2018. https://www.covenanthouse.org/sites/default/files/inline-files/Field%20Center%20Full%20Report%20on%20Human%20Trafficking%20Prevalence.pdf. Accessed 18 July 2019.
15. Administration for Children and Families. National youth in transition database data brief # 4. Washington, DC. 2014. Retrieved from http://www.acf.hhs.gov/programs/cb/resource/nytd-data-brief-4. Accessed 14 Oct 2019.
16. US Interagency Council on Homelessness. Preventing and ending youth homelessness: a coordinated community response. 2019. https://www.usich.gov/resources/uploads/asset_library/Youth_Homelessness_Coordinated_Response.pdf. Accessed 14 June 2019.

17. Dworsky A, Morton MH, Samuels GM. Missed opportunities: pregnant and parenting youth experiencing homelessness in America. Chicago: Chapin Hall at the University of Chicago; 2018.
18. Rafferty J, AAP Committee on Psychosocial Aspects of Child and Family Health, AAP Committee on Adolescence, AAP Section on Lesbian, Gay, Bisexual, and Transgender Health and Wellness. Ensuring comprehensive care and support for transgender and gender diverse children and adolescents. Pediatrics. 2018;142(4):e20182162. Accessed 14 Oct 2019.
19. Murphy LT. Labor and sex trafficking among homeless youth: a Ten-City study full report. New Orleans: Modern Slavery Research Project, Loyola University New Orleans; 2016. https://oag.ca.gov/sites/all/files/agweb/pdfs/ht/murphy-labor-sex-trafficking-homeless-youth.pdf. Accessed 20 Oct 2019.
20. Wolfe DS, Greeson JK, Wasch S, Treglia D. Human trafficking prevalence and child welfare risk factors among homeless youth: a multi-city study. The Field Center for Children's Policy, Practice and Research, University of Pennsylvania. 2018.
21. Bogard K, Murry V, Alexander C, editors. Perspectives on health equity and social determinants of health. Washington, DC: National Academy of Medicine; 2017. p. 127.
22. Bogard K, Murry V, Alexander C, editors. Perspectives on health equity and social determinants of health. Washington, DC: National Academy of Medicine; 2017. p. 16.
23. United States Interagency Council on Homelessness (USICH). Framework to end youth homelessness: a resource text for dialogue and action. 2013. https://www.usich.gov/resources/uploads/asset_library/USICH_Federal_Youth_Framework.pdf. Accessed 14 June 2019.
24. Auerswald CL, Eyre SL. Youth homelessness in San Francisco: a life cycle approach. Soc Sci Med. 2002;54:1497–512.
25. Gomez R, Thompson SJ, Barczyk AN. Factors associated with substance use among homeless young adults. Subst Abus. 2010;31(1):24–34. https://doi.org/10.1080/08897070903442566. Accessed 21 Oct 2019.
26. Maria DS, Padhye N, Yang Y, Gallardo K, Santos G-M, Jung J, Businelle M. Drug use patterns and predictors among homeless youth: results of an ecological momentary assessment. Am J Drug Alcohol Abuse. 2018;44(5):551–60. https://doi.org/10.1080/00952990.2017.1407328.
27. Auerswald, et al. Six-year mortality in a street-recruited cohort of homeless youth in San Francisco, California. PeerJ. 2016;4:e1909. https://doi.org/10.7717/peerj.1909. Accessed 24 Oct 2019.
28. Warf C, Clark L, Desai M, Rabinovitz S, Calvo R, Agahi G, Hoffman J. Coming of age on the streets: survival sex among homeless adolescent females in Hollywood. J Adolesc. 2013;46(2):S37–8.
29. Greeson JKP, Treglia D, Wolfe DS, Wasch S. Prevalence and correlates of sex trafficking among homeless and runaway youths presenting for shelter services. Soc Work Res. 2019;43(2):91–100. https://doi.org/10.1093/swr/svz001.
30. Hollywood Homeless Youth Partnership. Issue brief: exploring permanent connections for youth and young adults experiencing homelessness. 2016. http://hhyp.org/wp-content/uploads/2013/04/Exploring-Permanent-Connections-for-YYA-Experiencing-Homelessness.pdf. Accessed 14 June 2019.
31. US Interagency Council on Homelessness. Criteria and benchmarks for achieving the goal of ending youth homelessness. 2019. https://www.usich.gov/resources/uploads/asset_library/Youth-Criteria-and-Benchmarks-revised-Feb-2018.pdf. Accessed 14 June 2019.
32. US Department of Housing and Urban Development's Office of Community Planning and Development. Ending youth homelessness. Guidebook series: promising program models. https://files.hudexchange.info/resources/documents/Ending-Youth-Homelessness-Promising-Program-Models.pdf.
33. Street Medicine Institute. 2019. https://www.streetmedicine.org. Accessed 3 Oct 2019.
34. SAMHSA – Center for Integrated Care Solutions. https://www.integration.samhsa.gov/clinical-practice/trauma-informed.

35. HHS, Office of Population Affairs. What is positive youth development? https://www.hhs.gov/ash/oah/adolescent-development/positive-youth-development/what-is-positive-youth-development/index.html.
36. Catalano RF, Berglund ML, Ryan JA, Lonczak HS, Hawkins JD. Positive youth development in the United States: research findings on evaluations of positive youth development programs. Ann Am Acad Pol Soc Sci. 2004;591(1):98–124.
37. Department of Health and Human Services. What is positive youth development? https://www.hhs.gov/ash/oah/adolescent-development/positive-youth-development/what-is-positive-youth-development/index.html. Accessed 10 Nov 2019.
38. Hollywood Homeless Youth Partnership. Policy brief: towards a national housing strategy for homeless youth. 2013. https://www.chla.org/sites/default/files/atoms/files/HHYP_HOUSING_STRATEGY_2013.PDF. Accessed 25 Oct 2019.
39. Rice E. The TAY Triage Tool: a tool to identify homeless transition age youth most in need of permanent supportive housing. New York: Corporation for Supportive Housing; 2013. https://www.csh.org/wp-content/uploads/2014/02/TAY_TriageTool_2014.pdf. Accessed 25 Nov 2019.
40. Brown AF, et al. Structural interventions to reduce and eliminate health disparities. Am J Public Health. 2019;109(S1):S72–8. https://doi.org/10.2105/AJPH.2018.304844. Accessed 6 Dec 2019.

Chapter 5
Youth in Care: A Very High-Risk Population for Homelessness

Jimmy Wang and Eva Moore

Background

Over 440,000 children and adolescents are in foster care in the United States, and nearly 20,000 age out of care annually [6]. The foster care system is designed to protect abused and neglected children from further abuse; thus when the safety of a child cannot be reconciled within his or her home, the child is removed and placed by a government agency into a relative's home, foster home, group home, or residential treatment, all of which is referred to as *foster care* in this chapter.

Foster care ends at different ages depending on the jurisdiction. Legislation in recent years allows US states to extend foster care until age 21, although it may still end at age 17–19 for youth in certain states or for those who decline extended services. The United Kingdom has formally adopted 21 years as the upper age limit across the nation. Most provinces in Canada still end foster care at age 18 or 19, and most Australian states, where the term "out-of-home care" is also used, similarly end at age 17 or 18 [5]. However, very recently, there has been successful legislative advocacy in some of these jurisdictions to increase the age limit to 21.

Youth who have previously been in or are currently in foster care, collectively termed *youth in care*, make up a substantial portion of the homeless population. Youth in care have frequently had a lifetime of unstable housing, including frequent moves, nonfamily-based living situations such as group homes, and substandard or tenuous housing situations as young adults [16]. The pathway to homelessness for youth in care is distinct from other homeless youth.

J. Wang
Department of Pediatrics, University of British Columbia, Vancouver, BC, Canada

E. Moore (✉)
Division of Adolescent Health and Medicine, Department of Pediatrics, University of British Columbia, Vancouver, BC, Canada
e-mail: eva.moore@cw.bc.ca

C. Warf, G. Charles (eds.), *Clinical Care for Homeless, Runaway and Refugee Youth*, https://doi.org/10.1007/978-3-030-40675-2_5

Being a youth in care is a strong precursor for homelessness. One study that prospectively followed a large cohort of youth in care into young adulthood found that a sobering 36% of youth in care had experienced homelessness by age 26 [17]. In general, studies estimate that 12–46% of youth in care become homeless as adults [23], with many youth experiencing homelessness within just 6–12 months of leaving care [16, 18]. More alarmingly, youth in care have higher rates of eventual homelessness than adults who experienced abuse as children but who were *not* removed from their homes [21]. Former youth in care are more likely to be homeless compared to youth who grew up in poverty but were not removed from their homes [23].

As an added consideration, these rates likely also underestimate the true burden of housing instability, since most studies were limited to measuring shelter or street-based homelessness but did not include disguised forms of homelessness such as "couch-surfing" or staying with a friend. Conversely, from the perspective of people who are homeless, there is an overrepresentation of former youth in care. Shelters, street-based homeless populations, and programs for homeless mothers see high frequencies of former youth in care with most reports ranging between 20% and 35% [21]. Therefore, whether one looks at groups of homeless people or groups of former youth in care, a strong association exists between a history of being in care and risk of later homelessness.

"One study [...] found that a sobering 36% of youth in care had experienced homelessness by age 26."

Issues Affecting Youth in Care

Youth in care who become homeless commonly live unstable lives even before they are homeless. The impact of losing one's stable housing is exacerbated by a system that not only pushes youth in care to be socially and financially independent at an earlier age than is expected for the most other youth but also inadequately prepares these youth for independence. Youth in care can have unmet life skills, gaps in education, under-recognized health and developmental challenges, poor employability, and premature detachment from social supports. These youth commonly receive fragmented services, including housing, school, and healthcare, which seriously impede their healthy development and preparation for adult life [14].

Housing

Youth in care may be moved numerous times throughout their adolescent years, and these changes in residence commonly not only involve changing homes and caretakers but often also schools, primary care physicians, and peer groups, resulting in few relationships sustained over time. Former youth in care who become homeless are more likely to have been in group homes, had frequent moves, and had interactions with the juvenile justice system [16], indicating a pattern of trauma, loss, and instability starting before homelessness.

Group homes, where many struggling youth in care eventually find themselves, can come with their own challenges. The most striking testimonies reflect on the unforgiving rigidity of rules, the lack of privacy from surveillance, and the extent of peer-on-peer bullying in some group homes, which serve to undermine the healing and sense of security of traumatized adolescents. For girls and young women, being placed in one of the extremely rare female-only group homes can be invaluable in alleviating their constant vigilance against sexual assault [12].

Education

Youth with higher education outcomes significantly increase their earnings [23], but youth in care are less likely to attend post-secondary education, such as a college, university, or trades program. High school dropout rates can be over 50% in some provinces or states [20]. Too often youth in care have unrecognized learning disabilities, significant gaps in their education, and incomplete school files, revealing the pervasive systemic challenges confronting the current foster care system.

Poverty-related barriers to high school attendance, including school fees, uniforms or school-appropriate clothing, consistency of personal hygiene, and transportation, are exacerbated when youth are in care and trying their best to keep up with their education [12]. School truancy is often an unintended and disappointing sequelae of unstable housing. This is especially true in instances where a student may move foster homes multiple times during a school year or even slip in and out of homelessness.

"High school dropout rates can be over 50%..."

Employment

Unemployment and underemployment are big challenges for youth in care. Although many are employed when they leave care, half lose their employment within 3 years [23]. In addition, employed youth in care earn 50% less than their peers who are not in care [23]. Without a financial safety net from their parents or family, as many other youth have, youth in care can experience drastic consequences of what might be otherwise developmentally appropriate experimentation or exploration of new forms of employment and income-generation behaviors, being unable to turn to their parents during difficult times. They may lack skills and guidance for new tasks, such as paying rent and utilities on time and managing budgets.

Health

Many youth in care experience specific health issues that can impact their housing stability and well as their experience with homelessness. Their frequent childhood histories of loss; trauma; disrupted early attachment; household dysfunction; and emotional, physical and/or sexual abuse have serious implications for their health [17]. Physical and mental health symptoms, which often derive from the same sources of trauma, can interfere with regular employment and reaching out to social services.

Typically, physical and mental health deteriorate sharply following transition out of care. Within 18 months after leaving foster care, 30% of former youth in care had become young parents and 48% reported depression or other major mental health issues [24, 26]. At ages 17 or 18, these vulnerable youth are two to four times more likely to suffer from mental health disorders compared to those in the general population [19]; however, only a small minority receive professional help [19, 25]. These rates are unsurprisingly higher in those who become homeless [17]. Furthermore, adults formerly in care are consistently found to have higher rates of chronic health problems, such as asthma, diabetes, hypertension, and epilepsy [32].

Since youth with multiple childhood adverse experiences are more likely to experience adult health problems [17], youth in care may be at a lifelong disadvantage if they cannot navigate the adult healthcare system, which can often be unforgiving of youth. For example, a specialist clinic may terminate a doctor–patient relationship for reasons such as missed appointments. There are numerous obstacles in seeking healthcare for youth in care, including a lack of continuity in care, insufficient communication with healthcare providers, and insufficient training, information, and support provided for foster parents [22]. Child protection teams rarely have sufficient case management personnel to support even the children and youth with known chronic health conditions.

> "Within 18 months after leaving foster care, 30% of former youth in care had become young parents and 48% reported depression or other major mental health issues."

Social and Familial Attachment

Youth in care often lack consistent and strong family connections on whom to rely for support during tough periods of their life [16]. Young people entering care as adolescents are a high-risk subgroup, as they are frequently placed into group homes or independent living where there are fewer adult supports and attachments [16].

Youth removed from their homes and placed in foster care, even homes in which they had been victims of child abuse and neglect, commonly sustain strong attachments to their parents and caregivers from early childhood. Given these bonds, it is not unusual for youth in care to seek out and attempt reunification with their original family. In working with youth in care, it is essential to respect these relationships and to avoid prejudgment or negative characterizations of loved family members.

Marginalization

Indigenous and visible minority youth have long had a disproportionately high representation in developed nations' foster care systems. Racially discriminatory attitudes in their foster homes can drive youth in care to leave those unsafe and unsupportive homes and become homeless. In addition to their lived experience of targeted victimization, these youth are often distrustful of fostering due to historical victimization in the forms of colonialism, slavery, and child segregation, which is inherited through generational trauma [12].

Similarly, LGBT youth can experience discrimination in foster homes, group homes, and youth shelters. These youth often enter foster care as a result of fleeing homophobia in their home of origin. Schools and social services may also not be LGBT-friendly, which forces these youth into further vulnerability and disengagement and typically to conceal their LGBT identity as a survival mechanism [12].

> "[Youth in care] are often distrustful of fostering due to historical victimization in the forms of colonialism, slavery, and child segregation…"

Relations with Child Protection Services

Child protection services aimed solely at identifying safe living situations may not be adequately equipped to connect youth with needed mental health and counseling services, social supports, and developmental assessments that can be critical to their health [8, 10].

Parental neglect is by far the most prevalent reason for removal by child protection agencies from a family home. This stems from risk factors such as conditions of poverty, poor housing, parental incarceration or death, domestic violence, and parental substance abuse [28]. Consequently, many youth in care originate from families who may have similarly struggled with housing instability, frequent moves, and insufficient financial resources. The back and forth between inadequately stable housing and homelessness can be a destructive cycle that recurs through their childhood, adolescence, and young adulthood.

Understandably, many youth in care have a strong distrust of child protection services and related government agencies. This may introduce additional complexity in efforts to support their transition to independence.

Transition Out of Care

Transitioning out of care has been established as a period of great risk for an already marginalized group, which stems from an unrealistic expectation that they will become newly independent young adults with little to no support. A lack of coordination between multisystem services often means that youth "fall through the cracks" [8]. Youth can also become disconnected from services when they age out of care because they do not know or trust the new systems. As a consequence, despite youth service providers who may make every effort to facilitate connections, the history of trauma and disrupted relationships experienced by many youth in care creates barriers to following-up on such referrals [8].

One tragic case in Vancouver, Canada, that was subject of a government review illustrates the consequences that can befall youth in care as they abruptly transition out of care. On the last government agency note written for one youth who experienced frequently changes in foster homes as well as homelessness, her welfare worker wrote, "The child is one month from turning 19 and unfortunately she is still binge drinking heavily and appears not to be overly concerned about having anywhere to live at age 19." In contrast, an email from her foster parent expresses concern that "[the youth's] anxiety builds as her move out date approaches," implying that the youth's detached behavior recorded by the welfare worker was an expression of stress and worsening mental health. This youth subsequently died from an overdose 11 months later [31].

Accessing social services when a youth is still in care is often much easier than after they transition out of care, since the responsibility transfers from the welfare worker to the youth at the time of transition. In many jurisdictions, funding for psychological diagnostic investigations, which may be an avenue to qualify for necessary adult supports, is dependent on a youth's age and may be available only for those still considered minors. A former youth in care would be also simultaneously charged with new responsibility for finances, housing, food, and more, which can be overwhelming for a youth who may be living with a disability. Hence, there is a vicious cycle between disability and social needs.

Young adults seeking social services are not viewed any differently than adults seeking those same services, even though their needs are profoundly different from the needs of adults in the general population [31]. For example, a young adult attempting to access welfare income may have overwhelming difficulty trying to navigate the complexities of the system due to their inexperience with social services. Conflicting feelings about whether or not to access social services can also interfere with seeking help and following the multiple steps properly.

Adequately supporting the transition out of care is an essential component of preventing youth homelessness. The American Academy of Pediatrics emphasizes that during their period of transition, youth in care may innately have "difficulty assuming tasks of young adulthood which require rapid interpretation of information," such as key skills needed for employment and independent living [3].

Pediatricians and other physicians, nurses, social workers, and other professionals who work with youth in care play a vital role in supporting these youth and advocating for the transition services and resources that they need.

Promising Interventions and Strategies

Policy Changes

Extending foster care until age 21 has long been advocated by numerous social policy groups. The focus on extending the age of eligibility grew after convincing advocacy efforts demonstrated the benefits for youth in care, as well as for the government in fiscal savings. Currently, policies are beginning to shift in the United States and Canada, with more jurisdictions continuing some or all foster care services until age 21. It is not clear if extending foster care decreases homelessness in this population, but at the very least, it delays homelessness [17]. Since most youth in the general population rely on emotional and financial support from their families through young adulthood, this policy shift is a first-line effort to provide a better and more equitable life for youth in care.

However, even when available, extending foster care until age 21 is not enough. Policies that ensure adequate housing, fiscal availability, job readiness, and educational access are essential. Expert advocacy groups exist in the United States and Canada that provide extensive recommendations and creative ideas to plan for youths' transition out of care. These include interventions that interface more directly with youth, such as building savings accounts, assessing gaps in life skills, and facilitating connections with mentors and families.

Strong Foster and Adoptive Families

Though the numbers are sobering, there are many foster homes and foster parents who are, in many ways, a positive influence and transformative for youth who have had traumatic experiences. Healing from childhood adversity is a realistic possibility and requires time and attention. However, foster and adoptive families need the support of their government, team of professionals, and community resources to help break the cycle of trauma in which youth in care find themselves.

> "…foster and adoptive families need the support of their government, team of professionals, and community resources to help break the cycle of trauma…"

Nonprofit organizations, such as the Annie E. Casey Foundation, compile evidence-based strategies to support families to care for children and youth who have had to leave their families of origin [4]. Child welfare agency strategies and

Table 5.1 Effective or promising child welfare strategies

Increase support for families in crisis to avoid removal when possible
Support family and kinship relationships
Work toward permanent homes for all children
Promote expert frontline casework
Promote competent decision-making about placement and removals
Increase the pool of competent foster homes by supporting education, training, and support of potential families
Minimize disruptions in school

procedures can enhance the capacity of families to care for vulnerable youth (Table 5.1).

Focusing on family relationships, supporting kinship care through financial support, education, and mentoring of extended relatives and friends can provide less disruption when a child requires removal and also enhances the pool of strong foster families. A child needs a loving, supportive, permanent home as soon as possible, and child welfare agencies should feel a sense of urgency to address the problems that threaten the parents' ability to provide this or to find another stable and permanent alternative family.

Mentorship

A key factor that has been found to be significantly associated with better physical and mental health outcomes for youth transitioning out of care is mentorship. Mentored youth have improved outcomes in their transition to independence when they have had positive relationships to community professionals who, in a way, become the youth's surrogate family [2]. Young people have a number of formal and informal relationships that can help support them throughout their adolescent and young adult years as they navigate the foster care system and transition out of foster care. Research with youth formerly in care shows that youth may be more receptive to professional mentors at critical transitions, such as the move into or out of foster care [1]. These may be key times to target the introduction of professional supports. Facilitating youth's capacity to reach out and develop mentorship relationships may be an important life skill and should be integrated into transition planning for youth in care in their adolescent years.

Employment and Education Programs

Employment programs that provide paid training and work experience while engaging and providing mentorship in the work context are highly valuable for youth aging out of care. Trade programs or educational programs lasting 6–18 months may be more practical for youth who require a steady income and don't have others that they can lean on for housing and food that would allow for 4-year or more college or university experience. Job training programs such as Job Corps have been shown to increase earnings and educational attainment for vulnerable youth, but it does require significant governmental investment to run [27]. Similarly, governmental-sponsored programs in British Columbia, such as Intersections Media or Plea's Cue program for youth on probation, link youth with job placement under mentorship with positive feedback from youth and employers [13].

The Role of Healthcare Providers

How does a healthcare provider make a difference in the lives of these youth? Providers offer an important focus on health and well-being and can communicate those needs to others caring for the youth, including social workers, group home workers, foster parents, and counselors. Many pediatricians and adult providers are unfamiliar with the core issues affecting this demographic and may be intimidated by the social and systemic issues they face. However, this should not deter one from striving to provide the best possible care for these vulnerable youth, as there is much that providers have to contribute (Table 5.2) [30].

Providing a medical home that anticipates and responds to their specific needs, including medical, psychiatric, and neurodevelopmental, can improve outcomes for children and adolescents as well as newly fledged young adults [7]. Youth in care will almost universally need more frequent visits and close ongoing care coordination. For example, identifying concerns for a learning disability and advocating for appropriate psychoeducational and developmental assessments can transform a youth whose undiagnosed disability might otherwise be misinterpreted as a behavioral or disciplinary concern. Similarly, connection to appropriate trauma counseling and/or other indicated therapies can help avoid misdiagnosis of more severe psychiatric disorders, which can sometimes be the presentation of youth in crisis.

Table 5.2 Recommendations for healthcare providers caring for youth in care and former youth in care

Provide a medical home
Recognize the physical and behavioral effects of trauma and toxic stress
Incorporate trauma-informed care into your practice
Keep the youth involved in his or her medical care
Provide anticipatory guidance in preparation for the transition to adult care
Coordinate routine health assessments, including dental, vision, mental health, sexual health, immunizations, learning assessments, etc.
Be understanding of the youth when he or she misses or is late to an appointment or if he or she does not follow through on your recommendations
Work as an interdisciplinary team comprised of foster parents, social workers, psychologists, community resources, etc.
Advocate in your community and healthcare institution and, if possible, directly to your representatives in government

Some child protection jurisdictions have developed case management systems for youth in care, but the healthcare provider may need to advocate for connection to these services once a diagnosis is made. In other jurisdictions, care coordination is the responsibility of social workers who may have little health knowledge and are already overburdened with unrealistically high numbers of youth for case management. Many providers struggle with disrupted continuity of care and unpredictable placement changes that might impact treatment and follow-up plans.

Intervening early, prior to a youth aging out of care, yields the most benefit to the youth. Strong and positive attachments to communities are powerful determinants of better health outcomes [2, 9, 11]. Relationships between young people and service providers should be informed by an understanding of the youth's resiliency and self-sufficiency.

Conclusions

Youth in care are a distinct segment of the homeless youth population, and they require a larger safety net focusing on prevention and stabilization during the critical stage when they transition out of care. This safety net must include educational opportunities, secure employment, housing options, and fiscal strategies, as well as longitudinal supports involving family when possible, welfare workers, and healthcare professionals. Similar to other young adults, former youth in care often require these second or third chances when becoming independent to allow for setbacks that are inherent to their journey into adulthood. In this way, emergencies and times of crisis can be made tolerable, and homelessness can hopefully be avoided.

Looking ahead to the next decade, resources developed to support a youth's transition out of care should be transparent and easily accessible and facilitate a continuum of care from the services and care they received as children and adolescents. Vulnerable populations within this already high-risk population, including indigenous youth, visible minority youth, LGBT youth, and young women, will need dedicated consideration from all facets of the child welfare system. Healthcare providers can represent an important bridge during the transition out of care when the other professional supports, such as social workers, foster care, and group homes, fall away. In working toward effective advocacy for youth in care, we should remember that change needs to occur at all levels, whether it is involving the individual, family, school system, healthcare institutions, government housing and welfare system, or society at large.

References

1. Ahren KR, DuBois DL, Garrison M, Spencer R, Richardson LP, Lozano P. Qualitative exploration of relationships with important non-parental adults in the lives of youth in foster care. Child Youth Serv Rev. 2011;33(6):1012–23.

2. Ahrens KR, DuBois DL, Richardson LP, Fan MY, Lozano P. Youth in foster care with adult mentors during adolescence have improved outcomes. Pediatrics. 2008;121(2):e246–52.
3. American Academy of Pediatrics. Helping foster and adoptive families cope with trauma [Internet]. Elk Grove Village: American Academy of Pediatrics; 2016. [cited 2019 May 16]. Available from: https://www.aap.org/en-us/Documents/hfca_foster_trauma_guide.pdf.
4. Annie E. Casey Foundation. Ten practices: a child welfare leader's desk guide to building a high-performing agency [Internet]. Baltimore: The Annie E. Casey Foundation; 2015. [cited 2019 May 17]. Available from: https://www.aecf.org/resources/10-practices-part-one/.
5. Child Family Community Australia. Children in care [Internet]. Southbank: Australian Institute of Family Studies, Australian Government; 2018. [cited 2018 Dec 29]. Available from: https://aifs.gov.au/cfca/publications/children-care.
6. Children's Bureau. The AFCARS report: preliminary FY 2017 estimates as of August 10, 2018 – no. 25 [Internet]. Washington, DC: U.S. Department of Health & Human Services; 2018. [cited 2019 May 20]. Available from: https://www.acf.hhs.gov/sites/default/files/cb/afcarsreport25.pdf.
7. Christian CW, Schwarz DF. Child maltreatment and the transition to adult-based medical and mental health care. Pediatrics. 2011;127(1):139–45.
8. Collins ME, Clay C. Influencing policy for youth transitioning from care: defining problems, crafting solutions, and assessing politics. Child Youth Serv Rev. 2009;31(7):743–51.
9. Collins ME, Spencer R, Ward R. Supporting youth in the transition from foster care: formal and informal connections. Child Welfare. 2010;89(1):125–43.
10. Council on Foster Care, Adoption, and Kinship Care, Committee on Early Childhood. Health care of youth aging out of foster care. Pediatrics. 2012;130(6):1170–3.
11. Creighton G, Shumay S, Moore E, Saewyc E. Capturing the wisdom and the resilience: how the Pinnacle program fosters connections for alternative high school students [Internet]. Vancouver: University of British Columbia; 2014. [cited 2019 May 17]. Available from: http://apsc-saravyc.sites.olt.ubc.ca/files/2018/04/Pinnacle-Program-Evaluation-Report-Nov-18-WEB.pdf.
12. Czapska A, Webb A, Taefi N. More than bricks & mortar: a rights-based strategy to prevent girl homelessness in Canada [Internet]. Vancouver: Justice for Girls; 2008. [cited 2019 May 16]. Available from: http://www.justiceforgirls.org/uploads/2/4/5/0/24509463/more_than_bricks_and_mortar.pdf.
13. Department of Justice. Evaluation of PLEA programs [Internet]. Ottawa: Department of Justice, Government of Canada; 2015. [cited 2019 May 11]. Available from: https://www.justice.gc.ca/eng/fund-fina/cj-jp/yj-jj/sum-som/r22.html.
14. Doyle JJ Jr. Child protection and child outcomes: measuring the effects of foster care. Am Econ Rev. 2007;97(5):1583–610.
15. Drapeau S, Saint-Jacques MC, Lépine R, Bégin G, Bernard M. Processes that contribute to resilience among youth in foster care. J Adolesc. 2007;30(6):977–99.
16. Dworsky A, Courtney M. Homelessness and the transition from foster care to adulthood. Child Welfare. 2009;88(4):23–56.
17. Felitti VJ, Anda RF, Nordenberg D, Williamson DF, Spitz AM, Edwards V, et al. Relationship of childhood abuse and household dysfunction to many of the leading causes of death in adults. The Adverse Childhood Experiences (ACE) study. Am J Prev Med. 1998;14(4):245–58.
18. Fowler PJ, Marcal KE, Zhang J, Day O, Landsverk J. Homelessness and aging out of foster care: a national comparison of child welfare-involved adolescents. Child Youth Serv Rev. 2017;77:27–33.
19. Havlicek J, Garcia A, Smith DC. Mental health and substance use disorders among foster youth transitioning to adulthood: past research and future directions. Child Youth Serv Rev. 2013;35(1):194–203.
20. Kovarikova J. Exploring youth outcomes after aging-out of care [Internet]. Toronto: Provincial Advocate for Children and Youth; 2017. [cited 2019 May 20]. Available from: https://www.provincialadvocate.on.ca/reports/advocacy-reports/report-exploring-youth-outcomes.pdf.
21. Park JM, Metraux S, Brodbar G, Culhane DP. Child welfare involvement among children in homeless families. Child Welfare. 2004;83(5):423–36.

22. Pasztor EM, Hollinger DS, Inkelas M, Halfon N. Health and mental health services for children in foster care. Child Welfare. 2006;85(1):33–57.
23. Rosenberg R, Kim Y. Aging out of foster care: homelessness, post-secondary education, and employment. J Pub Child Welfare. 2017;12(4):1–17.
24. Rutman D, Hubberstey C, Feduniw A. When youth age out of care – where to from there? [Internet]. Victoria: University of Victoria; 2007. [cited 2019 May 18]. Available from: https://www.uvic.ca/hsd/socialwork/assets/docs/research/WhenYouthAge2007.pdf.
25. Sawyer MG, Carbone JA, Searle AK, Robinson P. The mental health and wellbeing of children and adolescents in home-based foster care. Med J Aust. 2007;186(4):181–4.
26. Scannapieco M, Connell-Carrick K, Painter K. In their own words: challenges facing youth aging out of foster care. Child Adolesc Soc Work J. 2007;24(5):423–35.
27. Schochet PZ, Burghardt J, McConnell S. Does Job Corps work? Impact findings from the National Job Corps Study. Am Econ Rev. 2008;98(5):1864–86.
28. Sinha V, Kozlowski A. The structure of aboriginal child welfare in Canada. Int Indig Policy J. 2013;4(2):1–21.
29. Smith A, Stewart D, Poon C, Saewyc E. Fostering potential: the lives of BC youth with government care experience. Vancouver: McCreary Centre Society; 2011. [cited 2019 May 19]. Available from: https://www.mcs.bc.ca/pdf/fostering_potential_web.pdf.
30. Szilagyi MA, Rosen DS, Rubin D, Zlotnik S, Council on Foster Care, Adoption, and Kinship Care, Committee on Adolescence, et al. Health care issues for children and adolescents in foster care and kinship care. Pediatrics. 2015;136(4):e1142–66.
31. Turpel-Lafond ME. On their own: examining the needs of B.C. youth as they leave government care [Internet]. Victoria: Representative for Children and Youth; 2014. [cited 2019 May 16]. Available from: http://www.rcybc.ca/sites/default/files/documents/pdf/reports_publications/rcy_on_their_own.pdf.
32. Zlotnick C, Tam TW, Soman LA. Life course outcomes on mental and physical health: the impact of foster care on adulthood. Am J Public Health. 2012;102(3):534–40.

Chapter 6
Refugee and Migrant Youth in Canada and the United States: Special Challenges and Healthcare Issues

Shazeen Suleman and Curren Warf

Background

The global community continues to see record numbers of displacement and mass migration, due to persecution, violence, and instability in home countries and increasingly due to climate change [1]. In 2017, the United Nations High Commissioner for Refugees (UNHCR) reported that there were 68.5 million people who were forcibly displaced from their homes, including 25.4 million refugees, 3.1 million asylum seekers, and 40 million internally displaced persons.[1] Of these, over half are children and youth under the age of 18, a number that continues to increase and includes at least 173,800 children and youth who are unaccompanied.[2] Today, 1 in 35 people is an international migrant [2].

Many families, children, and youth are economic or family immigrants, arriving in host countries seeking better opportunities. To qualify, families have often waited years before their name is chosen in a lottery system and their educational and professional qualifications carefully scrutinized.[3] In Canada, over 40% of children are considered first-generation or second-generation Canadian, the result of waves of

[1] UNHCR Global Trends 2017 report.

[2] UNHCR Global Trends 2017 report.

[3] https://www.canada.ca/en/immigration-refugees-citizenship/services/immigrate-canada/express-entry/works.html

S. Suleman (✉)
Department of Pediatrics, St. Michael's Hospital, Toronto, ON, Canada

Faculty of Medicine, University of Toronto, Toronto, ON, Canada

Li Ka Shing Research Institute, St. Michael's Hospital, Toronto, ON, Canada
e-mail: shazeen.suleman@mail.utoronto.ca

C. Warf
Department of Pediatrics (Retired), Division of Adolescent Health and Medicine, British Columbia Children's Hospital, University of British Columbia, Vancouver, BC, Canada

C. Warf, G. Charles (eds.), *Clinical Care for Homeless, Runaway and Refugee Youth*, https://doi.org/10.1007/978-3-030-40675-2_6

immigration, which is steadily growing.[4] In the United States in 2017, 25% of children (or 19 million) were either first-generation immigrants (born outside the United States) or second-generation immigrants (with at least one immigrant parent).[5] One in seven US residents is foreign born.[6]

The United Nations High Commission for Refugees defines *refugees* as "persons who are outside their country of origin for reasons of feared persecution, conflict, generalized violence, or other circumstances that have seriously disturbed public order and, as a result, require international protection" as per the 1951 Geneva Convention.[7] On arriving in their host country, refugees are then typically referred to as "resettled refugees." *Asylum seekers* or *refugee claimants* in the United States or Canada are individuals who make their claim for refugee status or asylum upon entering the respective country. The term "migrant" can be used to describe persons that move to a different country of residence, independent of their reason for moving or legal status; "irregular migrants" are essentially those who cross borders without documentation[8] and are referred to as "undocumented immigrants" in the United States; "immigrant" is often used to refer to individuals who have been legally permitted to gain permanent residency in another country, often for economic or family reasons.[9,10] While economic and family immigrants have their own unique needs, in this chapter, we will focus on refugees and migrants that may not have official legal status. We use the term "newcomer," an inclusive and welcoming term that encompasses all categories of individuals who have newly settled in their host countries.

Children and youth do not generally choose to be refugees or immigrants; they follow their families or are sent to seek safety and opportunity from social or civil violence or escape grinding poverty. However, this special population of youth faces specific challenges and are among the most vulnerable of young people. Adolescent refugee and immigrant health is of global relevance, affecting every country in the world. Internationally, the majority of refugees are hosted in developing countries, primarily in Asia and Africa, with Turkey hosting the largest number worldwide at 3.5 million refugees.[11] While the majority of refugees today come from three countries in the world – Afghanistan, Syria, and South Sudan – refugees and immigrants come from many home countries.[12] In the United States, most migrants originate

[4] https://www12.statcan.gc.ca/census-recensement/2016/as-sa/98-200-x/2016015/98-200-x2016015-eng.cfm

[5] Migration Policy Institute Data Hub. https://www.migrationpolicy.org/programs/data-hub/charts/children-immigrant-families

[6] Migration Policy. https://www.dhcs.ca.gov/services/medi-cal/eligibility/pages/medi-calfaqs2014b.aspx

[7] https://refugeesmigrants.un.org/definitions

[8] Institute of Migration. https://www.iom.int/key-migration-terms#Irregular-migration

[9] Ibid.

[10] https://www.dhs.gov/immigration-statistics/data-standards-and-definitions/definition-terms

[11] UNHCR Global Trends 2017 report.

[12] UNHCR Global Trends 2017 report.

from Central America and Mexico, though there are many from the Middle East, Somalia, Southeast Asia, and other regions.

It is important to recognize the ethno-geographic diversity of refugee and immigrant youth so that medical and health assessments can be tailored to specific needs. In this chapter, we discuss some health challenges affecting newcomer children in their host countries but recognize that this is not an exhaustive list. To support newcomer children and youth, challenges and their solutions must be framed in the context of their lives, beginning with themselves and encompassing their families, community, and other challenges (Fig. 6.1). Finally, we identify a framework for developing youth-centered solutions and discuss examples of successful programs that promote healthy development of immigrant and refugee youth.

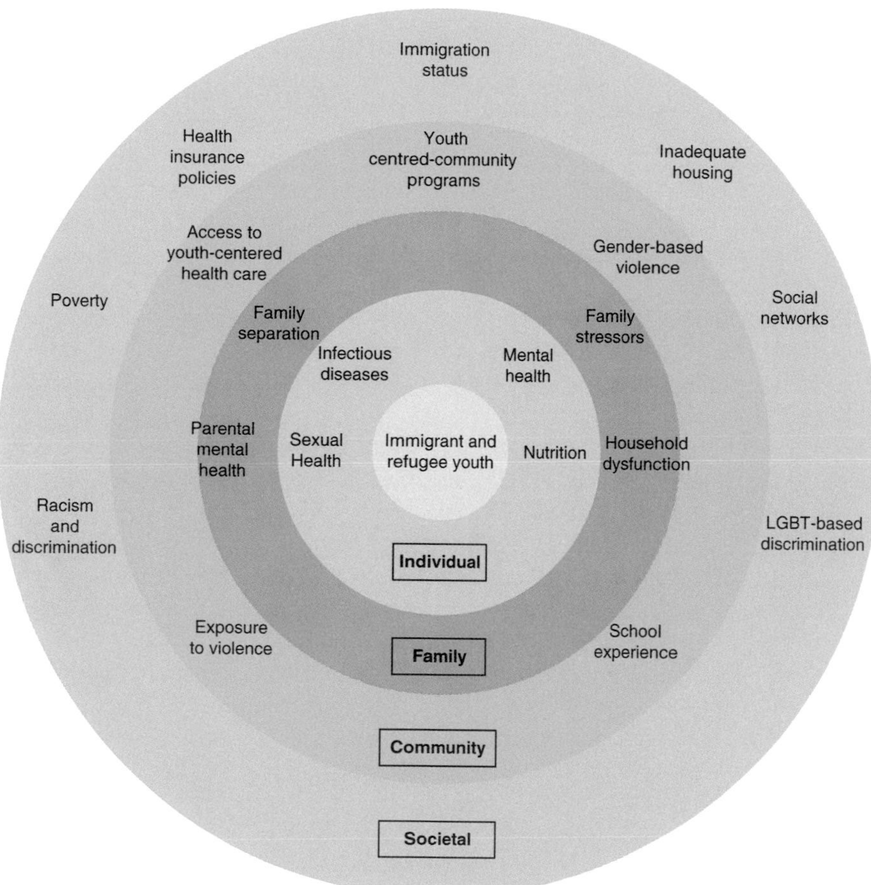

Fig. 6.1 A socio-ecological approach to health issues affecting immigrant and refugee youth

Individual Health Considerations for Immigrant and Refugee Youth

Infectious Disease Risk

Youth who are refugees or immigrants face unique and significant health risks, differing from both adults and young children in their exposure and treatment. Infectious diseases are seen in large numbers of refugee and immigrant youth, depending on the country of origin, with some studies reporting that more than half of all patients seen from sub-Saharan Africa are affected by infectious disease [3]. In addition to parasitic and vector-borne diseases like malaria and *H. pylori* infections, refugee and immigrant youth are at risk for exposure to preventable, sexually transmitted infectious diseases, such as HIV and hepatitis B [4, 5].

Non-infectious Health Challenges

Many refugee and immigrant youth faced inadequate nutrition prior to and during the resettlement process. Nutritional deficiencies common among newly arrived refugee and immigrant youth across the globe include iron deficiency anemia and vitamin A deficiency, a leading cause of worldwide blindness [6]. However, immigrant and refugee youth additionally face nutritional burdens following settlement, particularly when faced with acculturation burdens in Western countries. In a study of recently resettled Afghan youth, dyslipidemia was found in nearly one-third of patients [7]. Vitamin D deficiency is also prevalent, which can clinically present as rickets, and another preventable deficiency found in many refugees and immigrant youth. In the developing young adult, infectious diseases and nutritional deficiencies can have lifelong implications [7–10].

In addition, migrant children, youth, and their parents working in or residing near agricultural areas are commonly exposed daily to pesticides in air, food, dust, and soil and through agricultural product residues. For many children, their diet may be the most influential source. Unintended exposure at home may also come from clothing and footwear of agricultural workers. Children in cities may also be exposed through the use of insecticides in housing for urban pest control. Acute poisoning can take place through ingestion, skin exposure, or inhalation.[13] High-dose pesticide exposure can be devastating and lethal to children and youth.

Unfortunately, pediatric healthcare providers have a poor track record of recognizing the signs of pesticide exposure. The AAP has provided a clear chart on the clinical signs and symptoms and management considerations of exposure to common pesticides [11].

[13] Recognition and Management of Pesticide Poisonings, US Environmental Protection Agency. https://www.epa.gov/pesticide-worker-safety/recognition-and-management-pesticide-poisonings

Many pesticides are classified by the US Environmental Protection Agency as carcinogens. Chronic toxicity endpoints for children that have been documented in epidemiologic studies include preterm birth, low birth weight, congenital anomalies, pediatric cancers, neurobehavioral and cognitive deficits, and asthma. Case control studies and evidence reviews support a role for insecticides in risk of brain tumors and acute lymphocytic leukemia. Prospective studies link early life exposure to organophosphate insecticides with reductions in IQ and abnormal behaviors associated with ADHD and autism [11].

Food Insecurity

Famine and crop failure are increasing factors related to climate change driving migration; children and youth are particularly vulnerable to these negative consequences [12]. Rising temperatures and drought have affected food production, wiping out harvests and leaving families destitute. The World Bank concluded that climate change could lead to at least 1.4 million people to flee their homes in Mexico and Central America and migrate over the next three decades.[14]

Host countries must reduce the barriers faced by immigrant and refugee families to adequate nutrition without penalties. In the United States, certain categories of immigrants, specifically refugees, asylum seekers, and victims of human trafficking or domestic violence, have the same eligibility requirements for federal benefits as lawful permanent residents (LPRs)[15] and legally residing immigrant children, and families are now eligible for, and need to be enrolled in, Supplemental Nutrition Assistance Program (or SNAP) – formerly called food stamps[16] (legally residing immigrant children had been cut from food stamps in 1996 but restored in 2002). Unfortunately, undocumented immigrants, including Deferred Action for Childhood Arrivals (DACA) holders, have never been eligible for SNAP or food stamps and are ineligible for regular Medicaid or healthcare subsidies under the Affordable Care Act, Supplemental Security Income (SSI), or Temporary Assistance for Needy Families (TANF). Ominously, it was proposed in 2018 to permanently exclude from eligibility for legal status any undocumented or otherwise ineligible immigrant who had accessed public benefits, even if accessed legally, such as food stamps or Medicaid, so that they would be indefinitely subject to deportation. The resolution of this proposal remains unclear at the time of this writing. However, there are significant regional exceptions, for example, in California under Medi-Cal (California

[14] The World Bank, Internal Climate Migration in Latin America; Groundswell, Preparing for Internal Climate Migration, Policy Note No. 3.

[15] National Immigration Forum. https://immigrationforum.org/article/fact-sheet-immigrants-and-public-benefits/

[16] National Immigration Law Center. https://www.nilc.org/issues/economic-support/nutritionassistancechildren/

Medicaid), all undocumented immigrant children are eligible for food stamps and medical services and commonly need assistance in enrollment.

Mental Health Challenges

In addition to physical illnesses, many refugee and immigrant youth experience a disproportionate burden of mental health problems. Several studies show high rates of mental health disorders, including depression, anxiety, attention-deficit hyperactivity disorder (ADHD), oppositional defiant disorder (ODD), and post-traumatic stress disorder (PTSD) [13, 14]. However, prevalence rates of emotional trauma vary from 5% to 89%, suggesting that trauma is a ubiquitous part of the displacement experience which does not resolve readily on resettlement [15, 16]. Furthermore, the experience of trauma can present like many mental health diagnoses, making interviewing and diagnosis challenging. In a study of unaccompanied asylum-seeking youth, 89% of youth met criteria for psychiatric disorders 3 years after arrival in the host country [17] (Please refer Chap. 3).

Mental health is affected by external stressors, such a lack of social support, linguistic barriers in communication, limited navigation through the legal process, and the threat of, or actuality of, denial of asylum [18]. These problems are complicated, particularly in the United States, by policies enacted that involuntarily separate children and adolescents from their parents, their major emotional protection. Children (even infants) can be frequently moved hundreds or thousands of miles away into federal shelters while parents are held in involuntary detention or deported to their home countries, making it exceedingly difficult to reunite children with their parents [19]. In June 2019, the US Administration declared that it would restrict or cancel education, legal aid, and playground recreation for all migrant children and youth housed in government shelters; at the time of this statement, there were 13,200 migrant children, including adolescents, who crossed the border alone and young children who were separated from their parents, housed in more than 100 shelters across the United States – they had received English instruction, as well as math, civics, and other classes, and generally allowed access to a sports field, usually to play soccer, at least once a day [20]. Enactment of these policies has been highly traumatizing to thousands of children and youth, disrupted early attachment, and are a significant source of enduring childhood trauma [21, 22].

Conversely, evidence suggests that the receipt of legal status in the country of residence can lead to positive psychosocial functioning [23]. The major mitigating factor against mental illness and trauma is consistent attachment to the accompanying family, in particular parents when present but aunts, uncles, grandparents, older siblings, and family friends as well. Separation of children and youth from these critical attachment figures under circumstances of migration can be even more traumatic than the circumstances and experiences that led to migration [24].

Sexual Health

Sexual health and safety for refugee and immigrant youth are an area of vulnerability, further identified by youth themselves in consultations organized by the United Nations.[17] Menstruation continues to be stigmatized among some populations, with some women experiencing genitourinary infections from unsafe menstrual hygiene practices [25]. Young women have often never had preventative sexual healthcare, including contraception counseling and access, sexually transmitted infection prevention, and HPV vaccination. Stigma surrounding sexual health, particularly for adolescent women, places further barriers to accessing appropriate care. Many young women, and boys as well, have not had basic sex education and may be surprisingly naive. In particular, lesbian, gay, bisexual, gender-fluid, nonconforming, and transgender (LGBT) unaccompanied youth may have fled their home countries due to severe discrimination, trauma, persecution, or family rejection and thus require great sensitivity from healthcare providers. It is essential to appreciate the stigma these young people may have experienced and respect their boundaries and identify local LGBT-supportive resources. Refugee youth may have a history of sexual assault or being sexually trafficked; the shame experienced and internalized by these experiences and the perceived threat of social rejection may significantly inhibit disclosure of the experiences.

Benefits of Migration

Notwithstanding the multiple risks that the process of migration holds for children and youth, it is important to recognize that migration also is unavoidable at times and holds many potential benefits both for migrant children and their families, as well as the host countries where they bring their labor, skills, and talents. People move from one place to another in search of economic opportunity, to join family members, or driven by war, human rights abuses, and persecution. It will continue as long as economic imbalances and conflicts exist, and movement is an essential element in today's global economy [2].

There is some evidence for a "healthy immigrant effect," that is, many economic immigrants may have better health on arrival than the native populations, which has been attributed to both self-selection (educated, wealthy, and healthy people are more likely to have opportunities to migrate) and the exclusion of unhealthy migrants at immigration prescreening. However, this may not be seen in refugees, asylum seekers, and other forced migrant populations, since their migration is by definition involuntary, commonly occurs on short notice, and impacts all classes in a given community [26].

---

[17] UNHCR, Reproductive Health. https://www.unhcr.org/reproductive-health.html

Unaccompanied Migrant Youth

Many adolescents arrive in the United States, particularly in the Southwest, unaccompanied by parents. These young people may be traveling alone or with one or a few friends. Many lack fluency in English, money, and social supports, rendering these youth extremely vulnerable to poverty, poor health outcomes, and high-risk behaviors. There is growing evidence regarding the sexual exploitation of unaccompanied refugee children, including boys [27]. Unaccompanied refugee and migrant youth have significantly higher rates of mental health conditions, even when compared to refugee youth who are accompanied [28, 29]. Given their high state of vulnerability, unaccompanied youth should be identified and connected without delay to community agencies, stable housing, adequate meals, and food resources and be integrated into school or employment (see section "Contemporary Challenges for Refugee and Migrant Youth Entering the United States").

Exposure to Trauma and Adverse Childhood Events

Refugee and migrant youth may have had different exposures to adverse childhood experiences (ACEs), before and on arrival in their host country. In keeping with the "healthy immigrant" effect, many children accompanying their parents as economic or landed immigrants have reported fewer ACEs when compared to host country–born children [30–32]. However, refugee youth – many of whom are fleeing persecution and conflict – may have endured significant traumatic experiences and stress prior to arrival. Often, school staff are among the first to witness displays of trauma, such as externalizing behaviors, inability to focus in school, or social withdrawal.

It is important to consider the impact of household functioning on migrant and youth health. Many ACEs relate to household dysfunction, including having a parent with significant mental illness, witnessing intimate partner violence, parental incarceration, or parental separation due to divorce, deportation, or death [33]. Some adolescent children have experienced parental rejection secondary to their emerging sexual orientation or identity which may be highly stigmatized in their native culture. For adolescent migrants and refugees, there are additional ACEs specific to witnessing violence prior to migration, loss of community and social networks, loss of contact with extended family and caregivers, and potentially loss and involuntary separation from parents, grandparents, and other close attachment figures. Exposure to ACEs can result in toxic stress for the developing adolescent brain and may have long-standing, deleterious consequences.

Appreciation of Significant Family Stressors

The role of family stressors contributing to the mental health problems of adolescents cannot be overstated. Migrant parents have frequently undergone their own traumatic experiences and losses and may not have experienced the supports provided to their children; poor parental mental health can negatively affect well being and school performance in immigrant and refugee youth [34]. Parents need to survive in their new country, commonly working long hours at low-wage jobs that remove them from contact with their children. If they are undocumented, parents live with the constant threat of being apprehended and deported and being forced to leave their children behind and unattended; children and youth may have already experienced the abrupt deportation of one of their parents.

Parents may not have had the opportunity for basic education in their home country and may not be functionally literate even in their own language. As an example, indigenous refugees from Guatemala increasingly present at the border of the United States and enter in the United States, having been driven off their historic lands at home and fleeing violence by both police and private armed groups. This forced migration of parents and children, who are commonly not fluent in either Spanish or English and may not be literate in any language, poses significant challenges in settlement and education.

Parents also need to cope with the consequences of their displacement from home, the lack of a trusted social network, the lingering effects of trauma and loss on their own mental health, the lack of language fluency in their new home country, cultural continuity, poverty, poor employment opportunities, and a sense of despair about integrating into a new alien culture. All of these factors pose difficult obstacles to being the successful and effective parent for their children that they strive to be.

Children and youth often learn the language of the host country faster than their parents; for older adolescent siblings, this may also come with the expectation to carry out social roles that their parent otherwise would adopt. These increased responsibilities may shape the adolescent's overall well-being and acculturation, both positively and negatively. For some youth, taking on these roles as interpreter or bridge to a new culture may provide them a position of respect and value in the family. However, it is critical for clinicians to know the appropriate limits to using children and adolescents as interpreters for medical issues of parents or reporting parental traumatic experiences.[18] The use of trained interpreters who are respectful of confidentiality and culturally sensitive in assisting communication about more complex issues and in medical environments is essential to assure that children are not inadvertently further traumatized in the process of interviewing[19] and that the translation is accurate.

---

[18] https://www.cps.ca/en/documents/position/cross-cultural-communication

[19] https://www.cps.ca/en/documents/position/cross-cultural-communication

Prolonged Separation of Children from Parents

Migrant and refugee youth are highly resilient, with great strength and commonly with continuing ties to their family. Some data suggests that compared to their host country peers, migrant youth are more likely to live with a parent in the household and with extended family [35]. However, there are many adolescents who have been separated from their parents for years during early childhood and into adolescence; perhaps the parent has come to the host country to find employment years before them so that effectively, the parent does not have the expected influence and authority and the youth has not experienced the attachment that they would have otherwise.

Youth can experience a high level of anger at the absence of their parent, but this commonly wanes as they come to appreciate the demands and choices that the parent faced. In these cases, it is useful to have parents tell stories of their memories of when they had been with their child at a younger age, using photographs if available to tell and reinforce stories and details, and describe their earlier life together. This is a common concern for parents who had been separated from children during the formative years, while the parent migrated to send funds back home. It is also a very vulnerable period for families during which parents may separate and when the youth may feel disconnected and not experience a meaningful positive relationship with any adult. When possible it is useful to engage a social worker or family therapist experienced in working with immigrant families.

Commonly, newcomers from specific home countries or social groups may congregate in specific communities in the host countries. In these circumstances, there may be community agencies which can help welcome the newcomers including children and adolescents, provide an orientation, and facilitate integration. Cultural institutions such as the congregations of churches and mosques that attract specific immigrant populations may provide positive supports for distressed groups. In addition, engagement of children and youth in cultural practices consistent with their families' backgrounds can foster a sense of identity and belonging and be critical in building resiliency.[20]

Promoting Resiliency

As described above, ACEs are very common among refugee children and adolescents, and it is essential that clinicians, teachers, and others who interact with these survivors find ways for these experiences to shape characteristics of resilience and strength. Being resilient means being able to recover from adversity by adapting to

[20] https://www.nctsn.org/what-is-child-trauma/trauma-types/refugee-trauma/screening-and-assessment

change; promoting resilience in young newcomers is a key component in promoting their mental health.[21]

It is important that healthcare practitioners working with families who may have experienced trauma respect and encourage protective practices for children and youth, in particular promoting attachment to loving parents, grandparents, and other adults, siblings, and extended family members. Consistent relationships and support from at least one parent are the single most important factor in building and sustaining resiliency among displaced children and youth. Commonly, parents are best positioned to respond to the experiences that children have undergone. Continuation of family stories, including their own story of migration, family and cultural rituals, celebrations and holidays, continued preparation of meals from home, and exposure to culturally familiar music and literature can provide a sense of continuity for children and adolescents. Young people can also share in the grief that the parents have for their loss of loved ones and loss of home and culture; these are authentic experiences that families share and can build upon the connection and attachment that children experience. Parents commonly seek to protect their children by not discussing difficult issues, but this silence about core experiences can become a barrier to mutual understanding and appreciation. Resiliency can be promoted through nurturing close relationships (particularly family relationships), continuity with culture of origin, engagement in school, and successful development of skills in sports, arts, and other fields.

For unaccompanied migrant youth identification of extended family members, continued communication with family of origin when possible, and connection with local agencies working with migrant youth are stabilizing. It is essential that whenever possible, youth become promptly engaged in school, job training, and develop English fluency. Child protective services can commonly provide stabilization and housing for homeless migrant youth, in particular the younger adolescents.

LGBT youth can be connected to local agencies supportive of these youth; given the common level of distrust, it may be challenging initially to foster a trusting relationship. Parents, when possible, should be encouraged to accept their children for who they are; migrant parents face the same challenges of nonmigrants and commonly require time and multiple attempts to adjust to, and accept, their child's emerging identity; others may have already come to accept their child, have an understanding of what their child is going through, and anticipate barriers they may encounter.

It is essential that providers who care for and interact with children and youth appreciate that they are truly a work in progress and their future is filled with opportunities and potential. It is essential that their accomplishments and successes be recognized and acknowledged and that the young person not be labeled or characterized by mistakes or transient youthful behaviors. For clinicians, getting to know

[21] https://www.kidsnewtocanada.ca/mental-health/mental-health-promotion#risk-and-protective-factors

children, adolescents, and families over time and playing a role in their growth and development are one of life's most rewarding and memorable experiences.

Though every migrant youth needs to have their fundamental human rights respected, including the rights to safety and migration, it should also be recognized that immigrants have made and continue to make great contributions to host countries, including the United States and Canada. Though the road may never be easy, welcoming young people, supporting stability, providing education and healthcare, and ensuring that every person has a decent education, employment, and meaningful opportunity are the most realistic path toward integration and assuring that every person is provided the opportunity to contribute their fullest.

Host Community Considerations

Beyond the household, refugee and immigrant children and youth may face additional challenges in community programs, such as the educational system. Most migrant and refugee youth have experienced some kind of disruption in their formal schooling; some may never had the opportunity for formal schooling. Regardless, it is important that educators and child health practitioners support all immigrant and refugee youth in achieving the same educational outcomes as their peers, as studies show that their educational attainment is comparable when in a supportive, strengths-based environment [13]. From an educational perspective, school can be both a space of strength and difficulty for newcomer children in their host country.

The United Nations Convention on the Rights of the Child,[22] adopted by all countries of the world except the United States (but including Canada), clearly states that all children, regardless of immigration status, have the right to an education in the country in which they live. It is important that all child health practitioners in host countries advocate and support migrant and refugee youth in accessing formal education opportunities, such as helping with registration processes and identifying schools.

Risk factors for poor educational outcomes include poor parental understanding of educational systems and low teacher expectations. Furthermore, while trauma experienced prior to arrival in the host country can have negative influences on a youth's mental health, it is perhaps even more important to recognize that trauma following migration can have an even more deleterious effect [13]. This includes being bullied or ostracized in the school, which may superficially appear to be relatively innocent but are still forms of racist and xenophobic discrimination; the negative effects are even worse for targeted migrant and refugee youth who identify as LGBT, especially if they are unaccompanied or unsupported by their family, school, or community agencies. School staff may need support in developing a welcoming and accepting environment for migrant youth and need to make efforts to reach out to all students and their parents.

[22] UN Convention on the Rights of the Child. https://www.ohchr.org/en/professionalinterest/pages/crc.aspx

Special Concerns for Young Women Migrants and Refugees

The role of women varies greatly among different cultures. In contemporary Canadian and US culture, most healthcare professionals recognize and deeply support equal rights for women and men, and opportunities for boys and girls, and recognize that this equality of rights is central to the improvement of the health and well-being of society. In some cultures of origin, mixed socializing of men and women is uncommon or restricted to specific circumstances. It is important for providers to ask about and respect stated cultural preferences in clinical practice, such as a preference for male or female clinicians, while avoiding stereotyping, recognizing that there is great variability within the same cultural milieu.

Yet a critical facet of gender equality is for women, including adolescents, to have control over their reproductive lives, including the choice of who to marry, not to marry at all, the right to divorce, confidential access to family planning, contraception, safe and legal pregnancy termination, and access to prenatal care. Another facet is to be free from intimate partner violence and to be safe from threats of sexual assault or other forms of coercive sexual contact. Though generally accepted today, the integration of these principles into modern society is relatively recent and, in some sectors of the general population, still not universally accepted.

All adolescents, including irregular migrants and refugees, are entitled to safety and access to child protective services as needed in the case of sexual abuse, coercion, or exploitation.

Immigrant girls and women may come from societies with more patriarchal values and may have internalized these values. In some circumstances, they may have been in such desperate straits and with such limited options that they engaged in providing sex for survival needs for themselves or for their children. Immigrant girls and women may have been sexually assaulted in their home country or in transit, not uncommonly by police or soldiers, and may have an enduring distrust of police and soldiers. These experiences may be so stigmatized and incur such profound shame that they are not disclosed even with promises of confidentiality.

In some communities, female genital mutilation (FGM) or clitorectomy (sometimes called "female circumcision") is considered a religious or cultural practice. The World Health Organization recognizes FGM as a "violation of the human rights of girls and women. It reflects deep-rooted inequality between the sexes, and constitutes an extreme form of discrimination against women. It is nearly always carried out on minors and is a violation of the rights of children. The practice also violates the person's rights to health, security and physical integrity, the right to be free from torture and cruel, inhuman and/or degrading treatment…"[23] In Canada and in the United States, this practice is legally banned, irrespective of historic cultural or religious practices. A recent court case (November 2018) in the United States has put in question the legality of banning this practice as an infringement of "freedom of religion" [36]; nonetheless, it remains a legally banned practice.

[23] WHO, Jan 11, 2018. https://www.who.int/news-room/fact-sheets/detail/female-genital-mutilation

Surviving Gender-Based Violence

For centuries, young women have faced gender-based violence in the context of war, which continues in recent contexts, from Yazidi young women sold as sex slaves by Daesh to reports of the rape and torture of young Rohingya women fleeing ethnic cleansing in Myanmar to the mass kidnapping of school girls in Nigeria. It is essential to recognize the vulnerability of migrant and refugee youth to the experience of gender-based violence prior to migrating to the host country, or sometimes after arrival. The sequelae of these traumatic experiences last for years, if not for life, and therefore requires extending all facets of reproductive care in the host country, including facilitating access to affordable and safe emergency contraception; access to safe, legal, and confidential pregnancy termination; STI testing and prophylaxis; and ongoing supportive, trauma-informed counseling.

For sexual minorities, including LGBT youth, the risk of gender-based violence, persecution, or discrimination is even greater. It is important to explore their social support systems, as many youth find the lack of community support to be even further isolating. In addition, LGBT youth and adults may have experienced grave discrimination and persecution in their home country or during migration; in fact, this persecution may be the principal reason for migration. Contemporary scientific understanding of gender identity and sexual orientation appreciates that LGBT identities and orientation are within the spectrum of expected and normative human experiences and are found throughout the world. It is important that youth and adults identifying as LGBT hear these assurances from clinicians and that parents receive the support they need to come to an acceptance of their child's orientation and identity. It is also important for the youth and their parents to know that their child, regardless of gender orientation or identity, needs their love and acceptance and is entitled to the full protection of the law.

Importance of Inclusive Host Country Communities

The host country communities that are welcoming, inclusive, and supportive toward youth regardless of their culture or country of origin plays a critical role in supporting healthy child and adolescent development. Child health practitioners can ask about their patients' experiences of isolation and inclusion at school and identify programs and support systems in their local communities to promote the development of positive social circles; this is particularly important for unaccompanied adolescents. Helping newcomer youth retain positive traditions and customs of their home country or ethnic group while also developing ties to their new community is a protective factor in both educational success and preventing youth victimization by, or involvement in, violent behavior. As with other young people, youth who are disengaged from inclusive communities, out of school, without employment, and with a perception of poor future prospects may be vulnerable targets for inclusion in violent groups. Some studies have shown that a perceived lack of inclusion in their host countries, particularly school communities, have led to anger and frustration toward dominant social groups and was a driver for youth seeking out others that have had similar experiences [37].

Access to Healthcare of Migrants and Refugees in Host Countries

Perhaps of greatest relevance to healthcare practitioners is ensuring that migrant and refugee youth understand their rights and have access to appropriate healthcare and healthcare insurance. In Canada, asylum seekers receive healthcare coverage through the Interim Federal Health Program (IFHP), a separate insurance system from the universal, provincial health system that Canadian citizens and permanent residents enjoy. Although IFHP gives beneficiaries access to basic medical care and a wide array of supplementary and allied healthcare coverage, not all physicians are required to register or accept this insurance. Furthermore, physician knowledge of how to access services is weak, even in large tertiary centers. For health practitioners caring for migrant and refugee youth, it is important that they be aware of care coverage and support youth to know how to access the health services they are entitled to. Furthermore, practitioners can advocate to ensure that these services remain protected. In 2012, the Canadian government removed health insurance coverage for asylum seekers from designated countries. However, the Supreme Court overturned this policy, led by a group of physicians who challenged the federal government in this practice that violated the Canadian Charter of Rights and Freedoms.

In the United States, immigrant and refugee access to healthcare is even more problematical. There are barriers not only related to actual access but to the fears that commonly exist, sometimes based on real threats, that for migrants accessing publicly funded healthcare can create a future barrier to establishing legal residency or successful application for citizenship. There are also regional differences within the United States regarding restrictions to access of healthcare by migrants with some states being more accessible and others with higher barriers. In urban centers there are commonly youth-focused clinics that are funded through nonprofit agencies that can provide primary and secondary health services, in particular related to reproductive health for minors. Undocumented immigrants in the United States do not have access to Medicaid, the federally funded healthcare system, with the exception of emergency care. However, there are significant state-by-state differences and exceptions in eligibility requirements. For example, in California undocumented immigrants, both children and adults, are eligible for Medi-Cal (Medicaid in California) if they otherwise meet income eligibility requirements.[24] There is also a

[24] California Department of Health Care Services; Medi-Cal Eligibility and Covered California – Frequently Asked Questions. https://www.dhcs.ca.gov/services/medi-cal/eligibility/pages/medicalfaqs2014b.aspx

commonly held concern that information, including medical and mental health histories, may be accessible to immigration authorities and may be used to introduce unwarranted barriers to obtaining legal residency in the future, including for minors; this issue remains unresolved at this time.

Societal Considerations Impacting the Health of Newcomer Youth

Canada and the United States are often referred to as "nations of immigrants," countries colonized over several centuries by waves of immigrant settlers with the exception of Indigenous peoples and, in the United States, enslaved Africans and their descendants. Alarmingly, there are vocal sectors of the population and powerful political forces who politicize the issues and oppose immigration, falsely characterizing immigrants as a threat to safety or even as "criminals" or "terrorists" creating barriers to the health and well-being of children and youth.

Embedded in the anti-immigrant rhetoric is the confluence of both racist and xenophobic discrimination, both distinct yet each damaging [38]. Definitions by the International Labour Organization help explain the difference [39]. Xenophobia is defined as "attitudes, prejudices and behaviour that reject, exclude and often vilify persons, based on the perceptions that they are outsiders or foreigners to the community, society or national identity" whereas racism "assigns a certain race and/or ethnic group to a position of power over others on the basis of physical and cultural attributes, as well as economic wealth, imposing hierarchical relations where the purportedly 'superior' race exercises domination and control over others" [39, 40]. For refugee and immigrant youth, it is often the combination of xenophobic and racist discrimination that excludes them from the community (xenophobia) while asserting power and privilege (racism).

Historically, in the United States during periods of economic stagnation, prejudice against immigrants has increased as they are perceived as taking jobs. In addition, there is a long and tragic history of racism targeting African-Americans, Latinos, Asians, and others, particularly of non-Western European descent. People who hold these biases may put significant obstacles in the path of social integration for immigrants. As with xenophobia, there are political forces at work that foster, perpetuate, and take advantage of these irrational social biases. It is important to remember that while a minority of the population espouses explicit racial or xenophobic discrimination, which can be verbal, physical, or violent, others may hold implicit biases that are culturally reinforced but not openly expressed. It is equally important for all citizens, especially health practitioners, to be critical of policies that may endorse "pervasive, structural xenophobic discrimination"; for example, despite the appropriate qualifications and experience, many immigrants are denied the same job opportunities as their counterparts in their host country [38, 41].

Due to explicit and structural xenophobia and racism, as well as other issues, immigrants commonly face a degree of discrimination in multiple areas, most significantly in employment [41, 42]. This is greatly accentuated for immigrants with undocumented status. Lack of familiarity with or fear of social services, poor English fluency, and poor general education opportunities all play important roles in relegating many immigrants to employment where labor laws and minimum wage are not respected and other low-income employment, impairing their ability to emerge from poverty. Commonly, both parents must work to support the family, and at times, youth may also be financially supporting their family.

It is unsurprising then to learn that immigrant and refugee families are disproportionately affected by poverty. In a recent study in Toronto, heralded as one of the most multicultural cities in the world, one in two refugee children live in poverty.[62] While poverty decreased based on the length of time in Canada, the rate of poverty for immigrants remained at two to three times the rate of poverty for native-born Canadians, inferring an ugly truth that poverty exists along racial lines.[25] In the United States in 2011, children with an immigrant father, or immigrant father and mother, had poverty rates of 19.9% versus poverty rates of 13.5% among nonimmigrant families.[26] With poverty, many families are forced to live in shelters and inadequate, insecure housing, often with overcrowding and in neighborhoods threatened with violence. Unstable housing commonly is associated with changes in schools for children and obstacles in maintaining a stable group of friends, peers, and supportive adults or enrolment in a consistent school.

Contemporary Challenges for Refugee and Migrant Youth Entering the United States

Apprehension of Children and Adolescents at the US Border

Every year, thousands of unaccompanied children and adolescents arrive in the United States to escape persecution in foreign countries. For the past several years, most children arriving at the Southwest border of the United States are from Central America's Northern Triangle – El Salvador, Honduras, and Guatemala [43].

Fleeing crime, gang threats, violence, hunger, and ethnic persecution, these children and youth, alone or with families, endure perilous journeys to the United States. Often crossing several borders, children and adolescents travel hundreds of

[25] https://www.socialplanningtoronto.org/unequal_city_the_hidden_divide_among_toronto_s_children_and_youth

[26] Center for Immigration Studies, Immigrants in the United States: A Profile of America's Foreign Born Population. https://www.dhcs.ca.gov/services/medi-cal/eligibility/pages/medi-calfaqs2014b.aspx

miles by foot, by bus, by car, or atop dangerous freight trains. They endure weeks or months without sufficient food or medical care, without safe sleeping spaces, and a complete dependency on others for survival [44]. The absence of a parent or adult caregiver places unaccompanied children at higher risks of experiencing additional traumatic events, such as physical or sexual assault, during their trip to the United States.

Once they cross the border, many children are either apprehended or turn themselves in to the US Customs and Border Patrol (CBP) or other Department of Homeland Security (DHS) officers. Children and adolescents under age 18 who arrive without a parent or legal guardian are classified as "unaccompanied," even if they arrive with an adult relative or caregiver.[27] Once detained by a federal agency, unaccompanied children and adolescents must be transferred to the custody of the Office of Refugee Resettlement (ORR) within 72 hours.

ORR is the federal agency responsible for coordinating and providing the care and placement of unaccompanied children. Under the *Flores* Settlement Agreement, which has been in effect since 1993, ORR is required to detain children in the "least restrictive setting" and release children "without unnecessary delay" to a sponsor.[28] With limited exceptions, the Settlement requires ORR to place unaccompanied minors in nonsecure facilities that are licensed to care for dependent children.[29] Once a child or adolescent is in ORR custody, ORR is required to make "prompt and continuous efforts" to identify and screen potential sponsors (usually a parent, legal guardian, or close relative) and to plan for the child's release.[30] However, children may be detained for months or even years while they wait to be released to an adult sponsor, even if a sponsor is ready and willing to take custody.

Under the *Flores* Settlement Agreement, the *Flores* case remains open with active federal oversight of the parties' agreement. Under the Settlement, *Flores* class counsel have the ability to visit facilities and conduct interviews with detained children.[31] As a result of active monitoring efforts over the past two decades, *Flores* counsel have repeatedly uncovered violations of the Settlement Agreement and brought motions to enforce the Settlement in federal court. For example, *Flores* counsel recently uncovered numerous examples of children being administered multiple psychotropic medications without informed consent or appropriate oversight, in direct contravention of state law. In 2018, a federal court ordered ORR to comply with state law when administering psychotropic medications to children detained at a residential treatment center in Texas [45].

---

[27] *See* 6 U.S.C. § 279(g)(2) (2012).

[28] See *Flores* Settlement Agreement ("Settlement"), Case No. CV 85-4544-RJK(Px) (C.D. Cal. Jan. 17, 1997), ¶¶ 11, 14.

[29] Settlement ¶ 19.

[30] Settlement ¶ 18.

[31] Settlement ¶¶ 32–3.

Recent Family Separation Crisis Affecting Migrant Children and Youth Seeking Refuge in the United States

Children may become separated from their family at any stage during their migration – before they leave their home country, during the journey, at the border, or while detained in ORR custody. Recent governmental practices have called attention to family separation occurring at the Southwest border. Media reports in March 2017 that the Department of Homeland Security (DHS) was considering a policy of separating immigrant mothers from their children upon arrival at the US border alarmed the nonpartisan Society for Adolescent Health and Medicine (SAHM)[32] and the American Academy of Pediatrics (AAP) [24], as well as experts in child welfare, Juvenile Justice, and child development[33] who immediately spoke out against this proposed policy given the grave additional trauma on children that would be inflicted, augmenting the trauma already experienced.

In April 2018, DHS adopted a "zero-tolerance" policy, criminally prosecuting anyone who crossed the border illegally. Under that policy, federal authorities separated children from parents or legal guardians when they were apprehended by federal authorities – adults were prosecuted and held in the US Immigration and Customs Enforcement (ICE) custody, while the children were placed in ORR custody. New US governmental policies enabled indefinite separation of non-English-speaking children from their mothers and fathers, including infants and toddlers, as well as adolescents, and who at times have been put up involuntarily for adoption. These practices are sure to accentuate the grave trauma that these young asylum seekers had already experienced [46].

In June 2018, a Federal District Court ordered that all separated children must be reunited within 30 days, children under 5 within 14 days, and all parents must be able to speak with their children within 10 days [47]. Within this lawsuit, the government identified a class of 2737 children that they believed had been separated under this policy [48].

In November 2018, the United States held 16,000 immigrant children and adolescents who had been involuntarily separated from their parents, including 2700 apprehended over the summer of 2018 and held indefinitely in temporary camps on the Mexican border with thousands of others scattered around the United States in group homes and foster care settings [49, 50]. In January 2019, a report from the Office of the Inspector General of the Department of Health and Human Services found that an unknown number of children, potentially "thousands," were separated from parents and guardians at the Southwest border before June 2018 but hadn't been included in official government tallies of separated families [51]. The report

---

[32] SAHM Statement on Forced Family Separation. https://www.adolescenthealth.org/Advocacy/Advocacy-Activities/2018-Activity/SAHM-Statement-on-Forced-Family-Separation.aspx

[33] Renewed Appeal from Experts in Child Welfare, Juvenile Justice and Child Development to Halt the Separation of Children from Parents at the Border, June 7, 2018. http://www.adolescenthealth.org/SAHM_Main/media/Advocacy/2018/Opposition-to-Parent-Child-Separation.pdf

found that the government faced "significant challenges in identifying separated children, including the lack of an existing, integrated data system to track separated families" [51]. In February 2019, the *New York Times* reported that more than 11,000 toddlers, children, and teens were in federal custody as unaccompanied minors.

The tracking of child and youth migrants, separated from parents, and apprehended and detained were poorly recorded; thousands who had been taken from their parents even before the policy was announced were not disclosed [51, 52]. Government officials said there were no plans to attempt to reunite these children because "it would destabilize the permanency of their existing home environment, and could be traumatic to the children" [53].

In February 2019, it was found through documents released by the US Department of Health and Human Services Office of Refugee Resettlement that between October 2014 and July 2018, there were 4556 complaints of sexual abuse of immigrant youth in government-funded shelters; the Department of Justice received 1303 additional serious complaints including 178 allegations of sexual abuse by adult staff [54]. As of March 2019, over 11,000 unaccompanied children and adolescents remained in ORR custody nationwide [55]. In June 2019, the US Administration declared that it would restrict or cancel education, legal aid, and playground recreation for all migrant children and youth housed in more than 100 government shelters across the United States [20].

Unfortunately, the record keeping of young immigrants and asylum seekers has been negligent, with a federal judge in San Diego stating that they were treated "worse than chattel" and "under the current system, migrant children are not accounted for with the same efficiency and accuracy as property." This was illustrated by a report in January 2019 that thousands more children had been taken from their parents than previously reported and that record keeping had been so poor that the Department of Homeland Security's computers could not track them [52].

Prolonged detention becomes especially damaging when youth turn 18 years old. Once youth turn 18, they cease to qualify as "minors" and lose eligibility for many pathways for immigration relief. Recently, practices have been enacted to remove young people in ankle chains on their 18th birthday from federal shelters and transport them to adult detention facilities.[34]

Harms of Family Separation

In 2018 and 2019, the United States was met with worldwide condemnation for the separation of migrant children and youth from their families at the US–Mexico border and detained separately [49, 56]. The American Academy of Pediatrics (AAP) [57] and the Society for Adolescent Health and Medicine (SAHM),[35] along with many other child and youth health advocacy groups, opposed those detention

[34] NPR; Migrant Youth Go From A Children's Shelter to Adult Detention On Their 18th Birthday, February 22, 2019.

[35] SAHM Statement on Forced Family Separation. https://www.adolescenthealth.org/Advocacy/Advocacy-Activities/2018-Activity/SAHM-Statement-on-Forced-Family-Separation.aspx

practices for children and youth due to the known negative effects of family separation and toxic stress. The detention and separation of children from their families cause profound and long-lasting mental and physical harm. A long-standing body of research has established that detaining children interferes with healthy development, exposes youth to abuse, undermines educational attainment, makes mentally ill children worse, and puts children at greater risk of self-harm [58].

In Dr. Julie Linton's testimony before the US House of Representatives Committee on Energy and Commerce Subcommittee on Oversight and Investigations, she noted that "[H]ighly stressful experiences, like family separation, can cause irreparable harm, disrupting a child's brain architecture and affecting his or her short and long term health. This type of prolonged exposure to serious stress – known as toxic stress – can carry lifelong consequences for children. A parent or a known caregiver's role is to mitigate these dangers. When robbed of that buffer, children are susceptible to a variety of adverse health impacts including learning deficits and chronic conditions such as depression, post-traumatic stress disorder and even heart disease" [59]. A primary factor in recovering from such trauma is reunification with a parent or other trusted adult. Without the presence of trusted caregivers, children are often unable to cope with the psychological trauma and stress associated with separation and detention.

Recent governmental practices in the United States affecting children and youth seeking refuge with their parents may accentuate the trauma that children and youth experience. These children and youth, commonly with their parents, seek refuge from pervasive violence in Central America. They had already experienced high levels of trauma and loss, fleeing organized criminal gangs, civil conflict, or persecution of indigenous peoples by military governments.

There is renewed threat of more aggressive introduction of similar, even more aggressive policies to separate children from parents, refuse them basic education and recreational opportunities, and to incarcerate parents who are seeking asylum [60]. Children and parents seeking safety continue to confront insurmountable barriers to obtaining formal asylum, including gratuitous future barriers, to establishing legal residency if public benefits are utilized such as obtaining medical care through Medicaid-funded clinics or accessing food with food stamps. This tragic process remains unresolved and continues to unfold.

A Framework Toward Supporting Healthy Resettlement

In 2016, the United Nations High Commission for Refugees held a series of consultations with refugee youth around the world. In their report *We Believe in Youth: Global Refugee Youth Consultations*, ten challenges and seven core actions to support refugee youth were identified, many of which are described in this chapter [61]. Limited access to education, employment, and the ability to participate in decision-making; poor access to youth-centered healthcare, gender inequality and racist, xenophobic, and LGBT discrimination; and a lack of safety, security, and limited knowledge of rights and legal documentation were cited as core challenges facing refugee youth globally [61]. The seven core actions that advocate and host communities can take to mitigate these challenges include the following [61]:

1. Empowering youth through meaningful engagement
2. Recognize and utilize youth capacities and skills
3. Ensure refugee youth-focused protection
4. Support the physical and emotional well-being of refugee youth
5. Facilitate networking and information sharing among refugee youth
6. Reinforce the abilities of refugee youth to be connecters and peace builders
7. Generate data and evidence about refugee youth to promote accountability

We discuss some strategies to incorporate these actions into promoting health resettlement of refugee and migrant youth in the United States and Canada.

First, and most importantly, the strength and resilience of immigrant and refugee youth must be acknowledged. Schools can provide a critical stabilizing engagement for all youth, including unstably housed and many homeless youth. Many youth are pillars of support for their families, parents, and younger siblings, through their ability to adapt quickly to new surroundings while retaining a role as the cultural ambassadors for their families.

For the children of immigrants, accessing high-quality education is viewed as a principle opening for economic advancement. Many public schools in communities with high numbers of migrants have highly skilled and dedicated teachers who strive to help integrate the children and youth. It is essential that children and adolescents, including unaccompanied youth, be integrated into the public schools as soon as possible to continue their education.

As described earlier, it is important that child health providers recognize the impact of implicit or structural racism, xenophobia, and discrimination on immigrant and refugee youth. For many youth, it is the intersection of both racism and xenophobia that compounds the resultant discrimination, stress, and civic exclusion. From subtle indicators like a lack of interpreters to explicit federal policies that ban children and youth on the basis of their residency status or citizenship, healthcare providers must recognize the toll that these forms of discrimination can take. Newcomer children and youth must be given the opportunity to openly discuss negative experiences and receive support from their parents, teachers, healthcare providers, and other supportive adults. Furthermore, healthcare providers and community advocates alike must examine our own individual and institutional implicit biases and take action to challenge and improve these.

Providing opportunities for youth to engage meaningfully with their community is highlighted as a critical core action to promote healthy resettlement for immigrant and refugee youth. Programs that engage youth as partners – led by youth, for youth – with the opportunity to contribute and utilize their skills meaningfully enable the development of confidence in their own identities while sharing their lived experiences with others.

One such example is the Nai Syrian Children's Choir, led by CultureLink, a settlement organization that strives to promote equity healthy resettlement for newcomers in Canada. The chorus was founded in 2016, where youth participate in a weekly music program while their parents receive ESL classes, all without cost to youth or families. In this integrated model, both parents and children are able to participate in enriching opportunities simultaneously. Another example is the MusicBox Children's Charity, another arts-based education program in several cities in Canada. Since 2004, over 5000 children have come through their programs, with some children now achieving certifications for they themselves to be teachers.

Spotlight on MusicBox Children's Charity
MusicBox Children's Charity was developed by two young first-generation Canadians. Since launching in 2002, MusicBox harnesses the energy of young adults to provide high-quality music education programming to vulnerable youth across Canada. Multiple locations exist in partnership with local community agencies, such as the Ray-Cam Co-operative Centre (Vancouver), Inasmuch House (Hamilton), the YWCA and affiliated housing developments (Toronto), and Boys & Girls Clubs (Edmonton), among many others, that act as local hubs for children and youth in their neighborhoods.

Using a community- and asset-based model of delivery, MusicBox shapes programming based on student and community interest, offering programs in community spaces free of charge. Popular programs include private instrument lessons, such as guitar, piano, and drums; early childhood music education; and world music appreciation. However, programs are developed based on youth interests, which have led to more creative offerings such as DJ classes, drop-in "jam sessions," and drumming circles.

Evaluation of MusicBox programs has found that stakeholders perceive programming improved children's intrapersonal development, literacy, and kinesthetic skills. Parents expressed that music classes promoted mother–child attachment in shelter environments where children are facing adverse childhood experiences (ACEs).

One of the key strengths of MusicBox's programming is the investment in longstanding community partnerships and the development of positive relationships between youth. MusicBox has also partnered with medical schools to provide opportunities for medical students to engage in community-based service learning, witnessing the impact of community programs on children and youth facing difficult social circumstances.

The World Health Organization's Call for Universal Health Insurance for All Refugees and Migrants

Finally, ensuring timely, equitable, and accessible healthcare is an essential factor in promoting healthy resettlement of newcomer children and youth. The World Health Organization (WHO) has called for universal health insurance coverage for all refugees and migrants globally. Universal Health Coverage, according to WHO, is aimed at "ensuring that all people can use the promotive, preventive, curative, rehabilitative and palliative health service they need, and that these are of sufficient quality to be effective, while also ensuring the use of these services does not expose the user to financial hardship. Universal health coverage provides an opportunity to promote a more coherent and integrated approach to health, beyond the treatment of specific diseases for all populations, including migrants, irrespective of their legal and migratory status."[36,37]

United Nations Conventions on the Rights of the Child

The United Nations Conventions on the Rights of the Child states in Article 4 that "States Parties recognize the right of the child to the enjoyment of the highest attainable standard of health and to facilities for the treatment of illness and rehabilitation of health. States Parties shall strive to ensure that no child is deprived of his or her right to access to such health care services."

"States Parties shall pursue full implementation of this right and, in particular, shall take appropriate measures…to ensure the provision of necessary medical assistance and health care to all children with emphasis on the development of primary health care."[38]

A Practical Approach for Clinicians

Caring for migrant and refugee youth requires a comprehensive approach, beginning before the first visit and extending into the community. The following approach helps guide clinicians from before their first visit to supporting community programs.

Building a Healthcare Workplace and Environment Rooted in Trauma-Informed Care and Cultural Safety

To provide comprehensive care for migrant and refugee youth and their families, the entire medical team must be engaged in creating a workplace that is culturally safe.[39] Frontline staff like administrative or clerical support should know how to

[36] https://www.who.int/migrants/about/mh-qhc/en/

[37] WHO, Health of refugees and migrants. https://www.who.int/migrants/publications/PAHO-report.pdf?ua=1

[38] UN Conventions on the Rights of the Child. https://www.unicef.org/child-rights-convention/convention-text

[39] https://nam.edu/wp-content/uploads/2017/12/Perspectives-on-Health-Equity-and-Social-

welcome families and address questions like residency and insurance coverage in a safe and nonthreatening way. Allied health staff, including nurses, dietitians, social workers, and psychologists, are essential to caring for adolescents, especially unstably housed and many homeless youth.

Suggested organizational practices include the following:

- Placing clear signage for registration in English, Spanish, and other languages that are common in the area
- Ensuring access to high-quality health interpreters
- Providing written resources in multiple languages
- Creating a safe, welcoming physical space in the waiting room and office
- Promoting a culture of reflective practice, team huddles, and debriefs

For individuals, building skills in cultural competence, safety, and trauma-informed practice can enhance the quality of care newcomer youth can receive. The *LEARN (Listen, Explain, Acknowledge, Recommend, Negotiate)* mnemonic, promoted by the Canadian Paediatric Society, represents a useful approach for health-care providers to adopt in clinical encounters with families from diverse cultural backgrounds [62].[40] The goal is to develop respect and understanding between both the provider and patient and thus lead to improved patient care.

First, providers and patients *listen* to each other's understanding and explanation of the condition. For example, behavioral problems at school may be seen as due to stress by the patient and their family, while the provider and school may see this as symptomatic of ADHD. Next, the provider *explains* their understanding of the condition and *acknowledge* the differences in perspectives. Finally, the provider makes *recommendations* and *negotiates* a management plan collaboratively with the family. In the example above, the patient and their parents may first wish to explore ways to cope with stress and engage family, community, and social support, before considering medication.

During the encounter, there may be episodes of silence, which may express different feelings in various cultures. Cross-cultural communication includes respecting silence and reading nonverbal cues throughout the encounter. Allowing the patient and their family to speak – or not – as they so choose can facilitate trust and understanding. For more information, please refer to the position statement on promoting culturally relevant care by the Canadian Paediatric Society.[41]

Determinants-of-Health.pdf

[40] https://www.cps.ca/en/documents/position/cross-cultural-communication

[41] https://www.cps.ca/en/documents/position/cross-cultural-communication

The LEARN Model for Cross-Cultural Communication to Build Mutual Understanding and Enhance Patient Care Canadian Pediatric Society https://www.cps.ca/en/documents/position/cross-cultural-communication
Listen: Assess each patient's understanding of their health condition, its causes, and potential treatments. Elicit expectations for the encounter, and bring an attitude of curiosity and humility to promote trust and understanding.
Explain: Convey your own perceptions of the health condition, keeping in mind that patients may understand health or illness differently, based on culture or ethnic background.
Acknowledge: Be respectful when discussing the differences between their views and your own. Point out areas of agreement as well as difference, and try to determine whether disparate belief systems may lead to a therapeutic dilemma.
Recommend: Develop and propose a treatment plan to the patient and their family.
Negotiate: Reach an agreement on the treatment plan in partnership with the patient and family, incorporating culturally relevant approaches that fit with the patient's perceptions of health and healing.

Interviewing Youth and Promoting Positive Relationships

When interviewing young people, in particular for youth who are unaccompanied, it is important to focus on strengths and positive experiences and not focus entirely on problems. Stabilizing housing, engaging in education, and promoting engagement in environments where positive relationships with caring adults can be fostered are key building blocks toward promoting positive development for youth.

It is important for practitioners to be familiar with local resources, including shelters, alternative schools, and healthcare, that are accessible and available to these vulnerable youth. It may be necessary to engage social workers or others more familiar with community resources to facilitate these connections. It is important to identify and validate individual strengths including athletic or artistic talents, close interpersonal relationships, and positive aspirations for the future. For LGBT youth who commonly experience social and internalized stigma, it is important to assure that they are provided an accepting environment that will support self-acceptance and family acceptance when possible.

It is important for clinicians to be sensitive to differences between their own cultural background and their patients' cultural backgrounds; these differences can affect both verbal and nonverbal communication. The expectations and values of the practitioner can inadvertently communicate an "implicit bias" toward young people of other cultures or socioeconomic status. Ethnic and cultural groups are not homogeneous, and it is essential for clinicians not to overgeneralize, stereotype, or adopt other culturally biased assumptions. These are key components of providing culturally competent care.

If there are language barriers, it is important to use a professional medical interpreter; if not already available, it is important to find ways to make interpreters available, such as by telephone or online. Do not use children as interpreters, beyond narrowly circumscribed topics such as giving directions to locations.[42]

It can be difficult, overwhelming, and undesirable to attempt to get all of the desired information in one visit. It is usually easier to use multiple visits to complete a full history; engage other clinical staff such as social workers, nurses, or mental health providers; and explore the social determinants in more depth. Having multiple encounters allows the development of trust and rapport as well as identify and make available resources as their need becomes apparent. Regular follow-up visits help build relationships and trust with your patient and their family.

First Visit to the Office

The first visit can be daunting for both the provider and the patient. A comprehensive history and physical can be conducted over several visits, so cultivating trust and rapport with patients is essential.

It is important to note that some subjects covered in the interview are exceedingly sensitive areas for the youth and their family and potentially for the clinician as well. To respectfully explore these topics requires developing trust, taking time, and deeply respecting the boundaries and sensitivity of the young person and their families. The traditional structure of medical interviewing, using a "problem-based" approach, particularly regarding behavioral or social situations, can inadvertently derail a relationship with youth and their parents, as such approaches may leave families feeling misunderstood, judged, or unheard, with questions about problems interpreted as criticism. Worse still, an insensitive approach may leave patients believing that information disclosed may undermine their applications for immigration or protection.

Clinicians need to be prepared to be patient, to seek out and identify the young person's authentic strengths and positive attributes. It is important for clinicians to self-reflect on their personal skills and clinic structure and, in some cases, consider if another provider or clinic may be a better fit for the patient. Clinicians must remain nonjudgmental and positive, even as patients and families may have different values and opinions. In caring for newcomer children, an interdisciplinary and collaborative team of regular providers is ideal, particularly in clinical educational environments when rotating students, residents, or other trainees participate but are not available to develop a longer-term relationship. Please refer Chap. 3.

Taking a History

Important features of a comprehensive history, which may take place over several encounters, include the following:

[42] https://www.kidsnewtocanada.ca/mental-health/mental-health-promotion#risk-and-protective-factors

- Detailed past medical history, including any previous hospitalizations, surgeries, transfusions, or other medications.
- A travel history, detailing all countries in transit prior to arrival.
- Assess risk for exposure to contaminated water, agricultural pesticides, or other toxins.
- Reviewing immunization records; if records cannot be produced, consider a catch-up schedule for many preventable diseases. Many children have also received the BCG vaccine, which is important to note for tuberculin skin testing.
- Screening examinations for vision, dental, and hearing – many countries in the world do not have universal screening programs, which can lead to late diagnoses. Most children have not had adequate dental care and will need referral. Young people may not have been screened for visual refractive errors and will need referral for free or very low-cost corrective lenses.
- The adolescent interview and history: Depending on the adolescent, it may be worthwhile to explore portions of this history with the parent or caregiver in the room or with the adolescent alone. The parent may need time alone with the clinician as well and may offer great insights, particularly about early childhood experiences, that the youth is unable to articulate. It is important that the parent and youth understand the adolescent's right to confidentiality and the limits of confidentiality. This interview generally cannot be completed on the first visit as the young person may need time to develop trust and confidence. Given the sensitivity of many of the areas covered, it is important to be highly sensitive to, and respectful of, the boundaries of the youth and appreciate that sustaining a trusting relationship is more important that completion of all areas of the interview. It is important to keep in mind the differences in emotional development between early, middle, and late adolescence and frame inquiries accordingly. It is particularly important for LGBT youth that there be strict observance of confidentiality and an appreciation of the stigma the youth may encounter if information is disclosed; ideally, parents will come to accept their child's sexual orientation and identity, if they haven't already. In addition, traumatic sexual experiences are not uncommon among refugee youth, in particular girls, and may be highly stigmatizing within the family or to the youth himself or herself. It is essential to have available appropriate counseling services. (Please see Interviewing Homeless Adolescents in the Context of Clinical Care: Creating Connections, Building on Strengths, Fostering Resilience, and Improving Outcomes in this book.)
- Gynecological history for young women.
- Mental health screening, with the appreciation that mental health issues are likely to carry a high level of stigma and are conceptualized in widely different ways among cultures, as are acceptable approaches to management. Traumatic experiences from place of origin and during migration, disrupted attachments to family and community, and loss of culture of origin all play significant roles in what may be perceived as manifestations of mental illness. It is important to exercise patience, as the experience of trauma, stress, and other mental health challenges take time to unfold. If these become apparent, it is important to identify and involve additional community and mental health resources that are appropriate for the patient and their family.

Physical Examination

A full physical examination should also be conducted, including anthropometrics and a full set of vital signs. When considering diagnostic testing, specific attention should be paid to

- Features of chronic disease (i.e., diabetes, hypothyroidism)
- Infectious and communicable disease screening as indicated
- Inherited conditions (i.e., hemoglobinopathies)
- Oral health
- Nutritional markers, including vitamin and micronutrient status
- Screening for vision and hearing
- Sexually transmitted infection screening

There are several resources that can guide the history, physical examination, and recommended diagnostic and laboratory testing by country of origin. A useful resource is the Centers for Disease Control, which identifies the prevalence of communicable diseases by country of origin.[43] Another resource is the Caring for Kids New to Canada website produced by the Canadian Paediatric Society;[44] templates for history and physical examinations are provided.

Screening for and Addressing the Social Determinants of Health

In addition to a comprehensive history and physical exam, special attention should be paid to addressing the social determinants of health, especially housing and food insecurity. For unstably housed youth and families, this need must be addressed with urgency. In addition, it is essential that children and youth be engaged in school as promptly as possible. Allied health providers, including social workers and psychologists, are integral to providing comprehensive support to newcomer youth and their families. Some important elements for newcomer youth include

(a) *Immigration status and healthcare access*: In Canada, it is important for healthcare providers to know the patient's immigration status, to determine what type of health insurance and benefits they may be eligible for. However, this does not need to be documented in the medical record. For example, refugee claimants are eligible for the Interim Federal Health Program (IFHP), while government-sponsored refugees are covered under provincial health insurance plans. Families without status, including those on a visitor's visa, often have no access to health insurance which limits their ability to access basic medical and allied healthcare. Providers can learn about IFHP and how to access covered services through online resources.[45]

---

[43] National Notifiable Diseases Surveillance System (NNDSS). https://wwwn.cdc.gov/nndss/conditions/notifiable/2018/infectious-diseases/

[44] Caring for Kids New to Canada, Canadian Pediatric Society. https://www.kidsnewtocanada.ca/

[45] https://docs.medaviebc.ca/providers/guides_info/IFHP-Information-Handbook-for-Health-care-Professionals-April-1-2016.pdf

For families without documented status, this can be a particularly sensitive topic. Often, adolescents may not know their undocumented immigration status. With parents alone, healthcare providers can cautiously explore the length of time the child has been in the country and how they arrived. Parents may be extremely distrustful of the healthcare system, and providers should weigh these consequences carefully against the actual benefit of asking these questions, as the actual confidentiality of medical charts remains to be assured.

In the United States, it is useful to have resources for legal services to support youth with questions about immigration status. It is not necessary to document any concerning information regarding immigration status in the medical chart, given doubts about sustained confidentiality of electronic medical records. Though there has been an erosion of federal support in the United States for international migrants, including children and adolescents, it is important to know the resources available and accessible for migrant youth in one's own community, including schools, healthcare, family planning, nutritional support and food stamps, and shelters and housing. It is important to have staff who are knowledgeable regarding patient eligibility for healthcare as this varies state by state and is an ongoing area of negotiation and renegotiation. For example, migrant patients who meet income eligibility requirements are not eligible for federally funded Medicaid in most states; however, in California, home to many migrants, Medi-Cal (California Medicaid) is available to all who meet income eligibility requirements including documented and undocumented migrants.

(b) *Housing*: Housing is a core need for all children, youth, and families. Without stable housing, it is effectively impossible to address other social determinants of health. This is most acutely true for unaccompanied migrant adolescents. It is essential that agencies interacting with unaccompanied migrant youth be knowledgeable about accessible shelters and other resources. Commonly, local child protective services are very helpful in addressing this need for youth. In addition, there are nonprofit agencies with highly experienced staff that operate shelters and other resources in urban communities to which these youth can be referred; they may be able to send staff to healthcare centers to meet the individual youth and bring them to shelters. Many newcomer families live in insecure, crowded, and unsafe housing or with other families and friends. It is important to identify youth and families living in unsafe housing conditions and advocate for improvement.

(c) *Schools*: In Canada, education is under the mandate of the provinces and territories. As an example, in Ontario, Canada's most populous province, all youth under the age of 18 have the legal right to attend school, regardless of their immigration status. However, there may be variability between provinces and local school boards. Many families new to Canada struggle with the school registration process and school success. Healthcare providers can support youth and children with the school registration process, by helping to identify local schools and inform themselves and their patients about their right to education. Additionally, they can build relationships with local schools and advocate for educational resources and support to encourage a level playing field. In the United States, the Supreme Court ruled in 1982 that undocumented children and young adults have the same right to attend public primary and secondary schools as do US citizens and permanent residents. Public schools may not deny admission to a student on the basis of undocumented status, treat a student differently to determine residency, require a student or parent to disclose or document their immigration status, or require social security numbers from students or parents.[46] Many states, such as California, support enrolment of all children, regardless of immigration status, in public schools, and through the schools many other services are available to children and to their families.

(d) *Poverty*: As many newcomer families are at risk of living in poverty, healthcare providers can play a role in screening for and supporting families with accessing financial resources. Providers can support families with completing their taxes and other financial forms for which they are eligible. The Poverty Screening Tool,[47] developed by Canadian physicians, is a brief but useful tool to help physicians with screening and addressing poverty in the office. It is important to have available links to social workers to support negotiation of accessing services.

(e) *Food insecurity*: The Hunger Vital Sign [63] is a validated two-question screen to identify children and youth of food insecurity. Screening for food insecurity is therefore an essential component of caring for newcomer children and providing resources to access food in the community, such as food voucher programs, community food banks, and kitchens.

(f) *Adverse childhood experiences (ACEs)*: A number of short, validated screening tools for ACEs[48] exist, such as the Center for Youth Wellness ACE Questionnaire or the IHELLP screening tool. It is important to consider language and length of the tool when implementing in your practice but, most importantly, also to consider how to address issues that arise. For example, while screening for trauma it is important, it is even more critical that when identified, patients are able to access the age and culturally appropriate therapy and other resources that they need. It is critical to keep in mind that youth are resilient, they are not defined by their traumatic experiences, and that their strengths also need to be identified, acknowledged, and emphasized.

[46] Immigrant and Refugee Children: A guide for educators and school support staff. National Immigration Law Center. https://www.nilc.org/wp-content/uploads/2016/06/ICE-Raids-Educators-Guide-2016-06.pdf

[47] Poverty Screening Tool. https://cep.health/clinical-products/poverty-a-clinical-tool-for-primary-care-providers/?®ion=6

[48] https://screeningtime.org/star-center/#/screening-tools#top

Supporting Immigration Applications

Some families may approach their healthcare team to support their immigration applications. Providers may be asked to write a letter outlining the benefits of staying in Canada or the United States to the child or youth.

It is up to the individual discretion of the provider to choose to provide letters of support. Letters can be brief, summarizing the provider's relationship to the patient, their diagnoses, and the services and/or therapies they have been able to access in their host country. Based on the evidence available, the provider can briefly describe the potential detriment to the child if they – or their parents – were to return to their home country. Providers can share a draft of the letter with families to ensure that information is being conveyed respectfully and truthfully.

However, families may be reluctant to discuss immigration at all, for fear of being reported. The family's desires must be respected. Providers can help provide education to patients about their rights and connect them with legal aid support.

Community Advocacy

Perhaps most important is the role that providers play in community and broader advocacy. It is without question that refugee and immigrant youth continue to experience marginalization, as outlined earlier in this chapter. The voice of healthcare providers, including physicians, nurses, social workers, and others, is exceptionally powerful in paving the way forward for policies that improve the individual and community health of newcomer youth and their family. Advocacy can take place at the level of an institution, your community, or on city, county, provincial, state or federal platforms. It may look like training all providers to be skilled in trauma-informed care and cultural competence or advocating for better interpreter services at the respective institutions. Advocacy can include writing op-eds, speaking with elected officials, and standing up in the face of grave injustice. The American Academy of Pediatrics, the Canadian Paediatric Society, and the Society for Adolescent Health and Medicine are three professional medical organizations that have lent their voices to stand up for the rights of immigrant children and youth.

Conclusion

With growing migration worldwide, healthcare providers in the United States and Canada are increasingly likely to care for greater numbers of immigrant and refugee youth. While these youth may have faced a number of healthcare conditions, including infectious diseases, nutritional and mental health challenges, physical injuries, and more, they are incredibly resilient and often are anchors for their families in a new country; in fact, it is the hope of a better future that motivates many families to immigrate. Special considerations should be made to challenges affecting young immigrant and refugee women, unaccompanied minors, homeless, and LGBT and other sexual minority youth. Many newcomer youth face significant barriers through key social determinants of health, including food, housing insecurity, poverty, and discrimination.

For unaccompanied migrant youth in particular, it is essential that the highest priority be given to prompt housing stabilization, engagement in education, and provision of appropriate supportive services. Providers can play an important role in connecting youth to educational opportunities and community programs. Programs that are embedded in the community and led by youth for youth are often successful models to promote inclusion and acceptance. Successful care for migrant and refugee youth is built on the foundation of developing trusting, nonjudgmental relationships, built over time and integrated into community programs. Healthcare providers have the ability to be strong advocates for migrant and refugee youth, from the institutional to policy level.

In working with migrant youth who have experienced great trauma, loss, and challenges to obtaining the stability they so need, it is essential for clinicians and all healthcare providers to keep in mind their great resilience and that their future is not predetermined by the obstacles they have encountered. The same courage, inventiveness, and persistence that they have demonstrated through their personal migration process are also the seeds of their potential.

Appendix: Resources for the Care of Migrant and Refugee Children, Youth, and Families

The National Child Traumatic Stress Network, funded through the Center for Mental Health Services (CMHS), the Substance Abuse and Mental Health Services Administration (SAMHSA) and the US Department of Mental Health Services has produced best practices in Screening and Assessment specific to Refugee youth[49] and Families.[50]

The Canadian Paediatric Society has produced a free, web-based guide "Caring for Kids New to Canada: A Guide for Health Professionals Working with Immigrant and Refugee Children and Youth" (www.kidsnewtocanada.ca).[51]

Similarly, the American Academy of Pediatrics has produced an excellent resource "Immigrant Child Health Toolkit", also available online. https://www.aap.org/en-us/advocacy-and-policy/aap-health-initiatives/Immigrant-Child-Health-Toolkit/Pages/Immigrant-Child-Health-Toolkit.aspx.[52]

---

[49] https://www.nctsn.org/what-is-child-trauma/trauma-types/refugee-trauma/screening-and-assessment and https://www.nctsn.org/resources/refugee-services-core-stressor-assessment-tool

[50] https://www.nctsn.org/resources/measures-are-appropriate-refugee-children-and-families

[51] https://www.kidsnewtocanada.ca/mental-health/mental-health-promotion#risk-and-protective-factors

[52] Immigrant Child Health Toolkit. https://www.aap.org/en-us/advocacy-and-policy/aap-health-initiatives/Immigrant-Child-Health-Toolkit/Pages/Immigrant-Child-Health-Toolkit.aspx

References

1. WHO. Health of refugees and migrants. Regional situation analysis, practices, experiences, lessons learned and ways forward. WHO Western Pacific Region; 2018. Accessed Nov 2018
2. Bulletin of the World Health Organization. Well-managed migrants' health benefits all. https://www.who.int/bulletin/volumes/82/8/editorial20804html/en/.
3. Marquardt L, Kramer A, Fischer F, Prufer-Kramer L. Health status and disease burden of unaccompanied asylum-seeking adolescents in Bielefeld, Germany: cross-sectional pilot study. Tropical Med Int Health. 2016;21(2):210–8.
4. Paxton GA, Sangster KJ, Maxwell EL, McBride CR, Drewe RH. Post-arrival health screening in Karen refugees in Australia. PLoS One. 2012;7(5):e38194.
5. Cherian S, Forbes D, Sanfilippo F, Cook A, Burgner D. Helicobacter pylori, helminth infections and growth: a cross-sectional study in a high prevalence population. Acta Paediatr. 2009;98(5):860–4.
6. Woodruff BA, Blanck HM, Slutsker L, Cookson ST, Larson MK, Duffield A, et al. Anaemia, iron status and vitamin A deficiency among adolescent refugees in Kenya and Nepal. Public Health Nutr. 2006;9(1):26–34.
7. Sanati Pour M, Kumble S, Hanieh S, Biggs BA. Prevalence of dyslipidaemia and micronutrient deficiencies among newly arrived Afghan refugees in rural Australia: a cross-sectional study. BMC Public Health. 2014;14:896.
8. Campagna AM, Settgast AM, Walker PF, DeFor TA, Campagna EJ, Plotnikoff GA. Effect of country of origin, age, and body mass index on prevalence of vitamin D deficiency in a US immigrant and refugee population. Mayo Clin Proc. 2013;88(1):31–7.
9. Chernet A, Hensch NP, Kling K, Sydow V, Hatz C, Paris DH, et al. Serum 25-hydroxyvitamin D levels and intramuscular vitamin D3 supplementation among Eritrean migrants recently arrived in Switzerland. Swiss Med Wkly. 2017;147:w14568.
10. Aucoin M, Weaver R, Thomas R, Jones L. Vitamin D status of refugees arriving in Canada: findings from the Calgary Refugee Health Program. Can Fam Physician. 2013;59(4):e188–94.
11. American Academy of Pediatrics, Council on Environmental Health. Pesticide exposure in children, Table 2; Dec 2012. https://pediatrics.aappublications.org/content/130/6/e1757.
12. New York Times. Central American Farmers Head to the U.S., Fleeing Climate Change, Kirk Semple. Apr 13, 2019.
13. Graham HR, et al. Learning problems in children of refugee background: a systematic review. Pediatrics. 2016;137(6):e20153994.
14. Yalin Sapmaz S, Uzel Tanriverdi B, Ozturk M, Gozacanlar O, Yoruk Ulker G, Ozkan Y. Immigration-related mental health disorders in refugees 5-18 years old living in Turkey. Neuropsychiatr Dis Treat. 2017;13:2813–21.
15. Attanayakea V, McKay R, Joffres M, et al. Prevalence of mental disorders among children exposed to war: a systematic review of 7,920 children. Med Confl Surviv. 2009;25(1):4–19.
16. Bronstein I, Montgomery P. Psychological distress in refugee children: a systematic review. Clin Child Fam Psychol Rev. 2011;14(1):44–56.
17. Ehntholt KA, Trickey D, Harris Hendriks J, Chambers H, Scott M, Yule W. Mental health of unaccompanied asylum-seeking adolescents previously held in British detention centres. Clin Child Psychol Psychiatry. 2018;23(2):238–57.
18. Jakobsen M, Meyer DeMott MA, Wentzel-Larsen T, Heir T. The impact of the asylum process on mental health: a longitudinal study of unaccompanied refugee minors in Norway. BMJ Open. 2017;7(6):e015157.
19. Jordan M. Family separation may have hit thousands more children than reported. New York Times. Jan 17, 2019.
20. Jordan M. Migrant children may lose school, sports and legal aid as shelters swell. New York Times. June 5, 2019.
21. Linton J, Griffin M, Shapiro A. Detention of immigrant children. AAP Policy Statement. 2017. https://pediatrics.aappublications.org/content/139/5/e20170483.full.
22. AAP Testimony of Julie Linton. Examining the failures of the Trump Administration's Inhumane Family Separation Policy. Feb 7, 2019. https://docs.house.gov/meetings/IF/IF02/20190207/108846/HHRG-116-IF02-Wstate-LintonJ-20190207-U1.pdf.

23. Patler C, Laster Pirtle W. From undocumented to lawfully present: do changes to legal status impact psychological wellbeing among Latino immigrant young adults? Soc Sci Med. 2018;199:39–48.
24. Kraft C. AAP statement opposing the border security and immigration reform act. June 15, 2018. https://www.aap.org/en-us/about-the-aap/aap-press-room/Pages/AAPStatementOpposingBorderSecurityandImmigrationReformAct.aspx.
25. Das P, et al. Menstrual hygiene practices, WASH access and the risk of urogenital infection in women from Odisha, India. PLoS One. 2015;10(6):e0130777.
26. Kennedy S, Kidd MP, McDonald JT, Biddle N. The healthy immigrant effect: patterns and evidence from four countries. J Int Migr Integr. 16:317–32.
27. Frecerro J, et al. Sexual exploitation of unaccompanied migrant and refugee boys in Greece: approaches to prevention. PLoS Med. 2017;14(11):e1002438. https://doi.org/10.1371/journal.pmed.1002438.
28. Huemer J, et al. Mental health issues in unaccompanied refugee minors. J Child Adolescent Psychiatr Ment Health. 2009;3:13. https://doi.org/10.1186/1753-2000-3-13.
29. Norredam M, et al. Incidence of psychiatric disorders among accompanied and unaccompanied asylum-seeking children in Denmark: a nation-wide register-based cohort study. Eur Child Adolesc Psychiatry. 2018;27(4):439–46. https://doi.org/10.1007/s00787-019-01340-6. [Epub ahead of print].
30. Martin KJ, et al. Adverse childhood experiences among immigrants and their children. Pediatrics. 2018;142(1):753.
31. Vaughn M, et al. Adverse Childhood Experiences Among Immigrants to the United States. J Interpers Violence. 2017;32(10):1543–64.
32. Caballero TM, et al. Adverse Childhood Experiences Among Hispanic Children in Immigrant Families Versus US-Native Families. Pediatrics. 2017;140 (5):e20170297.
33. Felitti VJ, et al. Relationship of childhood abuse and household dysfunction to many of the leading causes of death in adults. Am J Prev Med. 14(4):245–58.
34. Patel SG, Clarke AV, Eltareb F, Macciomei EE, Wickham RE. Newcomer immigrant adolescents: a mixed-methods examination of family stressors and school outcomes. Sch Psychol Q. 2016;31(2):163–80. http://dx.doi.org.myaccess.library.utoronto.ca/10.1037/spq0000140
35. Landale N, et al. The living arrangements of children of immigrants. Futur Child. 2011;21(1):43–70. https://www.ncbi.nlm.nih.gov/pmc/articles/PMC3241619/
36. New York Times. Federal ban on female genital mutilation ruled unconstitutional by Judge. Nov 21, 2018. https://www.nytimes.com/2018/11/21/health/fgm-female-genital-mutilation-law.html.
37. Martinez Garcia JM, Martin Lopez MJ. Group violence and migration experience among Latin American youths in Justice Enforcement Centers (Madrid, Spain). Span J Psychol. 2015;18:E85.
38. Suleman S, et al. Xenophobia as a determinant of health: an integrative review. J Public Health Policy. 2018;39(4):407–23. https://doi.org/10.1057/s41271-018-0140-1.
39. International Labour Office. International migration, racism, discrimination and xenophobia. Geneva: ILO; 2001. Available from: https://publications.iom.int/system/files/pdf/international_migration_racism.pdf.
40. United Nations Education, Science and Culture Organization. Xenophobia. Updated 2017; cited 28 Apr 2017. Available from: http://www.unesco.org/new/en/social-and-human-sciences/themes/international-migration/glossary/xenophobia.
41. Tendayi Achiume E. Beyond prejudice: structural xenophobic discrimination against refugees. Georgetown J Int Law. 2014;45:323–81.
42. Marmot M. Social determinants of health inequalities. Lancet. 2005;365:1099–104.
43. Kandel WA. Unaccompanied alien children: an overview. Congressional Research Service. Jan 2017. https://fas.org/sgp/crs/homesec/R43599.pdf.
44. Desai N, Adamson M, Allwood M, Baetz C, Cardeli E, Issa O, Ford J. Primer for juvenile court judges: a trauma-informed approach to judicial decision-making for newcomer immigrant youth in juvenile justice proceedings. Feb 2019.
45. Schmidt S. Trump administration must stop giving psychotropic drugs to migrant children without consent, judge rules. Washington Post. July 31, 2018. https://www.washingtonpost.com/news/morning-mix/wp/2018/07/31/trump-administration-must-seek-consent-before-giving-drugs-to-migrant-children-judge-rules/?utm_term=.9a0e3cf3e8d6.

46. Testimony of Julie M Linton MD on behalf of the American Academy of Pediatrics. Examining the failures of the Trump Administration's Inhumane Family Separation Policy. Feb 7, 2019. https://energycommerce.house.gov/sites/democrats.energycommerce.house.gov/files/documents/Linton%20testimony%20FINAL_1.pdf.
47. American Civil Liberties Union. Ms. L v. ICE – order granting plaintiff's motion for classwide preliminary injunction. https://www.aclu.org/legal-document/ms-l-v-ice-order-granting-plaintiffs-motion-classwide-preliminary-injunction?redirect=ms-l-v-ice-order-granting-plaintiffs-motion-classwide-preliminary-injunction.
48. Rosenberg M. U.S. separated "thousands" more immigrant children than known: watchdog. Reuters; Jan 17, 2019. https://www.reuters.com/article/us-usa-immigration-children/u-s-separated-thousands-more-immigrant-children-than-known-watchdog-idUSKCN1PB209.
49. Gelernt L. The battle to stop family separation. The New York Review of Books; Dec 19, 2018. www.nybooks.com.
50. New York Time. At least 4500 abuse complaints at migrant children shelters. Associated Press; Feb 26, 2019.
51. U.S. Department of Health & Human Services, Office of Inspector General. Separated children placed in office of refugee resettlement care OEI-BL-18-00511. Jan 2019. https://oig.hhs.gov/oei/reports/oei-BL-18-00511.pdf.
52. New York Times. The lost children of the Trump administration. Jan 17, 2019.
53. Spagat E. US sees limitations on reuniting migrant families. Associated Press; Feb 2, 2019. https://www.apnews.com/48210bbf243e423ea151ff04e4878ce6.
54. New York Times. Thousands of immigrant children said they were sexually abused in U.S. Detention Centers, Report Says. Feb 27, 2019.
55. Kulish N, Barker K, Ruiz RR. Top officials resign from southwest key, shelter provider for migrant children. New York Times. Mar 11, 2019. https://www.nytimes.com/2019/03/11/us/southwest-key-migrant-shelters-resignations.html.
56. Zucker HA, Greene D. Potential child health consequences of the federal policy separating immigrant children from their parents. JAMA. 2018;320(6):541–2.
57. Kraft C. AAP statement opposing separation of children and parents at the border. May 8, 2018. https://www.aap.org/en-us/about-the-aap/aap-press-room/Pages/StatementOpposingSeparationofChildrenandParents.aspx.
58. Holman B, Ziedenberg J. The dangers of detention: the impact of incarcerating youth in detention and other secure facilities. Justice Policy Institute; 2006. http://www.justicepolicy.org/uploads/justicepolicy/documents/dangers_of_detention.pdf.
59. American Academy of Pediatrics. Testimony of Dr. Julie Linton before the U.S. House of Representatives: examining the failures of the Trump Administration's Inhumane Family Separation Policy. Feb 7, 2019. https://docs.house.gov/meetings/IF/IF02/20190207/108846/HHRG-116-IF02-Wstate-LintonJ-20190207-U1.pdf.
60. New York Times. Trump sees an obstacle to getting his way on immigration: his own officials, Eileen Sullivan and Michael Shear. Apr 14, 2019.
61. UN High Commissioner for Refugees (UNHCR). "We believe in youth" – Global Refugee Youth Consultations final report. Sept 19, 2016. Available at: https://www.refworld.org/docid/57ff50c94.html. Accessed 2 June 2019.
62. Berlin EA, Fowkes WA Jr. A teaching framework for cross-cultural health care. Application in family practice. West J Med. 1983;139(6):934–8.
63. Hager ER, Quigg AM, Black MM, Coleman SM, Heeren T, Rose-Jacobs R, Cook JT, Ettinger de Cuba SE, Casey PH, Chilton M, Cutts DB, Meyers AF, Frank DA. Development and validity of a 2-item screen to identify families at risk for food insecurity. Pediatrics. 2010;126(1):26–32. https://doi.org/10.1542/peds.2009-3146. https://childrenshealthwatch.org/public-policy/hunger-vital-sign/. Accessed 26 May 2019.

Chapter 7
Social Pediatrics: A Model to Confront Family Poverty, Adversity, and Housing Instability and Foster Healthy Child and Adolescent Development and Resilience

Christine Loock, Eva Moore, Dzung Vo, Ronald George Friesen, Curren Warf, and Judith Lynam

Introduction

The International Society of Social Pediatrics and Child Health (ISSOP) [1] defines social pediatrics as "a global, holistic and multidisciplinary approach to child health; it considers the health of the child within the context of their society…, integrating

C. Loock
Division of Developmental Pediatrics, Department of Pediatrics, British Columbia Children's Hospital, University of British Columbia, Vancouver, BC, Canada

E. Moore
Division of Adolescent Health and Medicine, Department of Pediatrics, University of British Columbia, Vancouver, BC, Canada
e-mail: eva.moore@cw.bc.ca

D. Vo
Division of Adolescent Health and Medicine, Department of Pediatrics, BC Children's Hospital & University of British Columbia, Vancouver, BC, Canada
e-mail: dvo@cw.bc.ca

R. G. Friesen
University of Saskatchewan, Saskatoon, SK, Canada

University of Victoria, Victoria, BC, Canada

Continuing Legal Education Society of BC, Vancouver, BC, Canada

C. Warf (✉)
Department of Pediatrics (Retired), Division of Adolescent Health and Medicine, British Columbia Children's Hospital, University of British Columbia, Vancouver, BC, Canada

J. Lynam
University of British Columbia, School of Nursing, Faculty of Applied Sciences, Vancouver, BC, Canada
e-mail: judith.lynam@nursing.ubc.ca

C. Warf, G. Charles (eds.), *Clinical Care for Homeless, Runaway and Refugee Youth*, https://doi.org/10.1007/978-3-030-40675-2_7

the physical, mental, and social dimensions of child health and development, as well as (health) care, prevention and promotion…" [2].

Social pediatrics initiatives target high-need populations to facilitate proportionate distribution of health resources and provision of services to meet the needs of children and youth living in poverty who are often at higher risk for developmental delay or poor physical or mental health, often miss out on routine screening, or do not benefit from diagnostic assessment, treatment, and/or early intervention [3–5]. Simply said, social pediatrics is most often about the children and youth "who we aren't seeing" in our traditional health-care settings [6].

Social pediatrics considers the needs of the whole child [7, 8]. Social pediatrics is an equity-oriented practice and philosophy that seeks to take action on the social determinants such as income, housing, education, social capital, and social environment, as critical mediators of child and youth health. It has been described as a primary health-care services "linked in and linked across" with both specialist health-care services and community services, providing a spectrum of services beyond the traditional health-care system [3]. In addressing the needs of vulnerable and low-income children, youth, and families, integrating extended families and community resources in support of youth, and confronting social determinants of health, social pediatrics offers a model to intervene early and prevent young people from becoming homeless and when they do become early stabilize them early and prevent acculturation to homelessness.

Following is a description of the origins of social pediatrics, a description of social determinants of health for homeless youth, the Vancouver RICHER Social Pediatrics Program, and associated Medical-Legal Community Partnership.

History of Development of Social Pediatrics

Social pediatrics in Canada, growing out of the innovative and foundational work over a 30-year period of Canadian pediatrician Dr. Gilles Julien and others, is an interdisciplinary approach to addressing inequities and social determinants of health, working with families, schools, communities, and youth to assure engagement in positive activities and promote supportive relationships [9]. The field of social pediatrics drew on longitudinal population-based data gathered in Britain [10] which linked poverty to poor health profiles over the life course. Studies in other countries have documented similar associations [11]. These studies and others have demonstrated that social conditions and health are inextricably linked, and negative consequences can accrue to children when attention is not paid to ensuring that the resources to foster children's development, including the provision of support of families, are in place. Social pediatrics is a model of practice that offers a means for holding these interests in the foreground as services are designed and delivered [6].

Social Pediatrics and the Social Determinants of Health

The World Health Organization (WHO) defines social determinants of health as "the conditions in which people are born, grow, work, live and age, and the wider set of forces and systems shaping the conditions of daily life. These forces and systems include economic policies and systems, development agendas, social norms, social policies and political systems" [12] The American Academy of Pediatrics (AAP) in its 2019 Policy Statement entitled "The Impact of Racism on Child and Adolescent Health" states that "racism is a social determinant of health that has a profound impact on the health status of children, adolescents, emerging adults, and their families" [13]. These health inequities are not the result of individual behavior choices or genetic predisposition but are caused by economic, political, and social conditions, including racism [14].

Children and youth grow and develop in the context of families and communities so that their social determinants of health mirror those of the adults and other children with whom they live:

> Child development is not just a reflection of private parenting patterns, or the resources that individual families have to invest in their children. It also reflects the broader social dynamics and institutions through which the entire citizenry organises itself economically, culturally, socially and so on…community conditions…create an environment for social care that moderates opportunities available to children as they mature [15]

Neglect, Rejection, and Maltreatment and Adolescent Homelessness

There are many paths to homelessness for youth, but commonly homelessness is the reflection of family poverty, adversity, and social inequities that have shaped their lives since childhood and in fact have shaped the lives of their families. These social inequities are commonly intergenerational, including the legacy of forced migration, coerced residential school placement, war trauma, slavery, genocide, incarceration, or other factors, and in some families may be reflected in parental capacity to provide a healthy environment for children. The experience of neglect, rejection, maltreatment, and abuse is tragically not uncommon in the lives of adolescents who runaway and end up homeless.

Parental mental illness or substance abuse may impair their ability to provide a supportive environment. Parents who themselves did not have the opportunity to learn positive parenting skills from their own parents may have limited ability to parent themselves. Rejection at home is commonly driven by family, parent, or step-parent negative response to the youth's expression of non-heteronormative sexual orientation or gender identity. The maltreatment that children and youth experience may bring them to the attention of child protective services where they may or may not find a safe and secure placement.

However, not all homelessness among adolescents is related to abuse, rejection, and maltreatment, and many young people who are homeless retain positive relationships with parents, remain in contact with them, and have a meaningful potential for reunification. Escalating rental costs, parental unemployment, poverty, homelessness, incarceration, or other factors may underlie the lack of capacity of parents to provide housing stability. Each situation needs to be evaluated individually, and those who work with homeless youth should be cautioned against making premature, unsubstantiated, and generalized assumptions about the sensitive subject of parental and other family relationships.

Homelessness of Adolescents in Rural Areas

Much of the research conceptualizes youth homelessness as an urban problem. "This exclusion has significant implications in that it marginalizes the rural homeless and hinders the development of social policy to address the issues that this population faces" [16].

Homelessness also looks different for youth in urban centers compared with those living in rural areas, and estimates for youth who experience rural homelessness reflect its invisible nature. Although it is commonly believed that youth have the option to migrate to urban centers for services [16], studies have shown that this is not ideal. In doing so, youth have to leave behind their network of informal social support and their sense of community.

Poverty, Youth, and Health Outcomes

The pervasive effects of poverty on health also have negative effects on health care:

> …poverty has long been associated with health disparities among young people. Adolescents who are poor report worse health outcomes, including higher rates of sexually transmitted infections and pregnancy, than higher socioeconomic status adolescents. They also have rates of depression and suicide and are more likely to be sexually abused or victims of homicide. Obesity is also higher among low socioeconomic status adolescents than those who are better off economically [17, p. 126]

> …poor families are most likely to experience the consequences of bleak economic times… poor families must deal with others' (often negative) assumptions about them and these assumptions create barriers to access… [18]

The profound impact of social context on disease continues during this era of advanced medical science:

> We cannot look at the status of a population's health without examining social context. Consider the risk of exposure, host susceptibility, course of disease and disease outcome; each is shaped by the social matrix, whether the disease is labeled "infectious," "genetic," "metabolic," "malignant" or "degenerative." The distribution of health and disease in human populations reflects where people live; when in history they live; the air they breathe and the water they drink…the status they occupy in the social order [19]

Disproportionate Impact of Inequities on Ethnic Minorities

The National Academy of Medicine's 2017 report on "Perspectives on Health Equity and Social Determinants of Health" states:

> "…subtle forms of inequity and discrimination are sometimes so deeply embedded in and accepted as societal practices that they may be difficult to uncover yet render many children and families hopeless. The interplay between and among relevant systems and the statuses accompanying power attributed to different ethnic, racial, cultural and socioeconomic groups affect both individuals and their social networks (e.g., family, neighborhood, and community). They are tied directly to and within institutional and structural hierarchies" [17, p. 16]. It goes on to state that "…systems produce very different lived experiences for entire categories of people who are embedded within complex webs and social networks at different levels (e.g., family, neighborhood, and community as well as institutional and structural). These lived experiences can either enhance or challenge the developmental pathways of children through adulthood and the ability of parents and families to ensure a positive trajectory for their children. They affect both the individual child and the networks and communities in which children live and grow and that define their access to resources" [17, p. 15]

Societal inequities are highly accentuated in the USA among adolescents who are African American, Indigenous or Native American, Latino, and migrants [17, p. 126] and in Canada among youth who are of Indigenous (First Nations, Metis, or Inuit) background, refugees, and new immigrants. Compared to white fifth graders, African American and Latino fifth graders have higher rates of exposure to violence, peer victimization, substance use, and terrorism worries; lower rates of seat-belt use, bike helmet use, and vigorous exercise; and lower self-rated health status and psychological and physical quality of life. The proportion of the US adolescent population is becoming increasingly diverse ethnically, with more Latino and Asian American youth and addressing racial and ethnic disparities will become increasingly more pressing in the next decade if progress is to be made towards health equity [17, p. 127]:

> "Racism is a core social determinant of health that is a driver of health inequities" [13, 20]. "Racism is a system of structuring opportunity and assigning value based on the social interpretation of how one looks (which is what we call 'race') that unfairly disadvantages some individuals and communities, unfairly advantages other individuals and communities, and saps the strength of the whole society through the waste of human resources" [21]
>
> Children experience the outputs of structural racism through place (where they live), education (where they learn), economic means (what they have), and legal means (how their rights are executed). Research has identified the role of implicit and explicit personally

mediated racism (racism characterized by assumptions about the abilities, motives, or intents of others on the basis of race) as a factor affecting healthcare delivery and general health outcomes. The impacts of structural and personally mediated racism may result in internalized racism (internalizing racial stereotypes about one's racial group). A positive racial identity mediates experiences of discrimination and generates optimal youth development outcomes. The importance of a prosocial identity is critical during adolescence, when young people must navigate the impacts of social status and awareness of personally mediated discrimination based on race [13]

Rather than focusing on preventing the social conditions that have led to racial disparities, science and society continue to focus on the disparate outcomes that have resulted from them, often reinforcing the posited biological underpinnings of flawed racial categories [22]. Although race used in these ways has been institutionalized, linked to health status and impeded our ability to improve health and eliminate health disparities [23], it remains a powerful measure that must be better measured, carefully used, and potentially replaced to mark progress in pediatric health disparities research [13]

Disproportionate Representation of LGBT Youth Among Homeless Youth

Lesbian, gay, bisexual, non-binary, gender fluid and transgender (LGBT) youth are particularly vulnerable to a range of health disparities and make up a disproportionate share of homeless youth, recently assessed to be between 20% and 40% [24]. LGBT adolescents and young adults have significantly worse health outcomes than heterosexual youth, including higher rates of mental health problems, chronic stress and depression, as well as suicide. These outcomes are significantly related to discrimination, harassment, and other forms of victimization, which takes place in families, schools and communities [17, p. 127]

Further complicating the access of LGBT youth to health care is the implicit heteronormative assumption present in many health-care environments, that is, despite good intentions, the underlying cultural assumptions may contribute to creation of an environment and experience for LGBT youth where they are unrecognized or experience stigma or neglect [17, p. 16].

To have a meaningful impact on homelessness among youth, it is essential that all agencies create a welcoming and nonjudgmental environment for all youth, inclusive of LGBT youth and migrants. It is essential that youth of all ethnicities be welcomed and supported in every health-care environment they encounter, from the physical environment to the language and behavior of staff.

Disproportionate Representation of Youth with Disabilities Among the Homeless

Poverty and disability are inextricably linked. Estimates of the number of persons living with a physical disability or mental illness run as high as 45% of the homeless population [25]. Children and youth with disabilities are twice as likely to be living in families receiving social assistance.[1] The causes of poverty related to disability are multifactorial and include both social and material poverty. Not only do the care needs have a direct impact on family income and employment, but there is a higher risk for social isolation and lack of inclusion for persons with physical and developmental disabilities. Children and youth with disabilities are at increased risk for bullying, abuse, and neglect. Youth with disabilities living in poverty are also at risk of being neglected by systems of care resulting in lack of inclusion and planning for their activities and participation in the community.

Conditions such as fetal alcohol spectrum disorder (FASD) and other neurodevelopmental disabilities are frequently recognized among the adolescent and adult homeless population [25]. Prenatal alcohol exposure and FASD are associated with a higher prevalence of intergenerational trauma and history of multiple adverse childhood experiences (ACES) [26].

Intergenerational Trauma

Communities that have had historical or contemporary trauma associated with colonization, racism, and social exclusion may also have increased prevalence of homelessness. Increased prevalence of homelessness is related to multigenerational discrimination and social exclusion and the historic disproportionate placement of children in foster care, residential schools, or juvenile justice removed from parents with interruption of early modeling and learning of parenting skills.

The American Academy of Pediatrics in the 2019 Policy Statement "The Impact of Racism on Child and Adolescent Health" states that:

> …it is important to examine the historical underpinnings of race as a tool for subjugation. American racism was transported through European colonization. It began with the subjugation, displacement, and genocide of American Indian populations and was subsequently bolstered by the importation of African slaves to frame the economy of the United States. Although institutions such as slavery were abolished more than a century ago, discriminatory policies, such as Jim Crow laws, were developed to legalize subjugation…Native Hawaiian, and Pacific Islander, Alaskan native, Asian American, and Latino American populations have experienced oppression and similar exclusions from society…remnants of these policies remain in place today and continue to oppress the advancement of people from historically aggrieved groups…Through these underpinnings, racism became a socially transmitted disease passed down through generations, leading to the inequities observed in our population today [13]

Poverty, increased rates of unemployment, and systemic barriers to access stable housing and other services contribute to family and parental instability and homelessness. Additional factors contributing to parental homelessness are lack of access to health care and social services and lack of prevention and early intervention

[1] Canada Without Poverty > Poverty > Just the Facts, http://www.cwp-csp.ca/.

services of substance abuse including treatment for addiction, alcoholism, and mental health, most notably for pregnant and parenting women and their partners [27].

Systems Change and Children's Social Determinants of Health

It is essential that health-care providers be cognizant of the profound impact of social determinants of health and intergenerational trauma on society, on the health and well-being of families, and on the development of children and youth and their inequitable opportunities for education and employment and ultimately their inequitable vulnerability to poverty, poor education, housing instability, and lack of opportunity. In the context of US society, it is essential to keep in mind that social determinants of health, intergenerational trauma, discrepancies in child and family poverty rates, vulnerability to long-term incarceration, and many other factors profoundly shaping the lives of children and youth in society are reflections of historic and pervasive racism [13].

Notwithstanding these challenging factors, which can seem overwhelming to practitioners working with impoverished communities, there have been a number of social policies enacted regionally and nationally that have led to meaningful improvement of the lives of children and youth in the USA and Canada. These social policies include the Food Stamp Program, the War on Poverty, efforts to improve education, housing opportunities, child health insurance in the USA and universal publicly funded health insurance in Canada, and environmental policies to decrease lead exposure and improve water purification. These positive efforts have led to decreased exposure to neurotoxins, improved health outcomes for injuries, asthma, and cardiovascular disease, and mental health problems as well as improved access to medical and dental care for African American, Hispanic children, immigrant, and low-income children. Policy initiatives have been far too modest and limited and have not addressed many critical social determinants, in particular unemployment, incarceration rates for adults and children in the US (particularly African American adults and youth), or income and extreme wealth inequality, but they do demonstrate that it is not beyond the capability of contemporary society to begin to address health issues within the lifetime of children who are alive today [13]:

> …the non-profit sector most frequently operates using an approach that we call "isolated impact." It is an approach oriented toward finding and funding a solution embodied within a single organization, combined with the hope that the most effective organizations will grow or replicate to extend their impact more widely…. Despite the dominance of this approach, there is scant evidence that isolated initiatives are the best way to solve many social problems in today's complex and interdependent world. No single organization is responsible for any major social problem, nor can any single organization cure it. In the field of education, even the most highly respected non-profits—such as the Harlem Children's Zone, Teach for America, and the Knowledge Is Power Program—have taken decades to reach tens of thousands of children, a remarkable achievement that deserves praise, but one that is three orders of magnitude short of the tens of millions of U.S. children that need help [28]

Addressing these factors substantively requires significant system change in multiple dimensions including housing access, access to education and improved quality of education, employment opportunities, support for families in need, improved treatment of children and families by child protective services, juvenile justice, the adult criminal justice system, and more. Our societies have struggled for generations with these historic factors, and we will continue to struggle with them into the foreseeable future. Nonetheless, recognizing the pervasive influence of these factors on the lives of children, youth, and families and the discrepant opportunities they are provided requires that system change be embraced in multiple dimensions and sustained over time so that future generations of children and youth encounter a more equitable world with greater resources and greater opportunities:

> Because the systems change process is necessarily a political one, with competition for scarce resources and priorities heightened at the time of change, the presence of individuals capable of successfully navigating these political waters is critical…Efforts to truly transform systems and change the status quo can encounter strong resistance and push back, stalling or terminating an initiative [29]

> Small wins are important first steps in significant change pursuits. By targeting smaller, more manageable problems stakeholders can become emboldened to take on more significant pursuits and are less likely to feel helpless facing insurmountable issues. Small wins can also promote well functioning action learning teams because they provide quick feedback on the effectiveness of strategies, offer immediate insights into system reactions, and generate member commitment to the effort [30, 31]

While these changes may start small through the strategy of enacting small wins, over time efforts can lead to more comprehensive and deep structural changes [32]. As opportunities arise to participate in changes fundamental to health, including improvements in access to preschool, quality education, after-school programs, affordable housing, food security, college education, trade school, and more, it is important that those providers closest to these children and families embrace and encourage these needed changes.

Accessibility and Engagement with Health-Care Services for Marginalized Patients

Ability to access health care is not determined simply as a matter of choice. People's decisions about where to go for health care are shaped by social determinants of health including income, health insurance status, transportation, housing, education, immigration status, gender, employment, legal status, safety, and primary health-care access.

Health-care access is shaped by how families and youth anticipate that they will be treated in community clinics, hospitals, or health provider offices. Barriers to health care access include the assumptions that patients feel will be leveled toward them when they seek care, and their worries that their health concerns will be dismissed because of these assumptions. Understanding these barriers can help shape the design of health services to be responsive to the complexities of health care access for those parents and their children who experience racialization and impoverishment [11, 33]. Implicit bias operating in the health-care environment creates significant barriers to access to health care for minority youth [34].

Advocating for Children and Youth at Risk for Homelessness

Clinicians have the opportunity to advocate on behalf of children and youth at high risk for homelessness by encouraging connections to immediate and extended families, home communities, and social networks. Maintaining these connections over time can encourage engagement and stabilization. Children and youth benefit from supportive environments that are inclusive of parents and caregivers, community agencies, and schools. These networks can also support youth living in higher-risk environments to continue to stay in school and to benefit from community resources, in particular youth centers. Recognizing that many youth leave home, or even home communities, because of traumatic experiences including neglect and maltreatment, it is essential that they have easy access to alternative schools, long-term connections with youth workers and social workers, and safe places to stay. Child protective services commonly have skilled social workers to provide youth and families with support and, if necessary, out of home placement.

Developmental Risk to Adolescents Experiencing Homelessness

Adolescence is a developmental stage of life in which youth learn social norms, coping skills, appropriate behaviors, life skills, and what it means to be an adult. This process involves a lot of trial and error as they "try on" different identities. Youth need to be able to experiment with opportunities and to be able to fail and try again in a supportive environment. In the absence of a stable home life, strong adult role models, or a supportive environment, the consequences for an adolescent of making mistakes can be life-altering. Survival on the street may become the extent of the life skills they learn, making it difficult for them to understand and function in mainstream society.

Promoting Resilience and Positive Youth Development

A robust body of research into youth resilience has led to consistent findings showing that protective factors can buffer risks and enable some adolescents to achieve good health and developmental outcomes even in the presence of significant risk factors [35]. Protective factors can be divided into two general categories: internal and external protective factors. Internal protective factors include an easy temperament and strong coping skills to manage stress. Many of the coping skills can be learned and enhanced with practice. External protective factors include a meaningful and trusting connection with a caring adult, which could be a parent or guardian, an older sibling, aunt or uncle, another caring adult in the family, family friend, or school or community worker.

Positive youth development [36, 37] is a strength-based approach that builds upon the abilities of youth and motivates and focuses on the development of skills to prepare a young person to achieve a successful adulthood. Positive youth development is based on the recognition that young people need to be prepared for their future independent life as adults and includes activities such as the arts, music, education, or physical activities depending on youth interests and staff capacities. Young people themselves can contribute to the development of resources for youth by becoming engaged in identifying program needs and in designing accessible programs for young people.

By identifying, offering, and strengthening internal and external protective factors, the practitioner can help support the adolescent's development toward a healthy life trajectory, fostering positive youth development and the life skills that youth will use throughout adulthood, including leadership and community involvement to continue to grow as adults, offering lifelong benefits.

Children and youth can have opportunities to develop resiliency and to achieve positive outcomes despite severe challenges when provided opportunities to grow in positive environments with responsive and high-quality schools, trade schools, community centers, after-school activities and employment, close relationships with stable peers and families, reliable and consistent support from youth workers, and opportunities to give back to their community. Young people who have experienced significant loss or undergone traumatic experiences, if given opportunities to explore these experiences in safe environments and find meaning, may utilize difficult experiences to grow and become surprisingly resourceful. This process may require engaging a psychologist or other mental health professional. If we care about positive youth development, we must also work to create environments which will enable youth to thrive. The resilience perspective gives powerful tools to the adolescent health practitioner that can have lasting impact, not only in the reduction of risk behaviors but supporting young people in achieving a viable and successful future [38].

Ginsburg describes seven qualities that adults can nurture in youth to support their optimum development. In nurturing these resilience strategies, adults need to believe in youth unconditionally, communicate high expectations, and model those behaviors in their own lives.

Competence: When we notice what young people are doing right and give them opportunities to develop important skills, they feel competent. We undermine competence when we don't allow young people to recover themselves after a fall.

Confidence: Young people need confidence to be able to navigate the world, think outside the box, and recover from challenges.
Connection: Connections with other people, schools, and communities offer young people the security that allows them to stand on their own and develop creative solutions.
Character: Young people need a clear sense of right and wrong and a commitment to integrity.
Contribution: Young people who contribute to the well-being of others will receive gratitude rather than condemnation. They will learn that contributing feels good and may therefore more easily turn to others and do so without shame.
Coping: Young people who possess a variety of healthy coping strategies will be less likely to turn to dangerous quick fixes when stressed.
Control: Young people who understand privileges and respect are earned through demonstrated responsibility will learn to make wise choices and feel a sense of control.
Ginsburg – from http://www.fosteringresilience.com/7cs.php

The Vancouver RICHER Social Pediatrics Model

The RICHER Social Pediatrics model in Vancouver, British Columbia, Canada was designed to complement existing tertiary and primary services and provide community-based health care to those children and youth who are most vulnerable and have high health-care needs. As with other social pediatrics models, the approach has focused on "groups of children and youth who are experiencing extreme difficulty on the physical, social, and psychological levels as well as families experiencing an alarming level of stress" [9]. Children, youth, their families, and their communities are understood to be "at risk" because of social, material, and cultural disadvantage. Children, youth, and their families require a distinct approach recognizing that the nature of their health concerns is different than those of adults and older members of their communities.

The RICHER Approach

The acronym RICHER represents:

- *Responsive* – the central importance of fostering enduring socially supportive relationships that mitigate risk for vulnerable children and youth and recognition of the competence of children, parents, and families and the continuities of care through childhood, school age, and adolescence

- *Interdisciplinary and intersectoral* – incorporates medical specialists, pediatricians, social workers, counselors, youth workers, community members, and others
- *Community-based* – nurtures local and enduring supportive relationships
- *Health* – recognizes the multiple determinants of health and wellness
- *Education* – for children, youth, parents, the community, and professionals
- *Research* – an imperative to assure that services are encompassing, effective, and compatible with contemporary understanding [11]

Created in partnership with Vancouver's inner city communities as part of the British Columbia Children's Hospital, the provincial-level governmental health system, and the University of British Columbia, this research-to-practice program was designed to develop new effective models together with the community to address inequities in health outcomes, engage families with increased vulnerability due to material and social factors, and bridge gaps in services for individuals and families. To address complex issues, RICHER Social Pediatrics promotes collaboration with government and nongovernment organizations and community agencies, including recreation centers, daycare, public schools, and community organizations.

Examples of grave challenges faced by parents and families that RICHER aims to address include the following:

- Parents who are homeless or face eviction and are unable to find suitable housing may find that apprehension of their children is the most readily available intervention offered by the formal system.
- Parents living in substandard housing who are told housing conditions (mold, standing water, lack of heating) underlie their child's repeated hospitalizations for compromised respiratory status and they risk being reported for neglect.
- The threat of eviction by their landlord if they complain about conditions.
- Youth living under orders of protection are given vouchers to access unsupervised inner-city single-room occupancy hotels with high-risk adult tenants instead of being accorded appropriate and supportive stable housing.
- Children and youth removed from their communities for protection concerns, but with the loss of community networks, experience disruption and loss of identity, culture, and stability.

Family and children's needs drive the RICHER program priorities, and the model is dependent on fostering strong relationships. Partnerships have developed that have increased access to health care, mental health, parent education and support programs, childcare programs, legal services, and more. Importantly, these services are distributed in local neighborhood spaces. Primary and specialist health-care providers share space in schools and community centers, thereby developing strong community connections and shared decision-making about care for children and families.

By breaking down invisible barriers of power, culture, and location and promoting care centered on relationships with families, children, and youth, the clinicians have effectively recognized and benefited from the community's expertise [6].

RICHER Social Pediatrics Clinical Care Model

Primary health care is delivered in the context of the community, in collaboration with embedded community agencies that have had long-standing engagement. The program is staffed by a team of nurse practitioners and includes a number of youth-focused models including school-linked services and clinics held simultaneously with parent engagement activities.

Other pediatric medical subspecialists that provide care in the community sites include child psychiatry, developmental pediatrics, adolescent medicine, ophthalmology, and dermatology. In addition, collaborative relationships have been developed with community-based youth workers (a publicly funded profession in BC developed to enhance engagement of homeless and insecurely housed youth) and publicly funded counselors.

Vancouver has a network of youth clinics that provide no-cost contraceptive services, and STI testing and treatment for adolescents. In addition, Vancouver has a network of youth centers that provide recreational activities, employment preparation and referral, resources and meals, tutoring, and other activities. Over the period of development, RICHER has contributed to several specialized youth engagement activities such as NAZKAR (Never Again Steal Cars –which teaches youth to work on cars with mentorship from police and college-level mechanical teachers), Hip Hop Drop (an urban youth-centered celebration of art and music), and the Eastside Boxing Youth Program (a noncontact physical activity program focused on youth engagement and self-discipline).

Through these accessible activities and with linkage to public agencies, in particular local schools, and with the engagement of skilled youth workers, resources are available to address youth who are tenuously engaged with school, on the streets, and not living at home. Other programs in these communities typically focus on adult needs and children and adolescents are too often excluded from programming as a means to protect their safety.

RICHER Community "Kitchen Table"

Community engagement and participation in health-care delivery is facilitated by weekly open "kitchen table" meetings that are held in a community center. Everyone is welcome, and the agenda is set at the meeting to allow for accessibility and responsiveness. The kitchen table meeting has created a forum for problem-solving and consultation with key community leaders and is well known and respected by long-standing nonprofit agencies and formal and informal community activists.

Following the open meeting, a confidential, case-based meeting for providers and clinicians allows for interdisciplinary discussions and case planning for individual patients and clients.

"Place-Based" Approaches Enhance Engagement, Relationships, and Trust

The success of the RICHER program has rested on a general philosophy that unifies the team. This is represented by (1) an explicit commitment to building respectful relationships as a key premise of the practice approach; (2) enacting practice through interprofessional partnerships that recognizes the community as the home and a key resource for children and youth, where families and cultural identity are central; and (3) an expressed commitment to work across organizational-jurisdictional service delivery boundaries in order to provide health care that is responsive to needs [18]:

> A place-based approach … aims to address issues that exist at the neighbourhood level, such as poor housing, social isolation, poor or fragmented service provision that leads to gaps or duplication of effort, and limited economic opportunities…[and] to make families and communities more engaged, connected and resilient.[2,3]

Through communicative and collaborative processes, shared goals are recognized: supporting children and youth to achieve their potential, recognition of the different talents each person or organization brings to the table, and a commitment to work together.

"Horizontal partnerships" and "horizontal communication" in which knowledge and power is shared by practitioners, partners, and families legitimize and validate community-based knowledge derived from lived experience and local conditions [39]. This is in keeping with analyses of primary health-care quality indicators about conditions that foster the broadest forms of engagement across individuals and organizations with differential power, in part because it recognizes and values different forms of expertise [39].

Addressing Adverse Childhood Experiences and Resiliency

The aim of RICHER has been to provide timely access to prevention and intervention services for children and youth at higher risk due to material and social poverty and adverse childhood experiences; to provide place-based care; to develop trust with community members, service providers, and vulnerable children, youth, and families; and to promote resilience.

Both primary care and specialist providers have identified a disproportionately high accumulation of adverse childhood experiences (ACEs), including violence victimization, physical and emotional neglect, and family dysfunction (addiction,

[2] https://www.ourplace-vancouver.ca

[3] https://ww2.rch.org.au/emplibrary/ccch/Policy_Brief_23_-_place-based_approaches_final_web.pdf

mental health, and incarceration) as recorded through clinical encounter forms. These findings mirror the recent findings from the Global Early Adolescent Study, with adolescents from low- and middle-income countries representing 14 urban communities [40].

RICHER has engaged with community organizations across service sectors to empower and support the development of resilience of children, youth, and families. These relationships create opportunities for children, youth, families, and community members through bridged trust to connect with services, such as the Medical-Legal Community Partnership/Circle of the Child initiative described below.

Medical-Legal "Community" Partnership

By engaging with a community characterized by ethnic diversity and established families, RICHER recognized the effects of family disruption, inequity in access, and social and material poverty. Challenges included lack of income, transportation, appropriate housing, education, legal services, primary care, and safety. Case studies focusing on families with a cluster of these challenges were developed. While anecdotal, consistently the challenges required multiple services including health, community, and legal services:

- Early work included establishing links with legal agencies and organizations and opening dialogue regarding interprofessional collaboration between health, legal, and community services.
- Further work included developing case studies that focused on families with a cluster of challenges that had led to family disruption and social isolation. Consistently the challenges required a multitude of services including health, community, and legal services to respond effectively. Without established interprofessional and community relationships, the complexity of responding was multiplied.
- As determined through community experience and research evidence, the cases that represented the most significant opportunities to reduce family disruption, improve access, and decrease system costs were seen as priorities.
- "Model" policies and processes were developed to resolve challenges identified in the case studies – consistently this required accessing expertise from the community and across multiple sectors.
- Evaluation assured that model policies and processes were working efficiently and effectively, and research could be conducted to determine implications for reducing family disruption, increasing access, and reducing costs. These processes were initiated with a small number of cases focusing on those that provided the most significant opportunities to reduce system costs.

Given existing health/community relationships through RICHER, early work focused on establishing links with legal services. The team explored the development of a medical-legal partnership (MLP) based on the work of Zuckerman et al. [41].

Development of the Medical-Legal Community Partnership (MLCP)

The Vancouver Foundation RICHER Medical-Legal Pilot Study

Committed to fostering health and human rights, the medical-legal pilot study was initiated to generate insights from within the community that would promote child/youth and family health equity. Research, funded by the Vancouver Foundation, was designed to examine the ways structural violence operated in the day to day lives of children, youth, and families living with marked social and material adversity in Vancouver's inner city. (Structural violence refers to "social structures – economic, political, legal – that stop individuals, groups, and societies from reaching their full potential." The idea of structural violence is linked closely to social injustice and the social machinery of oppression) [42].

By engaging with a community characterized by both ethnic diversity and established families, RICHER emerged with a recognition of the effects of family disruption, inequity in access, and social and material poverty. Challenges to the community included lack of income, transportation, appropriate housing, education, legal services, primary care, and safety. An acknowledgment grew that traditional approaches would be ineffective in dealing with complex problems.

Recognizing the importance of developing research-supported evidence to meet the standards of funders that would enable the building of successful and effective programs, RICHER initiated data collection to set priorities based on evidence and target high-risk families, particularly in areas such as access to housing, childcare, disability benefits, and justice. The goal of the research was to illustrate the impact of structural violence on health, child, and youth development and community well-being and to use this analysis to inform the design of a Medical-Legal Community Partnership (MLCP).

From the earliest stages, it was clear that legal services were a vital component of the health care/community team to facilitate direct service, influence institutions, and influence policy change.

The MLCP addressed the nonmedical, social determinants of health that have legal remedies and considered approaches that might assist the targeted community to address the systemic issues that contribute to poor health of children, youth, and families. As a result, the MLCP was an attempt to integrate the legal sector into existing RICHER social pediatrics relationships with sectors including health, education, social services, and housing.

In addition to including the legal sector, the community determined that a place-based strategy was desirable to mobilize supports at the community level given that "traditional systems of care simply do not serve marginalized communities or distressed neighbourhoods [whereas]… a place-based approach… builds on the capacity of our local community, eliminates inefficient service silos, and adapts to the unique challenges of living in the inner city."[4]

---

[4]Our Place, Promoting Local Access and Community Empowerment. https://www.ourplace-vancouver.ca/about/place-based-strategies.

Taking its cues from the community, the MLCP identified a place-based approach as fundamental to moving forward. Critical too was the addition of the legal sector to the strong interprofessional relationships between health and community that had been established through RICHER.

The medical-legal pilot study was initiated to illustrate the impact of structural violence on health, child, and youth development and community well-being and to inform the design of a MLCP to respond. Legal services were vital to facilitate direct service, transform institutions, and influence policy change to address systemic issues and structural violence, where the latter refers to "social structures – economic, political, legal – that stop individuals, groups, and societies from reaching their full potential" [42].

The next step was to identify possible models; the Child's Protective Circle model (or Circle of the Child) developed by the Fondation du Dr. Julien in Montreal was seen as the most appropriate model: "It involves collective know-how and cooperation between the community social pediatrics team and the child's family and social and institutional networks where the entire focus is placed on coming up with solutions together to best meet the child's needs."[5]

Adopting a "Circle of the Child (and Youth)" Approach: Intervention and Stabilization While Youth May Still Have Connections with Family and Community

A Circle of the Child model, which was adjusted for the community and extended to include youth and young adults, is being implemented in the Downtown Eastside (DTES) of Vancouver, one of the lowest-income neighborhoods in Canada. The Circle creates a family and community network around the child or youth to build on their strengths and help achieve their dreams.

The family network is determined with the child or youth supported by a facilitator and includes direct and extended family, foster family, other caregivers, friends of the child or youth, community members, elders, and others.

The community network includes a social pediatrics health-care provider, to ensure that developmental needs are identified, and may include school staff, child-care center workers, youth workers, elders, community members, housing, recreational center staff, community groups, health and social service providers, lawyers, legal aid services, and others. Ongoing relationships among the community network facilitate responsiveness and continuity. Not all members of the community network engage with every child, youth, or family: just those already connected and those most appropriate are involved. Because this is a place-based approach, the

[5] https://pediatriesociale.fondationdrjulien.org/en/about/quel-est-le-coeur-du-modele/la-cointervention/

relationships among the members of the community network are frequently preexisting.

In the Circle process, a facilitator (a lawyer with interest-based mediation skills) engages with the child or youth and their family and community network to create a plan to promote the child/youth's well-being and healthy development and to mobilize the network to implement the plan. The legal training of the facilitator is helpful in distinguishing which issues have legal remedies and directing those matters as appropriate.

It is a priority to foster and strengthen ongoing relationships among members of the community network including recruiting and training members so they understand the process, create ongoing relationships with other members, and quickly identify resources and implement actions to respond to challenges faced by the child, youth, or family.

The facilitator:

- Connects with the child or youth to understand their strengths, dreams, and challenges and to identify participants for the family network
- Connects with the family network to understand family dynamics, to frame conversations around supporting the child or youth's strengths, to identify what role each participant is able to play in supporting the child/youth, and to identify barriers
- Connects with both the family and community network to identify individuals who may be appropriate (and prepare them) to participate in a 1-day circle planning process to finalize a plan. The 1-day circle planning process is resource intensive and may not be required in all cases; however, building and mobilizing the network is critical in all cases.

The core principles of the Circle of the Child (and Youth) include the following:

- Recognition: The child/youth has a right to be heard and his or her views are to be taken seriously.
- Healthy development: The child/youth has the right to the best possible health and medical care and access to the information that will help his or her health.
- Family and community: Children and youth have the right to live with their family, unless it is a danger to them. If they cannot live with their family, they have the right to special protection and help. The entire community is responsible for child and youth health and well-being and will support them.
- Education and play: Children and youth have the right to an education that enables them to develop their abilities, character, and an understanding of their culture. They have the right to play and relax by doing the things they enjoy such as sports, music, arts, and drama.
- Best interests: All adults should make decisions in the child or youth's best interests.
- Rights: Children and youth rights can be enforced by law, and if poor or in need, they have the right to help from the government.
- Protection: Children and youth have the right to be protected from being hurt or treated badly.

The goals of the Circle of the Child (and Youth) are:

- To improve the well-being of children and youth, who are vulnerable in the context of social determinants of health, by developing a decentralized community-based mechanism for engaging in decision-making around difficult problems, separate from the current child welfare process
- To put the child or youth at the center of a network of supportive family and community resources
- To convene and mobilize the group to create a plan for the child or youth
- To empower the child or youth and family network by involving them as full participants and decision-makers in the planning process
- To build trust and connections among all participants in the child or youth's family and community networks including extended family, elders, friends, neighbors, other caregivers, community members, and service providers
- To reconvene and mobilize as appropriate to support adjustments to and effective long-term implementation of the plan

Professional Education on Social Pediatrics and the Care of Homeless Youth

Contemporary medical education has long been criticized for focusing disproportionately on tertiary hospital-based care that removes students and residents from meaningful engagement and connection with communities. This process leads not only to a lack of engagement but a lack of understanding or appreciation of the barriers that children, youth, and families encounter in their lived experiences. It also contributes to reinforcing a sense of identity of practitioners as separate and disconnected from the communities, families, and patients that they serve.

The American Academy of Pediatrics 2019 Policy Statement on The Impact of Racism on Child and Adolescent Development makes several recommendations for optimizing workforce development and professional education including:

- Advocate for pediatric training programs that are girded by competencies and sub-competencies related to effective patient and family communication across differences in pediatric populations.
- Encourage policies to foster interactive learning communities that promote cultural humility (e.g., self-awareness, lifelong commitment to self-evaluation, and commitment to managing power imbalances), and provide simulation opportunities to ensure new pediatricians are competent to deliver culturally appropriate and patient- and family-centered care.
- Integrate active learning strategies such as simulation and language immersion to adequately prepare pediatric residents to serve the most diverse pediatric population to date to exist in the USA and lead diverse and interdisciplinary pediatric care teams.

- Advocate for policies and programs that diversify the pediatric workforce and provide ongoing professional education for pediatricians in practice as a strategy to reduce implicit biases and improve safety and quality in the health-care delivery system [13].

In recognition of this dilemma and to promote greater understanding of the lives and communities of vulnerable patient populations, the chairs of the 16 departments of pediatrics at Canadian medical schools released a statement that argued:

> …that not only is the practice of social paediatrics evolving rapidly but, more importantly, it is time for a two-pronged approach. First, we need to ensure its inclusion in the mainstream of curriculum development in our medical faculties, using a broad interprofessional approach; second, the knowledge gleaned from the UNICEF and other reports should stimulate a vigorous child health advocacy strategy [43]

> Although the social context of children receiving care in children's hospitals is given attention in didactic lectures and bedside or clinic teaching, we contend that, to truly understand the social determinants of health, they must be experienced firsthand in community, school and home settings where they are brought into stark focus. These experiences move from the medical model of hospital care to an increasingly interprofessional sociological model as we move from tertiary through secondary and primary care to the public health issues affecting children and their families [43]

> We are training family practitioners, paediatricians and other health care providers, many of whom interact with children and their families for whom the social determinants of health have daily ramifications: food and lodging insecurity, inferior education and neglect and/or abuse. It is only through robust educational exposure that medical students will be prepared to address the needs of these children and youth. Preclerkship placements within the community agencies that deal with these groups is a first step, provided these are of sufficient relevance to the students' future medical practice, e.g., children's aid societies, youth centres and refugee health clinics. These learning opportunities should be an integral part of clinical training, not only for specialists who interact regularly with children and youth and their families (e.g., family physicians, paediatricians and psychiatrists), but also those dealing with chronic diseases impacted by the social determinants [43]

Resident's reflection after completing their requisite first year of social pediatrics rotation:

> I was struck on the first day of my Social Pediatrics rotation walking down the main street of the inner city for the first time, about how uncomfortable I felt. This was never somewhere I would have thought to visit; it is drastically different from the context in which I was fortunate enough to grow up. It was a little bit like entering a different world, characterized by extreme poverty and many among the most vulnerable people in the city. When I first entered medicine these were the contexts in which I was hoping to work, to make a difference, to work with the most vulnerable among us. Throughout medical training, my vision and direction were constantly directed towards tertiary care, large centers, and all the trappings that come along with it. Particularly in residency the work we do over long hours, evenings and weekends, becomes dissociated from that initial driving mission.
>
> As physicians we often expect patients to come to us while they are at some of their lowest points and interact with us on our turf, a place where we are familiar, and interact with us on our terms. It was a worthwhile experience to get out of my comfortable context, and spend time walking around the area where many of our patients actually live. Going on

to work, attending meetings seeing patients in school and alternate settings was a great way to interact with patients in their contexts, where they're more comfortable, and to do so more on their terms.

This kind of experience is something that had been lacking from my residency training so far. Many components of the social history seem like abstract concepts when discussed in a hospital ward, or even in the academic context in lectures. Seeing these determinants of health firsthand including, poverty and substance misuse, reinforces how overarching these loom in the lives of our patients.

Another easy misconception being within the tertiary care bubble is it can seem to us that we play an inflated role in our patients' lives. Having a chance to see some of the other major challenges our families face helped to re-contextualize the role we play in our patients lives. It reinforces that a degree of humility is essential, as our short clinic visits or ward stays are only a minor part of the rich, diverse and complex lives of our patients.

This has represented a different way to practice, mindful of the social determinants of health, community focused, meeting people where they are, and striving to help those among us who need the support most.

The integration of social pediatrics in the training of medical students and pediatric and family medicine residents has a rich potential to enable trainees to retain the ideals that brought them into medicine and better equip them to understand and to serve the needs of critical and vulnerable components of the population and have a deeper and more realistic appreciation for the underlying issues that are shaped by poverty, implicit and explicit bias, severe economic inequities, and other social determinants of health. This experience will help them care for the children, youth, and families who need their skills, commitment, compassion, and understanding.

Conclusion

Adolescent Health and Social Pediatrics

Community social pediatrics is a model well suited for adolescents in vulnerable families and distressed communities. Meaningful responses to inequities in health and opportunity require responsive interdisciplinary and intersectoral services with access to resource-rich, supportive social environments that foster resilience and development of social resources for all children and youth. The goal is to assure that youth rights, needs, and interests are respected, targeting not only psychosocial and physiological development but their growth in every area of life.

The social pediatrics model of care embraces the formation of intersectoral multidisciplinary teams to set up appropriate and tailored early intervention, treatment, and prevention programs that foster resilience and enable youth to grow up in good health, despite the potential of multiple early or ongoing life adversities. Social pediatrics respects the overall needs of children and youth in the community and considers the major determinants of health including income and social status, social support networks, level of education and literacy, employment and working conditions, social and physical environments, and the most fundamental interpretation for the rights of children and youth.

Through early intervention with connections to community social and family resources, the foundational supports and relationships are laid in place to address significant problems as they arise, engage the family and community supports, and avoid adolescent homelessness and social isolation.

References

1. Tyler I, Lynam J, O'Campo P, Manson H, Lynch M, Dashti B, Turner N, Feller A. It takes a village: a realist synthesis of social pediatrics program. Int J Public Health. 2019;64(5):691–701.
2. Spencer N, Colomer C, Alperstein G, Bouvier P, Colomer J, Duperrex O, et al. Social paediatrics. J Epidemiol Community Health. 2005;59:106–8.
3. Wong ST, Lynam JM, Khan KB, Scott L, Loock C. The social paediatrics initiative: a RICHER model of primary health care for at risk children and their families. BMC Pediatr. 2012;12:158.
4. Shonkoff J, Garner A, et al. The lifelong effects of early childhood adversity and toxic stress. Pediatrics. 2012;129(1):e232–45.
5. Power C, Atherton K, Strachan D, Shepherd P, Fuller E, Davis A, et al. Life-course influences on health in British adults: effects of socioeconomic position in childhood and adulthood. Int J Epidemiol. 2007;36(3):532–9.
6. Loock C, Suleman S, Lynam J, Scott L, Tyler I. Linking in and linking across using a RICHER model: social pediatrics and inter professional practices at UBC. UBCMJ. 2016:7.2(7–9).
7. Ford-Jones E, Williams R, Bertrand J. Social paediatrics and early childhood development: part 1. Paediatr Child Health. 2008;13(9):755–8.
8. Julien G. A different kind of care: the social pediatrics approach. Montreal: McGill-Queens University Press; 2004.
9. Julien G. A different kind of care: the social pediatrics approach. Montreal: McGill-Queen's University Press; 2004.
10. MacIntyre M. The black report and beyond: what are the issues? Soc Sci Med. 1997;44:723–45.
11. Lynam MJ, Loock C, Scott L, Khan KB. Culture, health and inequalities: new paradigms, new practice imperatives. J Res Nurs. 2008;13(2):138–48.
12. WHO. What are the social determinants of health? Geneva: World Health Organization; 2008. www.who.int/social_determinants/sdh_definition/en/.
13. Trent M, Dooley DG, Dougé J, AAP Section on Adolescent Health, AAP Council on Community Pediatrics, AAP Committee on Adolescence. The impact of racism on child and adolescent health. Pediatrics. 2019;144(2):e20191765.
14. The World Health Organization. Social determinants of health. Available at: www.who.int/social_determinants/thecommission/finalreport/key_concepts/en/.
15. Kershaw P, et al. Towards a social care program of research: a population level study of neighborhood effects on child development. Early Educ Dev. 2007;18:535–60.
16. Skott-Myhre H, Raby R, Nikolaou J. Towards a delivery system of services for rural homeless youth: a literature review and case study. Child Youth Care Forum. 2008;37(2):87–102.
17. Bogard K, Murry VM, Alexander C, editors. Perspectives on health equity and social determinants of health. Washington, DC: National Academy of Medicine; 2017.
18. Lynam MJ, Loock C, Scott L, et al. Social paediatrics: creating organisational processes and practices to foster health care access for children "at risk". J Res Nurs. 2010;15(4):331–47.
19. Holtz TH, Holmes S, et al. Health is still social: contemporary examples in the age of the genome. PLoS Med. 2006;3:1663–6.
20. Gee GC, Walsemann KM, Brondolo E. A life course perspective on how racism may be related to health inequities. Am J Public Health. 2012;102(50):967–74.

21. Trent M, Dooley DG, Dougé J, AAP Section on Adolescent Health, AAP Council on Community Pediatrics, AAP Committee on Adolescence. The impact of racism on child and adolescent health. Pediatrics. 2019;144(2):e20191765. Jones CP, Truman BI, Elam-Evans LD, et al. Using "socially assigned race" to probe white advantages in health status. Ethn Dis. 2008;18(4):496–504, pmid:19157256.
22. National Research Council. Measuring racial discrimination. Washington, DC: National Academies Press; 2004. https://www.nap.edu/catalog/10887/measuring-racial-discrimination (cited in AAP Policy Statement. The impact of racism on child and adolescent health).
23. Bhopal R, Donaldson L. White, European, Western, Caucasian, or what? Inappropriate labeling in research on race, ethnicity, and health. Am J Public Health. 1998;88(9):1303–1307 (cited in AAP Policy Statement. The impact of racism on child and adolescent health).
24. US Interagency Council on Homelessness. Preventing and ending youth homelessness: a coordinated community response, p. 3. https://www.usich.gov/resources/uploads/asset_library/Youth_Homelessness_Coordinated_Response.pdf. Accessed 14 June 2019.
25. Streissguth AP, Barr HM, Kogan J, Bookstein FL. Understanding the occurrence of secondary disabilities in clients with fetal alcohol syndrome (FAS) and fetal alcohol effects (FAE). Final report to the Centers for Disease Control and Prevention (CDC), August, 1996, Tech. Rep. No. 96-06. Seattle: University of Washington, Fetal Alcohol & Drug Unit; 1996.
26. Frankenberger DJ, Clements-Nolle K, Yang W. The association between adverse childhood experiences and alcohol use during pregnancy in a representative sample of adult women. Womens Health Issues. 2015;25(6):688–95. https://doi.org/10.1016/j.whi.2015.06.007.
27. Rutman D. Becoming FASD informed: strengthening practice and programs working with women with FASD. Subst Abuse. 2016;10(Suppl 1):13–20. https://doi.org/10.4137/SART.S34543.
28. Kania J, Kramer M. Collective impact. Stanf Soc Innov Rev. Winter 2011;9(1):36–41.
29. Foster-Fishman PG, Watson ER. The ABLe change framework: a conceptual and methodological tool for promoting systems change. Am J Community Psychol. 2012;49:503–16; Frost PJ, Egri CP. The political process of innovation. In: Staw B, Cummings L, editors. Research in organizational behavior, vol. 13. Greenwich; London: JAI Press; 1986. pp. 229–296.
30. Foster-Fishman PG, Watson ER. The ABLe change framework: a conceptual and methodological tool for promoting systems change. Am J Community Psychol. 2012;49:509.
31. Foster-Fishman PG, Nowell B, Yang H. Putting the system back into systems change: a framework for understanding and changing organizational and community systems. Am J Community Psychol. 2007;39(3/4):197–216.
32. Foster-Fishman PG, Watson ER. The ABLe change framework: a conceptual and methodological tool for promoting systems change. Am J Community Psychol. 2012;49:503–16.
33. Browne A. Discourses influencing nurses' perceptions of First Nations patients. Can J Nurs Res. 2005;37:62–87.
34. Young A. The character assassination of black males: some consequences for research in public health. In: Bogard K, Murry VM, Alexander C, editors. Perspectives on health equity and social determinants of health. Washington, DC: National Academy of Medicine; 2017. p. 47–61.
35. Ginsburg KR. The journey from risk-focused attention to strength-based care. In: Ginsburg KR, Kinsman SB, editors. Reaching teens: strength-based communication strategies to build resilience and support healthy adolescent development. Elk Grove Village: American Academy of Pediatrics; 2014.
36. US Dept of Health and Human Services, Family and Youth Services Bureau. Positive youth development. https://www.acf.hhs.gov/fysb/positive-youth-development.
37. American Academy of Pediatrics. Reaching teens. https://www.aap.org/en-us/professional-resources/Reaching-Teens/Pages/New-to-Reaching-Teens.aspx.
38. Ginsburg KR. The journey from risk-focused attention to strength-based care. In: Ginsburg KR, Kinsman SB, editors. Reaching teens: strength-based communication strategies to build resilience and support healthy adolescent development. Elk Grove Village: American

Academy of Pediatrics; 2014. ProQuest eBook Central. https://ebookcentral.proquest.com/lib/ubc/detail.action?docID=3000014.
39. Bradford N. Place-based public policy: towards a new urban and community agenda for Canada. Ottawa: Canadian Policy Research Networks; 2005.
40. Blum RW, Li M, Naranjo-Rivera G. Measuring adverse child experiences among young adolescents globally: relationships with depressive symptoms and violence perpetration. J Adolesc Health. 2019;65(1):86–93.
41. Zuckerman B, Sandel M, Smith L, et al. Why pediatricians need lawyers to keep children healthy. Pediatrics. 2004;114:224–8.
42. Farmer P. An anthropology of structural violence. Curr Anthropol. 2004;45(3):305–25.
43. Daneman D, et al. Social paediatrics: from "lip service" to the health and well-being of Canada's children and youth. Paediatr Child Health. 2013;18(7):351–2.

Resources

An excellent example of family-based work with homeless youth is Winlad DN, Gaetz SA, Patton T. Family matters: homeless youth and Eva's Initiatives Family Reconnect program. Toronto: The Canadian Homelessness Research Network Press; 2011.

Dolan C, Friesen A, Gallant A, Hughes K, Merchant J, Vincent D, Whyte C. Literature review and best practices for the housing and supports framework; Housing and supports initiative' and creating connections: Alberta's addiction and mental health strategy. 4 May 2012. https://canfasd.ca/wp-content/uploads/sites/35/2016/12/Housing-Literature-Review-FINAL-May-4-12.pdf.

Ginsburg KR. The journey from risk-focused attention to strength-based care. In: Ginsburg KR, Kinsman SB, editors. Reaching teens: strength-based communication strategies to build resilience and support healthy adolescent development. Elk Grove Village: American Academy of Pediatrics; 2014. ProQuest eBook Central. https://ebookcentral.proquest.com/lib/ubc/detail.action?docID=3000014.

Kann L. Youth risk behavior surveillance – United States, 2017. MMWR Surveill Summ. 2018;67(8):1–114. https://doi.org/10.15585/mmwr.ss6708a1.

Pittman KJ. The power of engagement. In: Youth today. Washington, DC: The Forum for Youth Engagement; 1999. https://forumfyi.org/. Accessed 22 June 2019.

Pope LK. Housing for homeless youth. Youth homelessness series brief no. 3. Washington, DC: National Alliance to End Homelessness; 2010.

Roth JL, Brooks-Gunn J, Murray L, Foster W. Promoting healthy adolescents: synthesis of youth development program evaluations. J Res Adolesc. 1998;8:423–59.

Shonkoff JP, Garner AS, Siegel BS, Dobbins MI, Earls ME, Garner AS, McGuinn L, Pascoe J, Wood DL, American Academy of Pediatrics. The Committee on Psychosocial Aspects of Child and Family Health, Committee on Early Childhood, Adoption and Dependent Care, and Section on Developmental and Behavioral Pediatrics. The lifelong effects of early childhood adversity and toxic stress. Pediatrics. 2012;129(1):e232–46. https://doi.org/10.1542/peds.2011-2663.

Trent M, Dooley DG, Dougé J, AAP Section on Adolescent Health, AAP Council on Community Pediatrics, AAP Committee on Adolescence. The impact of racism on child and adolescent health. Pediatrics. 2019;144(2):e20191765.

Chapter 8
Substance Use Among Young People Experiencing Homelessness: A Brief Motivational Enhancement Approach

John Howard

Introduction

There is abundant evidence from all continents that young people experiencing homelessness have significant preventable morbidity and mortality. Their difficulties may predate their homelessness or be exacerbated by or develop because of it. In particular, use of alcohol, tobacco and other drugs and substances, such as inhalants, among young people experiencing homelessness is associated with increased negative health and social consequences [1–16].

While boredom, curiosity and wanting to feel good (or better) may be reasons for initiating use of substances, other functions served by substance use can be to relieve hunger and pain, for peer/social acceptance, to keep awake or get to sleep, for increasing courage and pleasure. Most young people who experiment with various substances do not continue their use or develop significant problems. For those who do, many of the harmful consequences of substance use are determined by the interrelated cultural, legal, social and economic contexts within which they are consumed [17].

Unsafe sexual behaviour while intoxicated increases the likelihood of unplanned pregnancies and sexually transmitted infections (STIs). Road traffic and other accidents, often associated with alcohol use, are a major cause of mortality and injury among young people, and suicide and homicide are often associated with use of substances. To survive out of home, young people may put themselves at risk of violence by working in the illicit drug and commercial sex industries. Young people who inject drugs are more likely to be involved in riskier behaviours than those older, including from sharing injection equipment and exposure to HIV and other BBIs [18–20].

J. Howard (✉)
National Drug and Alcohol Research Centre, UNSW Medicine | Faculty of Medicine, University of New South Wales – Sydney, Sydney, NSW, Australia

C. Warf, G. Charles (eds.), *Clinical Care for Homeless, Runaway and Refugee Youth*, https://doi.org/10.1007/978-3-030-40675-2_8

In addition, significant harm results from the criminalisation of people who use substances, especially incarceration, which increases marginalisation and experience of stigma and discrimination. This, in turn, may decrease access to and participation in interventions to address their difficulties, including substance use-related harm [18, 19].

However, the burden of disease and morbidity tends not to be evenly distributed but falls on more heavily to those with increased vulnerability due to factors in addition to (or a cause or consequence) homelessness, for example, very young adolescents, sexuality and gender-diverse youth, minority populations/cultures, young people involved in sex work, those in juvenile justice/closed settings, indigenous young people and those with significant trauma histories [17].

Young women have specific issues, as they are often introduced to substance use by male partners and exacerbated if involved in commercial sex work by their 'pimps'. Homeless young women tend to exhibit greater levels of psychosocial distress and negative life events than do young men. Pregnancy is also a major issue, and young women who use substances are often viewed more negatively than young males [17].

Clearly, young people experiencing homelessness present with multiple, complex and interconnected needs and comorbidities that usually require contemporaneous management. Addressing substance use and related issues may assist with stabilisation of accommodation and participation in education, training or employment and improved mental health. However, how to deal with behaviours such as substance use that may be meeting a variety of needs, while exacerbating various social and health concerns, is challenging for primary and allied health workers, physicians, nurses, counsellors and youth workers (hereafter 'clinicians').

Stages of Change

Addressing substance use and related difficulties is a *process*, not an *event*, and total cessation/abstinence may not always be a necessary outcome. Young people who do not identify abstinence as their goal are not necessarily being resistant and unmotivated. Their goal may be to manage their lives more effectively – with our without substance use. Later, they may come to a realisation that such life management may not be possible without reduction of use or cessation. Engaging with them on a journey of change is possible, and motivational enhancement approaches aid such engagement.

Prochaska and DiClemente developed the 'transtheoretical model of behaviour change' to describe a process of change in the context of substance use and dependence [21]. See Fig. 8.1. Their stages of change are as follows:

- Precontemplation: not yet acknowledging that there is a problem behaviour that may need to be addressed
- Contemplation: acknowledging that there is a problem, but not yet ready or sure of wanting to make a change

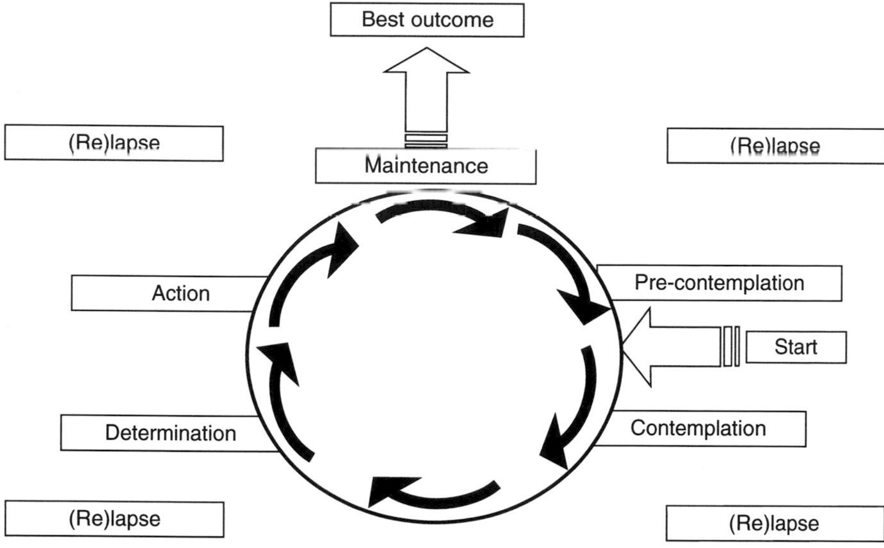

Fig. 8.1 Stages of change

- Preparation/determination: getting ready to change
- Action: change behaviour
- Maintenance: maintaining the behaviour change
- Termination: changes sustained

The motivational enhancement approach, developed by Miller and Rollnick [22], is useful in promoting self-reflection by a young person on their predicament and current 'stage' or readiness to change, identifying internal and external resources and supporting movement through the change process towards their desired outcomes. As, (re)lapse, returning to older behaviours and abandoning the new changes, is a most likely recurring event during the process of attempting to change most health-compromising behaviours, for example, diabetes, cardiovascular disease and obesity. Thus, identifying triggers and the development of relapse prevention strategies are important foci for interventions.

Motivational Enhancement Approaches to Assist Young People Experiencing Homelessness Address Substance Use-Related Difficulties

A major issue in the management of substance use-related difficulties in out of home/school, as in other settings, is how to engage young people in helpful conversations about the use of legal and illegal substances. Young people experiencing homelessness rarely self-initiate treatment for their substance use but may seek assistance for other issues, such as accommodation, physical health, poor sleep, anger, depression, anxiety, relationship issues or respiratory problems, and not mention that they use substances. In addition, substance use may be but one ingredient in a complex situation. Early detection of substance use-related issues is important in preventing escalating problems.

Clinicians may feel ill-prepared to engage in meaningful conversations with young people experiencing homelessness with regard to reduction or cessation of substance use. In addition, while some young people may avoid conversations about their substance use, others will be relieved that they did not have to bring it up themselves.

At a minimum, clinicians are encouraged to provide accurate information, and basic screening and detection are strongly encouraged. However, screening instruments do not replace an empathic conversation and history taking. Motivational enhancement approaches have proved to be useful with young people and tend to enhance more formal screening and assessment, as they aid the development of rapport and trust.

Brief, opportunistic motivational enhancement can be utilised in most settings and aim to engage with young people and explore their substance use and associated issues. Such settings can include where young person feels safe – open space (e.g. park), shelter common area through to more 'clinical' settings – from emergency room to office based. The approach fits with time constraints (for clinician and young person) and the short attention span of many young people. The approach emphasises collaboration, evocation of self-motivation and resources and autonomy (self-efficacy), rather than one focused on confrontation, education and authority vested in the clinician.

If it is within the role of the clinicians, use of any of the evidence-informed therapeutic approaches could follow, and it is likely that they may be more effective with initial attention to engaging with the adolescent using motivational enhancement. Alternatively, appropriate referrals could be provided.

A range of 'motivational enhancement' approaches have been evaluated in Australia, the Netherlands and the USA and have demonstrated reductions in substance use. They range from one off opportunistic encounters to two to three session and approaches that incorporate motivational enhancement with other models. Cannabis use has been the focus of a number of the studies, and participants came from a wide range of ethnicities including Hispanic, African American, Native American and Alaskan Indian [23–31].

The essentials of the motivational enhancement approach are as follows:

- Open-ended questions
- Reflective listening
- Affirmation
- Periodic summaries
- Eliciting self-motivation statements
- Recognising and dealing with resistance
- Recognising readiness for change

Motivational enhancement uses an engaging conversational style, ensuring respect and empathy, indicating an understanding that the young person's substance use is not mindless and that they recognise the 'benefits' and 'less good' aspects of substance use. The approach also indicates that the clinicians understand that change is difficult, and while possibly bringing benefits (never guaranteed), there are 'costs' associated with the change process, such as loss of peers and having to deal with problems their substance use might have hidden.

Essentially, the motivational enhancement involves consideration of five key questions and can take less than 10 minutes. The approach is illustrated below, using cannabis as the substance of focus, as adapted from Copeland and Howard [32].

Motivational Enhancement with Young People Who Use Cannabis: 'Five Key Questions'

The 'five key questions' usually take no more than 5 minutes to cover.

1. *So, what do you like/enjoy about your use of cannabis*? [exhaust reasons]
2. *Ok, and what do you like less about your use of cannabis*? [attempt to discount some, and give appropriate info as necessary]
3. *So, you say you like ..., but are less happy about....have you thought about what could be good about making a change in your use of cannabis?*
4. *OK, but what might be some less good things about making a change in your use of cannabis?*
5. (i) If young person is *not interested* in change at this stage: *'So, you don't seem too keen on making a change in your use of cannabis at this stage. Here is some info that you might find interesting or useful. Also, I am wondering what might lead you to re-think this decision at some stage?*

   Add: *Before we finish, I would like to give you some information that you might find helpful and some contacts where you might get some help in if you re-consider your decision, and remember I am happy to talk with you again about this if you want'.*

   or

   (ii) If young *person is interested in change: 'So we talked a lot about what you like and don't like so much about your use of cannabis, and what you might gain and lose from changing your use. Before we finish, I would like to give you some information that you might find helpful and some contacts where you might get some help in making the changes you are thinking about'.*

   If is it part of the clinician's role to provide brief interventions for young people wishing to address their substance use-related issues, they could then continue the conversation as follows:

   'We did not actually talk about how much cannabis you actually use .... so, can you tell me how many days a week you use....'

Clinical Vignette: Pedro Aged 16

Table 8.1 provides an example of the use of a conversational style of interviewing to cover the five key questions with Pedro, a 16-year-old male experiencing homelessness.

Table 8.1 An example of motivational enhancement

Role	Dialogue
C	[conversation begins after some general 'chat' Pedro has been having with the clinician/ youth worker] *…so, you were mentioning about using dope (cannabis)… I am wondering what YOU like about it – what are some of the things you get from it?*
P	I really don't know what to say … I like the 'high' …
C	*What else do you like about it?*
P	Well … it's something to do – fills the time… umm…I do it with me friends … we laugh
C	*So you have some fun times with friends and it fills the time… what else?*
P	I don't know … um … it helps me to get to sleep… I dunno
C	*It's hard for you to get to sleep without it*
P	Yep – sometimes… like when my head is spinning and it is giving me the sh##@!
C	*Ok, so it helps you to get to sleep too …. What else does the dope do for you?*
P	I dunno … it's fun … Better than being bored and with nothing to do … the streets can get hectic … and I can relax and chill…
C	*Sounds using dope gives you something to do, some fun times and then helps you sleep… Any more things you like about it?*
P	Hey … what else? I don't know – I just like it (Laughs)
C	*OK … I ask a lot of questions, hey? Are you OK?*
P	Yep …
C	*So, is there any 'down side' – things you don't like so much about dope?*
P	Hmmm (pause) … Well, umm … it's costing me a lot
C	*So, it's getting a bit expensive for you?*
P	Yep
C	*What else?*
P	Ah … sometimes I don't like what it does to my head – especially when I use it by myself… (pause)
C	*That must be tough … are there other things as well?*
P	Sort of … Like when I call Mum or Em (my sister) they keep saying – 'are you still using dope?', 'Are you stoned now?' It makes me angry and upset
C	*Upset?*
P	Yep – at them and me!
C	*Like?*
P	Like they think I am some sort of loser … they should talk!
C	*OK, so there is the cost, you head spinning, being a bit worried about what is happening to your head and how your mum and sister are treating you. Other things?*
P	… isn't that enough … Oh… it makes me lazy too – I don't look for work or a regular place to stay – I just sit with mates and get stoned ……
C	*Questions, questions …. But, seriously, are there other things you don't like so much about the dope?*
P	Nah … think they are the main ones – oh, and I think the cops are watching me

Table 8.1 (continued)

Role	Dialogue
C	*So, have you ever tried to cut down or stop?*
P	Yep – but it didn't work
C	*What did you try?*
P	Just tried to stop ...
C	*What happened?*
P	It didn't work
C	*What did you want to get from stopping or cutting down?*
P	I dunno ... Head quieter, some money for things ... family ... I don't know ... might get somewhere better to live, find a job, stop being lazy ...
C	*OK ... so you have some good ideas about what you wanted ... what about things that might be no so good about making a change?*
P	Hmmm, ... well guess my friends ... how they will treat me...
C	*Yes... that is something important ... what other things?*
P	Well ... getting bored ... what will I do.... there's nothing to do ....
C	*So, having something to do and coping with your friends and their reactions ... they will be hassles for you ... anything else?*
P	Nah... just being straight and handling things....
C	*Ok.... Let's see ...so you like getting stoned with friends, stops you getting bored, helps you relax and sleep, BUT on the other hand you are worried about what the dope might be doing to your head, it costs you lot, makes you lazy, not looking for accommodation and work, and your mum and sister hassle you*
P	Yep ... I guess that's it
C	*And, you think that if you cut down you might have more money and get on better with your family, get somewhere safe to live ... BUT you're worried that your friends might not be so happy with you, you might then have no friends and you will be bored*
P	Yep
C	*So what do you think? I have some information here about how you could try to cut down or quit by yourself... and some info on people or programs that could maybe help you if you would prefer that, or feel uncomfortable working with me ... some even on the web and there are some Apps ...*
	Option One: willing to change
P	I don't know ... what if I did want to try?
C	*Ok... and remember we'll support you with what you choose ... well let's look at this material (e.g. brochures from appropriate agencies) ----*
	Option Two: not so willing to make a change – at this stage
P	Hmmm, I'm not sure ... maybe too hard for me ... not sure I could do it
C	*OK, well at least you have had a good look at your situation – what you like and like less about dope and what might be good about change, but what also might be hard ... what about I give you this info here and you can look at it .... OK?*
P	Ok, yea...
C	*Good. Oh, and, one last thing ... I just wanted to leave you with a question ...'What do you think could happen that might make you think again about making a change?'*
P	I don't know ... maybe getting busted by the cops?... I don't know
C	*That could be a big thing .... OK – let's hope that does not happen ... if you do think again about what we have been talking about today ... you know where we are – and I'm more than happy to have another chat? OK?*
P	Ok – thanks ----

C = clinician/youth worker; P = Pedro aged 16

The themes evident in this scenario include the following:

- The clinician is attempting to build motivation for reflection on Pedro's predicament and easing Pedro to a point where he can make a 'decision'.
- The clinician tries to exhaust 'good things' about use, and not overreact to 'less good things', thus letting Pedro know that he or she understands that Pedro uses cannabis for specific reasons, is not merely engaging in delinquent behaviour and is aware of the impact of his cannabis use. It is important not to attempt to deal with all issues raised; the main task is engagement and enhancing motivation for change.
- The clinician tries to elicit Pedro's views about 'good and less good things' about reducing or ceasing use.
- The clinician summarises and attempts to have Pedro reflect on this and make a decision about attempting change or staying where he is.

If Pedro is ready to contemplate change, further intervention could be offered within the initial consultation, and/or over time if engagement with Pedro strengthens and is actively maintained via sensitive and appropriate reminders, possibly text messaging based. Key components of these might include the following:

- Providing further feedback linking cannabis use with current and potential health problems.
- Elaboration of cannabis use: patterns, amount of use alone and with others, times of day, locations of use, age mix of those they use with, any coercion and any risks associated with their cannabis use – e.g. location, mix of co-users, sharing of means of use – bong or joint.
- Provision of harm reduction strategies.
- Discussion aimed at eliciting change talk. For example, discuss Pedro's level of confidence that he can change their substance use if he wants to. If confidence is low, encourage Pedro to recount other changes he has made or the personal qualities that would help him to make changes in his cannabis use.
- Assisting Pedro to identify his personal strengths/resources.
- Raising specific options to assist change (a menu of options). For example, identify high-risk situations, triggers and strategies to avoid them. Triggers for use include moods/feelings; people (family, friends, peers, others); places; odours, for example, room and clothing not cleaned; implements and waste left around; visual stimuli such as posters linked to cannabis, its use and famous cannabis users; mixing bowls; and certain prodrug use songs.
- Identifying other pleasurable activities.
- Helping Pedro decide on his goals.
- Encouraging Pedro to identify people who could provide support and help for the changes he wants to make.
- Assisting Pedro develop a realistic relapse prevention plan, that will be regularly reviewed.
- Providing self-help resources, youth-friendly written information and web links to reinforce what has been discussed.

- Inviting Pedro to return to discuss his progress and offering further help or information as necessary.
- Connecting Pedro to appropriate accommodation, education/training or employment providers.
- Considering a family work approach.

Clinical Vignette: Emma Aged 14

Emma
is a 14 year-old female who lived with her mother and a younger brother, until she left home after an increase in conflict with her mother. She decided to see a doctor at a youth health service to obtain contraception. She had become sexually active at age 13. She told her doctor that she had been using cannabis and methamphetamine occasionally and did not see it as problematic. Her doctor did not share this view, but when she began to explore Emma's cannabis and methamphetamine use, Emma became rather hostile and attempted to close off the issue. However, the doctor was able to employ a motivational enhancement style of interviewing.

Emma eventually revealed that she liked methamphetamine and said that it made her feel excited and happy. She was using once or twice a week with a loose group of males and females aged 14–24. She often stayed out late and roamed streets and parks. Her 'boyfriend' is 18 years old, probably methamphetamine dependent and occasionally injecting. He also uses cannabis daily, drinks heavily and is unwilling to use condoms. Emma believed that she had no difficulties with her methamphetamine use and that she was doing well at school, when she attended, even if her grades were not as good as they had been.

Her mother, who had used cannabis in her youth, appeared to have a laissez faire view of parental control, limit setting and behaviour. She knew that Emma had tried cannabis, but not methamphetamines, and was sexually active, but not to the extent of either activity. She had been sexually active in her mid-teens and experimented with drugs and believed that cannabis was a 'soft drug'. Emma's father appeared to be somewhat stricter as a parent but had been minimally involved with Emma over the past 3 years.

To aid the development of a functional therapeutic or working relationship with Emma to address issues raised in the vignette, the five key questions illustrated in the case of Pedro could be helpful. After using the motivational enhancement approach, undertaking a more detailed exploration of her relationship with methamphetamine and cannabis would follow, and then consideration of the following:

- Determining what ongoing approach would be best, for example, CBT, supportive therapy, any involvement of her mother and brother, an approach that also engaged her peers and other systems, such as education and youth activities
- Whatever the approach taken, the development of a realistic relapse prevention plan for identifying and managing triggers that could result in a return to problematic substance use, takes time. Change is usually an uneven process
- Addressing child protection and mandatory reporting issues
- Connecting Emma to an appropriate and youth-friendly sexual and reproductive health service, if not provided by current service
- Connecting Emma to a suitable education provider
- Gaining Emma's agreement to meet with her mother, if deemed appropriate, taking into account any child protection service involvement
- Exploring the possibility of working with Emma and her boyfriend, if she wishes to maintain the relationship

Motivational enhancement fits with the FRAMES approach recommended by the WHO [33–35]. FRAMES refers to providing *F*eedback, promotion of *R*esponsibility, providing *A*dvice and a *M*enu of options, as necessary and appropriate, employing an *E*mpathic approach and supporting *S*elf-efficacy. This approach can guide ongoing work with young people with substance use-related difficulties [36].

It is important to discuss the symptoms of withdrawal, as they can trigger (re) lapse. For example, cannabis withdrawal symptoms typically emerge after 1–3 days of abstinence, peak between days 2 and 6 and typically last from 4 to 14 days with sleep difficulties often taking some weeks to ameliorate. The most common symptoms include nightmares and strange dreams, difficulty getting to and staying asleep, night sweats, irritability and diminished appetite.

Likewise, cravings should be addressed and can occur within the context of the actual consultation by enquiring about the effect the conversation is having on the young person in real time. Strategies to manage cravings, such as delaying, decatastrophising, distracting, de-stressing and drinking water can be discussed.

It needs to be remembered that change is a 'process', not an 'event'. This is especially the case with young people experiencing homelessness and who have multiple and complex needs; there will be many moves backwards as well as forward. The clinician needs to be sturdy enough to withstand the onslaught, be well supported by colleagues, have regular supervision available and find time to ensure interventions being provided have an evidence base. Also essential is having positive working relationships with relevant services such as education (formal or informal); training; employment; housing; mental, sexual and reproductive health (if not provided by the clinic/service within which they are located) and welcoming and appealing youth activity programs.

Some links to online resources and training on motivational interviewing and enhancement are provided below.

Conclusion

Clinicians occupy unique and trusted positions and, by virtue of this, can provide opportunities for young homeless and runaway youth to address behaviours that can impact on them at multiple levels – physical and mental health, academic performance, family relationships, sport and other social and recreational activities and engagement in activities prohibited by law. Being comfortable in engaging in helpful, motivating conversation about substance use and strategies to address their concerns is one such opportunity to assist them in managing their lives effectively.

References

1. MacKenzie D, Flatau P, Steen A, Thielking M. The cost of youth homelessness in Australia. Melbourne, Vic.: Swinburn University of Technology: 2016. https://doi.org/10.4225/50/5722A58AE5600.
2. National Health Care for the Homeless Council. Substance use among youth experiencing homelessness. Heal Hands. 2016;20(2):1–9. Available: https://www.nhchc.org/wp-content/uploads/2016/09/healing-hands-substance-use-among-youth-experiencing-homelessness-v2-web-ready.pdf
3. Narendorf S, Cross M, Maria D, Swank P, Bordnick P. Relations between mental health diagnoses, mental health treatment and substance use in homeless youth. Drug Alcohol Depend. 2017;175:1–8. https://doi.org/10.1016/j.drugalcdep.2017.01.028.
4. UNICEF. Experiences form the field: HIV prevention among high risk adolescents in Central and Eastern Europe and the Commonwealth of Independent States. Geneva: UNICEF; 2013. Available: http://www.youngpeopleandhiv.org/files/ExperiencesFromTheField2013.pdf
5. Woan J, Lin J, Auerswald C. The health status of street children and youth in low- and middle-income countries: a systematic review of the literature. J Adolesc Health. 2013;53(3):314–21. https://doi.org/10.1016/j.jadohealth.2013.03.013.
6. Al-Tayyib A, Rice E, Rhoades H, Riggs P. Association between prescription drug misuse and injection among runaway and homeless youth. Drug Alcohol Depend. 2014;134:406–9. https://doi.org/10.1016/j.drugalcdep.2013.10.027.
7. Embleton L, Mwangi A, Vreeman R, Ayuku D, Braitstein P. The epidemiology of substance use among street children in resource-constrained settings: a systematic review and meta-analysis. Addiction. 2013;108:1722–33. https://doi.org/10.1111/add.12252.
8. Gomez R, Thompson S, Barczyk A. Factors associated with substance use among homeless young adults. Subst Abus. 2010;31(1):24–34. https://doi.org/10.1080/08897070903442566.
9. Johnson K, Whitbeck L, Hoyt D. Substance abuse disorders among homeless and runaway adolescents. J Drug Issues. 2005;35(4):799–816. https://doi.org/10.1177/002204260503500407.
10. Mitra G, Wood E, Nguyen P, Kerr T, DeBeck K. Drug use patterns predict risk of non-fatal overdose among street-involved youth in a Canadian city. Drug Alcohol Depend. 2015;153:135–9. https://doi.org/10.1016/j.drugalcdep.2015.05.035.
11. Njord L, Merrill R, Njord R, Lindsay R, Pachano J. Drug use among street children and non-street children in the Philippines. Asia Pac J Public Health. 2010;22:203–11. https://doi.org/10.1177/1010539510361515.
12. Nyamathi A, Hudson A, Greengold B, Slagle A, Marfisee M, Khalilifard F, Leake B. Predictors of substance use severity among homeless youth. J Child Adolesc Psychiatr Nurs. 2010;23(4):214–22. https://doi.org/10.1111/j.1744-6171.2010.00247.x.

13. Roy E, Robert M, Fournier L, Vaillancourt E, Vandermeerschen J, Boivin J. Residential trajectories of street youth – the Montréal Cohort Study. J Urban Health. 2014;91(5):1019–31. https://doi.org/10.1007/s11524-013-9860-5.
14. Salomonsen-Sautel S, Van Leeuwen J, Gilroy C, Boyle S, Malberg D, Hopfer C. Correlates of substance use among homeless youth in eight cities. Am J Addict. 2008;17:2224–34. https://doi.org/10.1080/10550490802019964.
15. Towe V, ul Hasan S, Zafar S, Sherman S. Street life and drug risk behaviors associated with exchanging sex among male street children in Lahore, Pakistan. J Adolesc Health. 2009;44:222–8. https://doi.org/10.1016/j.jadohealth.2008.09.003.
16. Wincup E, Buckland G, Bayless R. Youth homelessness and substance use: report to the drugs and alcohol research unit, Home Office Research Study, vol. 258. London: Home Office Research, Development and Statistics Directorate; 2003. Available: http://citeseerx.ist.psu.edu/viewdoc/download?doi=10.1.1.473.1664&rep=rep1&type=pdf
17. Ball A, Howard J. Psychoactive substance use among street children. In: Harpman T, Blue I, editors. Urbanization and mental health in developing countries. Aldershot: Avebury; 1995. ISBN: 1856289710.
18. Degenhardt L, Hall W, Lynskey M. The increasing global health priority of substance in young people. Lancet Psychiatry. 2016;3:251–64. https://doi.org/10.1016/S2215-0366(15)00508-8.
19. Hall W, Patton G, Stockings E, Weiner M, Lynskey M, Morley KI, Degenhardt L. Why young people's substance use matters for global health. Lancet Psychiatry. 2016;3:264–79. https://doi.org/10.1016/S2215-0366(16)00013-4.
20. Barrett D, Hunt N, Stoicescu C. Injecting drug use among under-18s. London: Harm Reduction International; 2013. ISBN: 978-0-9927609-1-5. Available: https://www.streetchildrenresources.org/wp-content/uploads/2014/01/injecting_among_under_18s_snapshot_WEB1.pdf
21. Prochaska J, DiClemente C, Norcross J. In search of how people change: applications to addictive behaviors. Am Psychol. 1992;47:1102–14. https://doi.org/10.1037//0003-066x.47.9.1102.
22. Miller W, Rollnick S. Motivational interviewing: helping people change. London: Guilford Press; 2012. ISBN: 9781609182274.
23. D'Amico E, Miles J, Stern S, Meredith L. Brief al interviewing for teens at risk of substance use consequences: a randomized pilot study in a primary care clinic. J Subst Abus Treat. 2016;35:53–61. https://doi.org/10.1016/j.jsat.2007.08.008.
24. Davis J, Houck J, Rowell L, Benson J, Smith D. Brief motivational interviewing and normative feedback for adolescents: change language and alcohol use outcomes. J Subst Abus Treat. 2016;65:66–73. https://doi.org/10.1016/j.jsat.2015.10.004.
25. Department of Families, Housing, Community Services and Indigenous Affairs. Literature review: Effective interventions for working with young people who are homeless or at risk of homelessness. Canberra: Australian Government Department of Families, Housing, Community Services and Indigenous Affairs, Canberra; 2012. Available: https://www.dss.gov.au/sites/default/files/documents/06_2012/literature_review.pdf
26. Dickerson D, Brown R, Johnson C, Schweigman K, D'Amico E. Integrating motivational interviewing and traditional practices to address alcohol and drug use among urban American Indian/Alaska Native youth. J Subst Abus Treat. 2016;65:26–5. https://doi.org/10.1016/j.jsat.2015.06.023.
27. Dupont H, Candel M, Kaplan C, van de Mheen D, de Vries N. Assessing the efficacy of MOTI-4 for reducing the use of cannabis among youth in the Netherlands: a randomised controlled trial. J Subst Abus Treat. 2016;65:6–12. https://doi.org/10.1016/j.jsat.2015.11.012.
28. Martin G, Copeland J, Swift W. The adolescent cannabis check-up: randomised trial of a brief intervention for young cannabis users. J Subst Abus Treat. 2008;34:407–14. https://doi.org/10.1016/j.jsat.2005.06.005.
29. Slesnick N, Guo X, Brakenhoff B, Bantchevska D. A comparison of interventions for homeless youth evidencing substance use disorders: results of a randomized clinical trial. J Subst Abus Treat. 2015;54:1–13. https://doi.org/10.1016/j.jsat.2015.02.001.

30. Tucker J, D'Amico E, Ewing B, Miles J, Pedersen E. A group-based motivational interviewing brief intervention to reduce substance use and sexual risk behaviour among homeless young adults. J Subst Abus Treat. 2017;76:20–7. https://doi.org/10.1016/j.jsat.2017.02.008.
31. Xiang X. A review of interventions for substance use among homeless youth. Res Soc Work. 2013;23(1):34–45. https://doi.org/10.1177/1049731512463441.
32. Copeland J, Howard J. Cannabis use disorders. In: Rosner R, editor. Handbook of adolescent addiction. New York: Wiley-Blackwell; 2013. ISBN: 978-0-470-97234-2.
33. WHO. Brief intervention: the ASSIST-linked brief intervention for hazardous and harmful substance use: for substance use: manual for use in primary care. Geneva: WHO; 2010. ISBN: 978-92-4-159939-9. http://www.who.int/substance_abuse/publications/assist_sbi/en/
34. WHO. ASSIST: the alcohol, smoking and substance involvement screening test (ASSIST): manual for use in primary care. Geneva: WHO; 2010. ISBN: 978-92-4-159938-2. http://www.who.int/substance_abuse/activities/assist/en/
35. WHO. Self-help strategies for cutting down or stopping substance use. Geneva: WHO; 2010. ISBN: 978-92-4-159940-5. http://www.who.int/substance_abuse/publications/assist_self_help/en/
36. Marsh A, Dale A, Willis L. A counsellor's guide to working with alcohol and drug users. 2nd ed. Perth: Alcohol and Drug Office, Government of Western Australia; 2007. ISBN 9781876684211. http://fundassist.flinders.edu.au/uploads/docs/Outcome_Indicators_WA.pdf

Online Resources for Motivational Interviewing and Enhancement

American Society for Addiction Medicine.: https://www.asam.org/education/live-online-cme/fundamentals-of-addiction-medicine/additional-resources/motivational-interviewing

Motivational Interviewing Network of Trainers.: http://www.motivationalinterviewing.org

Oregon Health.: http://www.oregon.gov/oha/HPA/CSI-TC/Resources/Online%20MI%20Training%20Resources%201-22-18.pdf

Portico. Canada – Centre for Addiction and Mental Health: https://www.porticonetwork.ca/treatments/treatment-methods/motivational-interviewing/mi-resources-and-training

PsyMontréal.: https://psymontreal.com/resources-motivational-interviewing/?lang=en

SAMHSA-HRSA – Centre for Integrated Health Solutions.: https://www.integration.samhsa.gov/clinical-practice/motivational-interviewing

Chapter 9
Building an Effective System of Care for Adolescents Following Opiate Overdose: Stabilization Care, Residential Secure Care, Family and Community Engagement, and Ethical Concerns

Tom Warshawski, Grant Charles, Eva Moore, Alice Virani, Nina Preto, Amanda Pollicino, and Curren Warf

Introduction

Opiate overdose is now the leading cause of death for adults under 55 years old in the United States and Canada. In British Columbia and in other areas, opiate overdose is now the leading cause of death for persons aged 10–59 years [1, 2], killing

T. Warshawski
School of Social Work, University of British Columbia, Vancouver, BC, Canada

Child and Youth Network, Interior Health Authority, Kelowna, BC, Canada

G. Charles
School of Social Work, University of British Columbia, Vancouver, BC, Canada

E. Moore
Division of Adolescent Health and Medicine, Department of Pediatrics, University of British Columbia, Vancouver, BC, Canada
e-mail: eva.moore@cw.bc.ca

A. Virani
Ethics Service, Provincial Health Services Authority, Vancouver, BC, Canada

Department of Medical Genetics, University of British Columbia, Vancouver, BC, Canada

N. Preto
Ethics Service, Provincial Health Services Authority, Vancouver, BC, Canada

A. Pollicino
Vancouver, BC, Canada

C. Warf (✉)
Department of Pediatrics (Retired), Division of Adolescent Health and Medicine, British Columbia Children's Hospital, University of British Columbia, Vancouver, BC, Canada

C. Warf, G. Charles (eds.), *Clinical Care for Homeless, Runaway and Refugee Youth*, https://doi.org/10.1007/978-3-030-40675-2_9

more than suicide, car accidents, and homicide combined. The principal opiate involved is fentanyl, followed by heroin [3].

Relative Incidence of Unnatural Causes of Death in BC

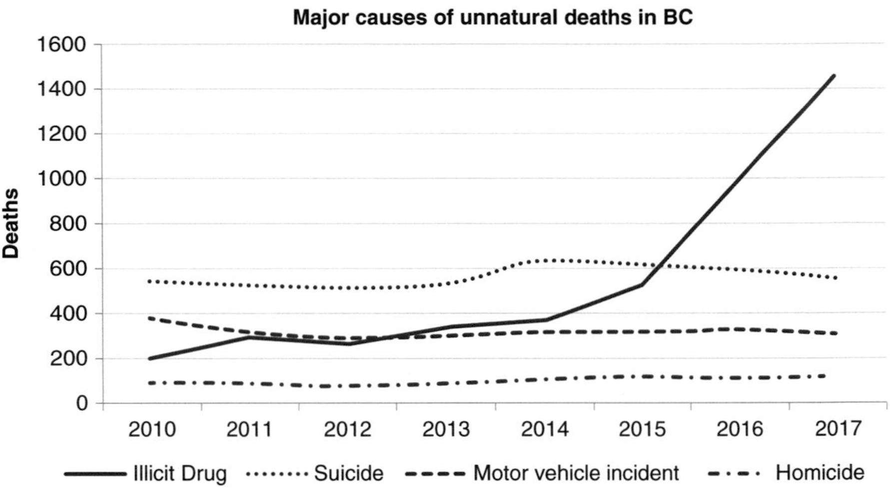

BCCDC, BC Coroners Service, Illicit Drug Overdose Deaths in BC, Jan 1, 2008–Feb 28, 2018

Many if not most of these deaths are unintentional exposures through the contamination with fentanyl of other non-opiate drugs including amphetamines and cocaine [4]. Fentanyl and its illicit analogues are particularly dangerous as they have between 40 and 100 times the potency of heroin. However, a significant portion of deaths are from deliberate fentanyl use that exceeded tolerance or fentanyl contamination of other opioids. Regardless of how the overdose occurred, adolescents who have presented to an emergency department with an opioid overdose are at exceedingly high risk of dying from a subsequent overdose in the near future.[1] Assertive, effective intervention among youth who present with an opioid overdose can mitigate the risk of subsequent overdose. Youth who had deliberately used opioids can potentially be motivated to abstain or shift to opioid agonist therapy in order to avoid long-term opioid use and entrenched addiction. Youth who inadvertently consumed opioids are also at high risk for subsequent overdose due to their unsafe pattern of substance use, and efforts should also be made to move them away from substance use or to consume more safely. Those determined to continue using need coaching on how to consume in a safer fashion.

[1] Preventing Death After Overdose: BC Coroners Service Child Death Review Panel. A Review of Overdose Deaths in Youth and Young Adults 2009–2023. Report to the Chief Coroner of British Columbia. January 2016. http://www.llbc.leg.bc.ca/public/pubdocs/bcdocs2016/591444/overdose-death-young-young-adult-report.pdf

Fentanyl Detected in Over 80% of BC Overdose Deaths

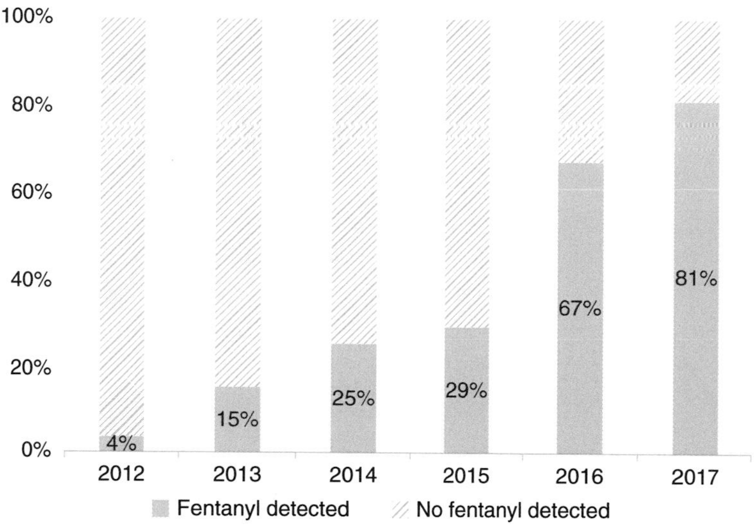

BCCDC, BC Coroners Service Fentanyl-Detected Apparent Illicit Drug Overdose Deaths, 2012–2017

In this chapter we will review emerging early intervention models for adolescents who present to the emergency department with opioid overdose or who are developing dangerous levels of opiate or other drug use, acknowledging their special vulnerability and great promise, and offer new approaches to management. We will explore the rationale for assertive intervention to help youth who present with an opioid overdose and serious substance abuse and discuss the ethical questions which arise with compulsory intervention. Assertive interventions are feasible, realistic, and interdisciplinary and commonly include family engagement approaches that are particularly applicable for many homeless or runaway youth.

These approaches are not meant to take the place of harm reduction strategies that are critical in addressing the use of opiates by adults who have a longer history of opiate use; nor are these approaches meant to take the place of outpatient approaches such as cognitive-behavioral therapy for adolescents for less dangerous substance abuse.

In view of the growing threat to life that synthetic opioids have for both adolescents and adults, we need to look critically at the actual interventions that now exist, evaluate how effective they have actually been, and be open to new approaches to interrupt the patterns of addiction that leave young people so vulnerable to lethal overdose.

Following are sections elucidating the arguments for new approaches to intervention, including hospital-based certified stabilization care after acute overdose and certified and mandated residential secure care for more prolonged treatment.

We will discuss the importance of effective engagement of adolescent patients with parents and/or other supportive adults as well as engagement of social work and other supportive community agencies. As with any mandated treatment, whether of adolescents or adults, ethical questions that arise must be addressed clearly and openly. The questions arising from certification and involuntary hospitalization for stabilization and placement in residential secure care will also be explored.

The Threat of Opiates to the Life and Well-Being of Adolescents

Over the last decade, youth aged 18–25 have had the highest increase in rates of use of heroin.[2] The majority (86%) of young urban injection drug users interviewed in 2008–2009 disclosed that they had first used opioid pain relievers obtained from family, friends, or personal prescription [5]. The incidence of heroin initiation was 19 times higher among those who reported nonmedical use of prescription opioid pain relievers than among those who did not [6].

Many youth experiment with illicit drugs and approximately 5–15% of these will go on to develop substance use disorders (SUDs). [7] Serious substance use disorders are more common among street-entrenched youth [8]. Regular illicit drug use is of concern as it often adversely affects development, family relationships, education, and employment and may lead to significant medical complications and even death.

Many adults addicted to opiates began their use as adolescents; it should be appreciated that the opiate use that one encounters among young people, whether prescription or heroin, may be the beginning of a long-term addiction and derailment of their life's potential.

Chronic or even episodic opioid use carries significant risks. The most severe outcome is death from overdose. North America is in the midst of an opioid overdose crisis; in 2017, there were 3996 apparent opioid-related deaths in Canada, of which 73% involved fentanyl or fentanyl analogues [9]; in the United States in 2017, there were 70,237 drug overdoses, with 47,600 (67.8%) deaths involving use of opioids, nearly a 600% increase since 1999.[3] In the United States and in Canada, opiate overdose is now the leading cause of death for adults under 55 years of age. Almost 60% of these deaths involved synthetic opioids. Youth under the age of 25 years accounted for 8.7% of opioid deaths[4]with 2% of deaths occurring in persons aged 19 years and younger [10].

[2]National Institute of Drug Abuse. What is the scope of heroin use in the United States? www.drugabuse.gov https://www.drugabuse.gov/publications/research-reports/heroin/scope-heroin-use-in-united-states

[3]National Institute of Drug Abuse https://www.drugabuse.gov/related-topics/trends-statistics/overdose-death-rates. Accessed March 4, 2019

[4]Lawrence Scholl, PhD1; Puja Seth, PhD1; Mbabazi Kariisa, PhD1; Nana Wilson, PhD1; Grant Baldwin, PhD1 L Scholl, P Seth; M Kariisa; N Wilson; G Baldwin. MMWR/January 4, 2019/Vol. 67/Nos. 51 and 52

Spectrum of Effects of Substance Use

- *Overdose death is the most extreme negative outcome of drug use.*
- *Neurological, mental health, and cognitive impairment.*
- *Physical health from infection, accidents, violence, sexual assault, and exploitation.*
- *Social functioning: school failure and dropout, conflict with peers and family, homelessness and street involvement, and interface with police or criminal justice system.*
- *Failure to meet adult responsibilities: parenting and employment.*

Chronic use of opiates such as heroin, fentanyl, OxyContin, and others has significant effects on health and development of youth. Use is associated with poor social functioning, school failure and dropout, conflict with peers and family, homelessness and street involvement, and interface with the police and criminal justice system. Physical health is affected by serious infections including endocarditis, risk of HIV, injuries from accidents and violence, and victimization by sexual assault and sexual exploitation. Long-term developmental problems are also affected including failure to meet adult responsibilities, sustain employment, and parenting children.

Street Supply of Fentanyl

Fentanyl on the streets is usually imported from illicit amateur manufacturers, commonly originating overseas. The product is generally of unknown potency and may include several types of synthetic opioids. A mailed envelope can contain 100,000 doses or even more. Kilograms of fentanyl have been found by police in individual shipments or in transit. Under these circumstances, fentanyl of unknown concentration is commonly introduced deliberately to methamphetamine or cocaine supplies to increase sales by providing an extra kick or simply through sloppy preparation. These are among the circumstances contributing to inadvertent fentanyl overdoses.

Harms Posed by Opioid Abuse

Infectious complications are well known and include HIV and hepatitis C through needle sharing, as well as septicemia, endocarditis, and multiple abscesses through contaminated intravenous injections and equipment. Although all substance abuse is concerning, perhaps the most dangerous of the illicit drugs are opioids, in particular fentanyl.

It has been long recognized that experiencing a nonfatal opioid overdose is a significant risk factor for subsequent fatal overdose [11, 12] and the risk seems to have significantly increased over the past decade. Given the growth of use of opiates since 1995 (including prescribed opiates such as OxyContin) and the dramatic increase in deaths from synthetic opiates (in particular fentanyl) since 2013,[5] the current approaches to prevention and early intervention are clearly inadequate.

Current Management of Adolescents with Opioid Overdose

Within North America, there is no standard management practices for adolescents after presentation to the emergency department with an illicit drug overdose. Fentanyl and other synthetic opioids are so potent that the drug screens available to hospital emergency departments are not sufficiently sensitive to detect the drug during the acute overdose treatment period, leaving the physicians no option but to treat based on clinical presentation without laboratory guidance. Laboratory test results may be reported after several days; it is not known if they are capable of detecting other very high potency opiates. Practices vary considerably among institutions and between individual providers.

Currently, when a youth presents to hospital with an opioid overdose, parents or legal guardians are generally not contacted, nor is the teen admitted for stabilization, as the youth typically refuses to consent to either. The operating principle is that the youth emerging from overdose is competent to make these decisions regarding admission or parental notification. It is often assumed that it is safe to discharge an opioid overdose victim, including an adolescent, as little as 1 hour after having been revived by naloxone administration, as the risk posed by the presenting overdose is thought to be minimal [13]. Many teens are discharged after 1 or 2 hours of observation, often alone or with another minor. This practice and the assumptions underlying them need to be questioned.

The practice of early discharge of youth after opiate overdose contrasts sharply with the approach to adults who have received therapeutic opiates in hospital settings for day surgery. These patients must be discharged into the care of a responsible adult and are advised to wait at least 24 hours before making important decisions out of recognition of the impact of opioids, including therapeutic use of opioids, on the judgment of adults.[6]

Although the risk of immediate death after naloxone resuscitation is low, the 12-month risk of overdose death is extremely high. Adults who present to the emergency department with a nonfatal opioid overdose have up to a 10% risk of dying within 1 year [12]. The risk is likely similar for youth, or higher, as many of them have a propensity for risk-taking [14] or are homeless [8] or may have overdosed as a manifestation of a concurrent mental health issue with suicidal ideation [15].

[5] The age-adjusted rate of drug overdose deaths involving synthetic opioids other than methadone increased by 45% from 2016 to 2017.NCHS Data Brief No. 329, November 2018. https://www.cdc.gov/nchs/products/databriefs/db329.htm

[6] Guide: Planning for my Outpatient Day Surgery, https://www.ottawahospital.on.ca/en/documents/2017/01/p084-english.pdf/ (accessed May 21,2019)

Despite these hazards, many youth who have just survived an overdose are discharged into the same circumstance from which they have been admitted and with less oversight than adults who have received opioids for surgical day procedures [16].

Given the extreme risk of subsequent death facing youth who have experienced even a single opioid overdose, as well as the opportunity to intervene at a relatively early point in the developing opiate addiction in youth, there is an urgent need for health professionals to develop a coherent strategy to care for them and improve their safety after discharge. In formulating a management strategy, special consideration must be given to the unique developmental aspects of the teenage brain, the effects of opioids on cognition, the role of concomitant mental health disorders on decision-making, the neurocognitive pathology underlying SUD, and the availability of social supports for the adolescent including parents, older siblings, extended family, and social services.

Development and Capacity for Decision-Making of Children and Youth

Most Western nations recognize that for some decisions, children and youth are competent to provide informed consent. Studies which demonstrate the ability of children and youth to exert sound judgment gauge competence on whether the child demonstrates the ability to understand information and then make what the assessors deem to be an appropriate choice. This principle evolved from a landmark British ruling on a child's right to consent to treatment which defined a competent child as one "who achieves a sufficient understanding and intelligence to enable him or her to understand fully what is proposed and has sufficient discretion to enable him or her to make a wise choice in his or her own interests." [17] In a study which used clinical scenarios to assess the capacity of children and youth grouped in age clusters of 9-, 14-, 18-, and 21-year-olds, the 14-year-olds were as competent as the two adult groups in that they were as likely to come to "reasonable outcomes, ...the choice a hypothetical reasonable person might make." [18] However, the authors caution that the "generalizability of these findings be tempered by the fact that subjects were ...of high intelligence ….and not influenced by psychological disorder or ...confusion, depression, or anxiety...."

In contrast with the "reasonable outcome" approach, others have proposed that competency should not rest solely on whether or not the assessor agrees with the decision but whether or not the reasoning that explains and justifies it seems to be valid [17]. This point of view departs from the requirement that the decision be "wise"; however, evaluating both the reasoning behind a choice and the wisdom of the choice is subjective. There must therefore be an operating principle with which to weigh the benefits of autonomous decision-making versus the accompanying risks.

Most agree that under optimal conditions, children and youth are capable of informed consent, and this right is often granted when the risks associated with consent, or refusal, are of minor consequence. However, when the ramifications of withholding consent are severe, and perhaps life-threatening, the developmental stage of the child or youth as well as their global cognitive capacity must be taken into account. In addition, the judgment of the child or youth must not be impaired by delirium, delusion, or depression [19]. If these factors are present, there is good reason to doubt capacity. It must also be noted that a person's capacity, in particular an adolescent's capacity, may fluctuate and may require multiple assessments over time.

Although many adolescents have adult levels of working memory, and verbal and visual comprehension, their reasoning processes, and therefore their capacity, may be affected by peer pressure, impulsivity, and risk-seeking behaviors [20]. Youth are also affected by "hot cognition" and "cold cognition," [21] that is, youth in calm, supportive environments who are not intoxicated, angry, or in conflict are capable of making thoughtful assessments and decisions similar to adults, while the same youth when angry, intoxicated, and under high levels of peer influence may take thoughtless, impulsive, and dangerous actions.

The prefrontal cortex (PFC) is the area of the brain most involved in attention regulation, inhibition of impulses, and anticipation of the consequences of actions [22]. The PFC develops slowly, with much individual variability, and continues to develop and mature at least through the mid to late twenties [21]. In general, a 25-year-old has greater reasoning capacity than a 15-year-old in that the older brain is less impulsive and more resistant to peer influence and emotional impulses. This reasoning ability is heavily influenced by the social and peer environment, in addition to the influence of intoxicants.

The pubertal surge in testosterone, estradiol, and DHEAS results in the development of the secondary sexual characteristics which herald adolescence and exert profound effects on the brain [23]. These hormones trigger structural changes in areas such as the prefrontal cortex [24], ventral striatum, amygdala, and hippocampus [25] which themselves have estrogen and testosterone receptors. These structural changes coincide with significant behavioral correlates. Many adolescents tend to underestimate risks and overvalue rewards [14], discount adult direction in favor of peers [26], and are disproportionately influenced by emotions [22]. Youth in whom these problematic traits are present to a high degree are predisposed to substance misuse [27]. These attributes tend to improve in most young people by age 20–25 years.

There has been a long-standing "common sense" that many youth do not possess adult levels of judgment, and this is reflected in our laws which set the legal age to drink alcohol and to smoke tobacco at age 18–21 years, depending on the region. Advances in neuroscience support this view. Adolescents are not merely inexperienced adults; they have unique developmental vulnerabilities.

By virtue of their developmental stage, many adolescents may be impulsive, show poor decision-making, and have difficulty following through with treatment despite the best of intentions. This is greatly accentuated while acutely intoxicated and during the period immediately afterward. Problems are qualitatively magnified when there is an absence of an involved and responsible supportive adult relationship and when the youth is left unsupervised with peers. Knowledge of the unique vulnerability of adolescents must guide all interventions aimed at them, but this is especially true when life and death decisions are being made.

Persistence of Neurological Effects of Opioids Following Overdose

Even in the absence of frank delirium or delusion, acute intoxication with opioids can significantly impair an individual's cognitive and behavioral capacities [28]. Once an individual who has suffered an opioid overdose is given naloxone, they "are unlikely to seek and engage wholeheartedly in addiction treatment .... [as they] will be having intense cravings to use opioids." [29] Naloxone is very effective in countering the respiratory depression of individuals with opiate overdose but has little or no effect on the cognitive and emotive impairments associated with addiction. Individuals who have had an opioid overdose may display significant cognitive deficits in memory [30] and problem-solving [31]. Even in the absence of a recent overdose, in the days following opioid abstinence, there are demonstrable deficits in complex working memory, executive function, and fluid intelligence [32]. This dysfunction is partially transient with relatively rapid improvement over 1–2 weeks [32, p. 8]. However, chronic opioid users display prolonged cognitive dysfunction [33], and it has been suggested that many require significant help in medical decision-making [34].

Mental Health and Decision-Making

Individuals with disorders such as ADHD [35], anxiety [36], or depression [37] often demonstrate significant cognitive difficulties, and there is a high incidence of mental health disorders among youth with SUD [38]. Cognitive impairment that may accompany some mental health conditions can combine with drug-induced cognitive impairment to significantly impair an individual's ability to evaluate treatment options and appreciate the risks of continued drug use. Perhaps even more concerning is the observation that among street youth in particular, drug abuse "appears to be a form of indirect suicide that manifests in repeated accidental overdoses." [15]

The combination of SUD and one or more mental health conditions is a significant risk factor for repeat overdose and death [39]. It is therefore imperative that youth who present with an opioid overdose be carefully assessed for concurrent mental health disorders and that treatment be initiated when mental health disorders are identified. This assessment requires amassing a complete picture of the youth's circumstances, a process which generally requires days to complete.

Increased Adolescent Vulnerability to Addictive Patterns of Drug Use

Modern science has transformed our understanding of substance use disorders. Substance use disorders "were once viewed largely as a moral failing or character flaw but are now understood to be chronic illnesses characterized by clinically significant impairments in health, social function, and voluntary control over substance use." [40]

There is good evidence that the repeated use of illicit substances "produce changes in brain structure and function that promote and sustain addiction and contribute to relapse." [41] The areas most affected by illicit drug use include the prefrontal cortex, ventral striatum, and amygdala [41, pp. 2–5]—areas which normally undergo significant changes with puberty. It has also been noted that "as individuals continue to mature between 13 and 21 years, the likelihood of lifetime substance abuse and dependence drops 4-5% for each year that initiation of substance use is delayed." [7] Teens seem particularly vulnerable to the addictive properties of illicit drugs. This observation raises the concern that illicit drugs may hijack normal pubertal brain development and predispose to addiction. It would appear that early and assertive intervention to prevent and minimize drug use in teens is warranted.

The modern view of substance use disorders is that they result from drug-induced brain impairment rather than a series of voluntary hedonistic acts [42] and this may be particularly true for youth. This understanding of a substance use disorder must be kept in mind when evaluating whether an individual is exercising freedom of choice when they continue to use illicit drugs despite obvious harm. It becomes more problematic to take this view when continued drug use carries a significant risk of death.

The modern understanding of addiction and the neurological effects of opiate and other substances of abuse, as well as the very real dangers posed to adolescents, lay the basis for the development of new approaches to management of youth with life-threatening substance use disorders.

Assuring the Safety of Youth After Medical Presentation with Opiate Overdose

Many youth who present after an overdose are unwilling to consent to emergency department staff contacting family and caregivers to gather vital information. Given the evidence regarding cognition after opioid overdose, it is inappropriate to expect a youth who has just received naloxone for a drug overdose to be capable of informed consent regarding notification of their parent or legal guardian to gather vital information and ensure a safety plan for discharge and what follows. Failure to contact a legal guardian, or alternatively to engage supportive services, may result in the youth being discharged with only another minor (who may be no more competent than the patient) or on their own and left to their own devices. It is equally inappropriate to expect the youth to be fully competent to consent to, or more significantly to refuse, treatment options.

Prior to discharge, the youth's mental well-being needs to be formally reassessed and documented, and cognitive functioning must be at a sufficient level to meaningfully discuss treatment options and harm reduction strategies, family and community supports contacted and engaged, and ancillary information gathered to confirm the history.

This shift in our management strategy mandates that we consider the complex ethical issues that are involved in implementing certified stabilization care and residential secure care which are explored later in this chapter.

Implications for Shaping Clinical Evaluation and Management

Youth who present with a nonfatal overdose are at high risk for a subsequent fatal overdose in the near future and ethically deserve a thorough briefing of their treatment options at a time when they are capable of understanding and engaging in the process [43]. A fully informed discussion regarding treatment options and the provision of a safety plan cannot be adequately completed until there has been significant improvement in global cognition. A clinical dilemma then arises as most youth who have suffered an overdose are uncooperative, refuse admission, and will not consent to the notification of caregivers. A rational solution is to involuntarily admit the youth until cognition significantly improves. Unfortunately, the scientific literature provides little guidance as to when to conclude that cognition is sufficiently cleared to embark upon a fulsome discussion of the risks of continued opioid use and treatment options.

Involuntary Admission and Treatment of Adolescents for Other Medical Conditions

Within North America many jurisdictions have guidelines which recommend involuntary admission and treatment for youth with eating disorders if voluntary admission is refused and if the "patient with an eating disorder is at serious medical risk to the extent that they are in jeopardy of dying." [44] Yet these same jurisdictions do not have similar guidelines for the involuntary admission of youth with life-threatening substance use disorders. There appears to be inconsistency between the criteria for competency for those with serious SUD as opposed to mental health disorders such as severe depression or eating disorders despite the fact that those who survive an overdose have a 1-year mortality rates as high as 10%, considerably higher than that of either anorexia nervosa or unipolar depression [45].

Stabilization Care: An Evolving Model of Care for Adolescents Presenting with Opioid Overdose

Given the greatly increased numbers of youth experiencing opioid overdose, including fentanyl overdose, and the rapid growth in mortality from these overdoses, several hospitals in British Columbia are developing a more assertive approach to youth who present with an opioid overdose. These new initiatives are iterative processes, best viewed through the lens of quality improvement and have developed through interdisciplinary collaboration of the staff and leadership of the emergency department, pediatrics and adolescent medicine, child psychiatry, nursing, medical ethics, hospital-based social work, and local child protective services. The management of adolescents presenting with opiate overdose is one important component of improving the hospital care of adolescents, in particular homeless youth and adolescents in other high-risk situations.

Change in practice requires a collaborative approach. All stakeholders must be engaged and find common ground in order to move forward. In British Columbia, concern about the opioid crisis in regard to youth and the role of the hospital arose among three separate working groups that had come together years earlier. One working group was an intersectoral community—hospital working group coalesced to address unaccompanied youth (youth without a responsible adult) presenting to the emergency department. Another working group was an initiative of the British Columbia Pediatric Society (a chapter of both the Canadian Paediatric Society and the American Academy of Pediatrics) that brought together a regional group of experts working with youth to evaluate the current policies and practices for adolescents with serious life-threatening substance use in British Columbia. A quarterly community-organized group, consisting of diverse front-line and decision-making individuals working with youth, was formed following the tragic death of a young person from overdose. As the opioid crisis progressed, the youth needs also changed, and individuals working closely with these youth recognized the urgency of the issue and the gross lack of developmentally appropriate services. The combination of regional, provincial, and community efforts fueled a change in the medical approach to youth when they present to the hospital with serious, life-threatening substance use.

Once the urgency and need were agreed upon among this interdisciplinary group of champions, the problem and its urgency were presented to medical leadership at various levels across British Columbia. Steering committees and working groups were established with a focus on education, procedure development, and engagement of direct service providers. From here, an approach was developed called "stabilization care."

Stabilization care is an approach in which a youth is admitted to the hospital following a life-threatening overdose requiring resuscitation in the field or the emergency department. Presentation of a youth to the emergency department with a life-threatening illicit drug overdose is an extremely dangerous situation as well as a window of opportunity for intervention. The process of stabilization care may take 5–7 days or more and generally proceeds as follows:

1. In the emergency department, every youth who is clinically evaluated to be at risk for illicit drug exposure is ordered a urine toxicology screen for drugs of abuse, including heroin and fentanyl.
2. Based on clinical findings and independent of toxicology findings, the patient is treated with naloxone, repeatedly as necessary.
3. Youth is then admitted to the hospital, involuntarily if necessary. Parents and guardians are notified and asked to participate in the hospitalization and discharge planning.
4. Every effort is made to support and engage the youth in a developmentally appropriate way and to enable the youth to develop insight over the dangers of their substance use.
5. If the youth experiences withdrawal or other discomfort in the hospital, appropriate monitoring for opioid withdrawal is employed, and opioid agonist therapy is initiated using state-of-the-art protocols as indicated.
6. Youth who have concurrent medical complications such as pneumonia, abscesses, or trauma are evaluated and treated promptly.
7. Hospital-based and community-based services, such as social work, child protective services, indigenous cultural liaisons, and counselors, are involved and encouraged to engage while in hospital.
8. Once mentation is sufficiently cleared, usually within 48–72 hours, psychiatric assessment is provided along with thorough gathering of ancillary information from family and counselors.
9. A team meeting is organized and ideally occurs within 72 hours of admission.
10. The youth meets with a drug and alcohol counselor to evaluate treatment options, and the youth and family are thoroughly briefed on harm reduction strategies.
11. If possible, connections are re-established with family, mental health clinicians, and drug and alcohol workers.
12. If treatment is accepted, either community or residential treatment is facilitated with an aim for direct transfer whenever possible.
13. Discharge is offered when withdrawal plan is managed, mental health concerns are addressed, suicidality is assessed, shelter is arranged, and connection with drug and alcohol counselors is arranged. This may be after 5 days to 2 weeks of hospital admission; it is significantly longer if there are major medical complications.
14. Potential transfer to longer residential or inpatient substance use treatment as available and indicated.

New and innovative approaches for intervention for youth with serious life-threatening substance use such as stabilization care and other approaches need to continue to be developed and evaluated. Rates of fentanyl deaths in Western provinces, such as British Columbia, are increasing at the same rate among youth as other age groups, and it is now the leading cause of death for ages 10–18 [1, 2]. Youth should not be expected to receive services for serious substance use disorders at adult treatment facilities. Youth require services tailored to their specific developmental needs that include approaches for engagement of families and youth-specific services, including parents when appropriate and realistic, as well as child protection, schools, and peer mentorship.

Given that this is an unprecedented epidemic, new interventions need to be based on the understanding of the development of drug addiction in adolescents and on the best evidence available, but actions will also need to be taken in the context of limited guiding evidence. It is important that there be continual quality improvement, following of cases over time, processes for external monitoring, and continued community engagement. As with any new initiative, research and evaluation need to be part of the process.

In parallel with treatment of opiate and other serious drug abuse among adolescents, it is important that there be ready access to low-barrier harm reduction approaches for those with more entrenched opiate abuse including supervised consumption sites, availability of clean needles and syringes, and in some circumstances availability of clean and unadulterated opiates, including heroin. Training for opioid overdose response and naloxone distribution is needed for all substance users and their family and friends. Supervised consumption sites and other places of interface with people addicted to opiates need to have readily available access for detoxification and substance abuse treatment which make opioid agonist therapy readily available in non-stigmatizing environments with appropriate supports.

Secure Care

While the term secure care is widely used across jurisdictions, there is not a universally agreed-upon definition. Indeed, there is a significant variation on how the term is used ranging from short-term crisis and substance misuse interventions to second-tier mental health services to criminal justice interventions. This variability in terminology makes comparisons about outcomes, research findings, policies, and legislation difficult. It also means that people who are not familiar with the different uses of the terms make false assumptions about any number of aspects in any discussion on the topic. As a result, one can come to conclusions that are often based on a shallow and selective interpretation of what is meant by secure care, making informed decision-making quite difficult and resulting in the delay of development of a badly needed intervention in some jurisdictions.

While in many US jurisdictions secure care often refers to criminal justice programs, in Canadian jurisdictions, it refers to two general categories of secure interventions: secure treatment and secure care. Both have significant legal safeguards built into their enabling legislation to ensure that the human rights of the young people are respected while at the same time ensuring that they are made safe. These intervention programs are not utilized loosely and are applied only to young people who are at significant risk of serious harm. The legislation acknowledges that young people have the same right as adults for protection from inappropriate confinement. This includes an appeal process and review mechanisms.

Secure treatment programs tend to be of a longer term than secure care, ranging from up to 90 days to more indefinite periods of time based upon the perceived needs of the young person. Generally, secure treatment programs serve young people who have significant mental health issues, who are at high risk for harm to self or others, and who often have a long history of absconding from community-based interventions.

Secure care programs are the more common intervention in Canada. While they often serve a range of young people, in the case of youth who misuse substances, they tend to focus on offering stabilization, assessment, and detoxification services.

A primary focus of secure care is upon the safety and stabilization of the young person. The purpose of the stabilization function is to provide a short-term period of time-out to young people whose lives are out of control. By stabilizing the young person in a locked setting, it is possible to assist in the current and overwhelming crisis the young person is experiencing. This provides the young person with the time and the structure to experience psychological and emotional regulation while also having their medical needs met. The safety and security of the setting allows for the young person to access their existing strengths and begin to interact with their world in a nonreactive manner. For those who are involved in substance misuse, it provides a safe environment in which to detox. As importantly, secure care allows the young person's family/caregivers, and those professionals supporting them, to themselves have a time-out from the effects of trying to help a young person who is experiencing a significant, and often long-term, ongoing crisis.

Seven of the ten Canadian provinces have legislative provisions for the use of secure care or treatment. All of the larger provinces, with the exception of British Columbia, have legislative provisions for secure, residential interventions. The other two provinces that do not offer secure care or treatment, Prince Edward Island and Newfoundland and Labrador, have significantly smaller populations and probably could not financially justify such a specialized intervention.

British Columbia appears to object to the provision of secure care options on philosophical grounds, seemingly based more on opinion than evidence. Within the jurisdictions that offer secure options, the legislation in four of them allows for secure care or treatment for young people with serious substance misuse issues, within a more general framework. Three provinces (Alberta, Manitoba, and Saskatchewan) have specific legislation for the provision of substance misuse secure interventions.

It should be noted that one serious consequence of not having secure care or treatment services is that in order to access safe environments for the young people, they may be labeled with mental health diagnoses or criminal justice charges and placed in the acute mental health or criminal justice settings. This pathologizing or criminalizing of young people is the only way they can be safely confined in order to deal with their self-destructive behavior. These practices can result in long-term stigmatization that could well have consequences for individuals throughout their lives. It is a classic example of fitting young people into system boxes rather than having services that are specifically designed to ensure their safety and well-being.

Risks and Efficacy of Stabilization and Secure Care for Adolescents with Severe Substance Use Disorders

Involuntary treatment for severe life-threatening substance use disorder, also termed "secure care," can range from brief civil commitment of 5–7 days to prolonged mandatory treatment of up to 90 days. Critics cite three major concerns as sufficient cause to oppose involuntary treatment of SUD. The first is the increased risk of overdose posed by enforced abstinence, the second is the assertion that involuntary treatment is ineffective, and the third that it is unethical to subject an individual to involuntary treatment given the first two premises. All three criticisms warrant closer scrutiny and are discussed below.

There is good evidence that loss of opioid tolerance increases the risk of overdose for both those placed in involuntary treatment [46] and for those in voluntary treatment [47]. The risk of dangerous intolerance appears to increase proportional to the days of abstinence, with evidence that there is little risk of fatal loss of tolerance in those who were abstinent less than 9 days [47], suggesting a window of safety. Of note is that the risk of fatal overdose following prolonged voluntary treatment may be as high as 10%, similar to, but not exceeding, the risk of death following opioid overdose recently observed in Massachusetts [12]. There are no studies available of risk to adolescents involved in involuntary treatment who would likely have shorter-term experience, potentially lower level of use, and greater potential to engage parents and other social supports.

These facts underscore the continuing need for harm reduction strategies such as opioid agonist therapy and supervised injection sites for individuals who are unable or unwilling to abstain from drug use. These facts do not negate the value of treating opioid addiction among adolescents with the goal of abstaining from drug use and the restoration of health and resumption of a normal developmental trajectory.

There is no evidence that involuntary opioid treatment carries a higher risk of death of posttreatment overdose compared to voluntary treatment or no treatment after opiate overdose. Opioid use is highly risky, particularly risk of death from subsequent overdose after treatment, regardless of whether use follows a period of abstinence or not. Contamination of the drug supply by fentanyl and its analogues means there is a variability in the amount one is taking making the exposure to highly potent synthetic opioids unpredictable, even if one is attempting to use a previously tolerated dose.

Youth drug use is also quite different than adult drug use. Youth are more likely to engage in poly drug use, which means less consistent opioid dosing and potentially less physical tolerance. They may not meet criteria for severe substance use disorder even with highly dangerous behavior due to a more experimental and opportunistic approach to substance use. Coroner's data suggests that youth who die of overdose are using polysubstances and it is the combination of toxic substances that contributed to their fatal overdose [48]. Therefore, youth at risk of fatal overdose may not have the same level of opioid tolerance as adults at risk. Youth-specific research and data are required to guide overdose prevention efforts in youth that may need to be distinct from an adult approach.

These facts underscore the need for harm reduction strategies such as opioid agonist therapy and supervised consumption sites that are youth specific to reach youth that are unable or unwilling to abstain from drug use. These facts do not negate the value of treating substance use with the goal of abstaining from drug use and the restoration of health and resumption of a normal developmental trajectory.

The second assertion by critics of secure care is that it is ineffective. This is not a fair assertion; in fact, the evidence for or against secure care is very limited. Systematic reviews of the literature on involuntary care for adults with severe SUDs conclude that evidence is limited and inconclusive [49–52]. There is no consensus on whether involuntary treatment is an effective alternative to voluntary substance use treatment, although one review found evidence to suggest that short-stay involuntary commitment may be effective as a harm reduction/crisis stabilization mechanism [52]. Evaluating the literature is difficult given that there is no consistent operational definition of involuntary treatment for individuals with SUDs, conflation of civil and criminal commitment outcomes [49, 51], and inconsistent uses of comparators across studies [51–53].

Despite limitations, a number of important findings have emerged in peer-reviewed literature to suggest that a closer look at a secure care approach for youth is important. Completion of involuntary treatment has been associated with reduced risk of mortality [54, 55] and self-reported improvements in quality of life [56]. Involuntary care can result in at least short-term improvements in drug-use behavior after discharge [57, 58]. A common theme across studies assessing involuntary treatment is the need to improve post-discharge treatment plans and continuing care [59, 60]. It is important to appreciate that the available studies are of interventions with adult substance users, not adolescents, and may not have applicability for young people; however, given the presumed shorter-term use of addictive substances of adolescents and the greater availability of parents, family, and other social supports, there may be greater impact than with adults.

The third argument against involuntary treatment is a concern about imposing involuntary treatment and confinement. This issue is explored at length later in this chapter in the section "Ethical Concerns Regarding Involuntary Treatment of Adolescents for Opioid Overdose and Other Serious Substance Abuse Problems."

Although the literature does not prove that compulsory treatment is effective, a lack of proof of effectiveness is not proof of ineffectiveness. Few would suggest that involuntary treatment is superior to voluntary treatment but that is not the choice confronting caregivers and clinicians. As one study comparing compulsory treatment (CA) to voluntary drug treatment stated in its conclusions:

> Voluntary treatment for substance use disorders generally yielded better outcomes; nevertheless, we also found improved outcomes for compulsory treatment patients. It is important to keep in mind that in reality, the alternative to compulsory treatment is no treatment at all and instead a continuation of life-threatening drug use behaviours. Our observed outcomes for CA patients support the continuation of compulsory treatment. [61]

Building Community Capacity and Family Support for Youth with Substance Abuse Problems

Few would dispute that social stressors can create the conditions leading to addictions which in turn lead to adverse health outcomes; however, the current biomedical focus of the healthcare system means that treatment for acute medical concerns is often provided without addressing the root causes of social and environmental stressors. Social and environmental stressors are external conditions or events occurring at the home or community level that negatively influence a youth's well-being including family conflict, poor relationships with peers, poverty, housing insecurity, food insecurity, engagement with child protection, racism, and other forms of discrimination [62]. Social stressors, particularly low socioeconomic status, are also known to be associated with an increase in suicidality, substance use, and substance-related injury or fighting [63, 64]. Many youths present to the emergency department with acute medical concerns related to addictions—which are the product of severe social stressors. While ED staff can acknowledge that the youth's environment is a significant risk factor leading to their presentation in the ED, resolving those circumstances is beyond the scope of an ED's capacity. As a result, those social and environmental stressors need to be addressed within the young person's community and family.

Unfortunately, in many jurisdictions, there is an overall shortage of community-based mental health and substance use disorder prevention and treatment programs for young people. [65] The fragmented nature of social, medical, mental health, and substance use services means that no one agency or ministry has the mandate or capacity to provide or coordinate the necessary services, resulting in many youth not receiving the community- and family-based resources they need [65]. The lack of integration, the lack of effective communication, and the insufficient levels of resources can also mean that intake processes and waitlists for services are barriers to access for youth. Often the services youths want are not available when they want them, resulting in missed opportunities for intervention and creating a further distrust in the medical and social service systems [65]. The limited community-based supports and resources that do exist are typically offered on weekdays during "regular business hours"—but most young people tend to experience crises at night or on the weekend. These service shortfalls have signaled the need for increase in family- and community-based supports that are designed to meet the needs of youth.

Many youth with addictions are viewed as "service resistant" or "noncompliant" by child protection and other community agencies if they do not access the resources or services set up as part of care plans. However, many care plans for youth were developed in a patronizing manner, prescribing resources with little to no involvement from the youth themselves. Youth were expected to conform to requirements (such as age restrictions, time of access, sobriety) if they wanted to receive services. Some professionals would argue that youth do not want to engage with the development of care plans, but many youth distrust the medical and social service systems due to negative past experiences. Furthermore, by calling youth "service resistant," the onus is put on the youth themselves to find help when they have already experienced a high level of abuse and trauma [65].

Ethical Concerns Regarding Involuntary Treatment of Adolescents for Opioid Overdose and Other Serious Substance Abuse Problems

Based on the sum of the evidence regarding risk of subsequent overdose death and impaired cognition, it seems logical that consideration of assertive management of youth who present with an opioid overdose is warranted. In most circumstances, immediate notification and engagement of the youth's legal guardian, as well as admission to hospital for stabilization, involuntarily if necessary, is the most responsible first step in keeping the youth safe while allowing time to craft a care plan. Such a plan includes a thorough evaluation of mental health status, identification and optimization of community supports, discussion of substance use intervention and treatment programs, and the implementation of a harm reduction strategy.

This chapter raises a number of compelling arguments supporting assertive interventions for certain youth presenting with opioid overdose, including involuntary treatment for those with serious or life-threatening substance use disorders. However, overriding autonomy by means of involuntary treatment should never be taken lightly, as this too can cause significant harm. As has been outlined earlier, evidence supports that many youth possess the capacity to make their own healthcare decisions, sometimes even those healthcare decisions requiring a high level of capacity (e.g., where the risks associated with the available options, including refusing treatment, are high). It is also recognized, though, that individuals with severe substance use disorders may struggle to follow through on decisions to reduce or abstain from substance use due to the neurobiologic effects of addiction—leading to actions that go against their authentic values or best interests. The question of whether an individual (be they youth or adult) with a severe substance use disorder can be capable of making autonomous decisions with respect to their substance use and treatment is unsettled. Decision-makers must therefore balance the potentially coercive effects of addiction against the authoritative act of involuntary treatment.

In the context of youth engaged in high-risk substance use, it may be extremely tempting to intervene, even without the youth's consent or over their express objections, in order to prevent serious harm and high risk of death. Given the risk of significant harm, including death, and potentially compromised capacity related to serious substance use disorders, intervening against a youth's wishes for short-term stabilization purposes or in order to compel longer-term treatment could be ethically justifiable in some cases. In the following section, the circumstances under which involuntary treatment for youth with substance use disorders may be ethically justified are considered, drawing on an ethics framework describing five criteria rooted in key bioethics principles [66].

The Intervention Is Effective (Beneficence)

Any involuntary intervention must have documented efficacy to be ethically justifiable.

Healthcare providers have a professional obligation to promote the patient's best interests, specifically determining the option that has the highest net benefit by evaluating interests in each option and discounting risks [67]. This concept does not invalidate the principle of autonomy and may vary over time. In addition, consideration of best interests must be broad and evaluate medical and other factors including social and emotional well-being and intersubjective factors. This duty is rooted in the principles of beneficence and non-maleficence and requires the healthcare provider to act in ways that optimize benefit for patients (and families) and to avoid options and actions that are likely to result in more harm than benefit for the patient. Before involuntary stabilization or secure care is considered, the nature and goal(s) of the intervention, as well as individuals for whom it is likely to be effective, must be identified. The weaker or more limited the evidence is supporting the effectiveness of secure care in meeting treatment goals, the more such infringement on youth autonomy is ethically problematic. Similarly, consideration of potential harms that might ensue from mandating involuntary care must be considered. Such harms include, but are not limited to, mistrust of healthcare providers and public institutions more generally, trauma in relation to restriction of freedom and "being admitted involuntarily," negative impacts on outside relationships, etc.

The question of evidence is challenging in this context. As has been described earlier in this chapter, while there is some evidence regarding the effectiveness of involuntary treatment for severe substance use disorders, it is noted to be limited and inconclusive and may not be applicable to youth. However, if, as some have argued, the alternative to involuntary treatment is in fact no treatment, it must be acknowledged that this option too raises profound concerns particularly given our societal duty to protect the most vulnerable.

In medicine and healthcare, as in other fields, there are often circumstances in which we must invoke the precautionary principle and act in the face of uncertainty and in the absence of clear evidence in order to at least try to address or mitigate harms that are unfolding around us. Even in these situations, those in the privileged position of implementing change are ethically obligated to be as informed as possible, be clear and transparent as to the basis on which decisions are being made, evaluate the intervention, and support methodologically, scientifically, and ethically sound research when appropriate to support evidence-based interventions moving forward. Applying this to the current question highlights the importance of being as clear as possible as to the basis on which a measure is implemented, including specific goals of the intervention. By way of one illustrative example, if a key goal of secure care is determined to be enhancing capacity and there is evidence that opioids take 5–7 days for the most acute neurological effects to improve, then a justified intervention period for youth whose capacity is compromised by substance use may be 5–7 days. If, on the other hand, the intervention period implemented was either longer or shorter, then the basis for this would need to be clearly articulated and justified (e.g., to address the continued impact of substance abuse and addiction).

It is also important to consider the ethical justifiability of treatment options, after the most acute drug effects have improved, as clearly significant risks to the youth continue. For example, the chronic disease approach to addiction calls for comprehensive assessment; stabilization; coordinated treatment of multifactorial issues related to personal, environmental, social, and psychological status; treatment of comorbidities; and longer-term care. Thoughtful consideration to evaluate the risks and benefits of different treatment models, length of such treatment models, and voluntariness of treatment models is warranted. [68]

Intervention Is the Least Intrusive Yet Effective Option (Respect for Persons/Autonomy)

Respect for persons refers to our duty to support individuals to make autonomous decisions and to treat them with dignity. For individuals with capacity to make their own healthcare decisions, this means respecting those decisions even where the decisions go against what is medically recommended and have negative implications for the health and well-being of the patient. Individuals deemed to lack decision-making capacity are still owed respect, and their wishes and preferences honored to the extent possible. In the context of involuntary interventions, this means, for example, using the least restrictive/intrusive intervention that will be effective and also supporting the individual to make those decisions they have capacity to make, both in terms of their healthcare and more generally.

Determining whether a patient has the capacity to make a medical decision refers to the patient's ability to perform a set of cognitive tasks, including (1) understanding and processing information about diagnosis, prognosis, and treatment options; (2) weighing the relative benefits, burdens, and risks of the therapeutic options; (3) applying a set of values to the analysis; (4) arriving at a decision that is consistent over time; and (5) communicating the decision. As alluded to above, decisional capacity is specific to a particular healthcare decision. The level of capacity required varies according to the complexity and seriousness of the decision at hand; decisions that are more complex and have higher stakes (e.g., life or death) require a greater degree of decisional capacity than less complex and less serious ones. When minors lack the capacity to make a specific healthcare decision, the appropriate substitute decision-maker (typically a parent) is given the responsibility of making the treatment decision and is held to a best interest standard in making such decisions.

In many cases, the capacity of youth (specifically in relation to treatment for SUD) with serious substance use disorder is likely significantly diminished, particularly in times of crisis. As has been discussed earlier in this chapter, addiction has been described as an impediment to informed decision-making regarding treatment for substance use disorders, and given the changing structure of the brain, such an addicted individual could well be said to be "coerced" into their drug-seeking and drug-taking behaviors by their addiction [69–71]. From an ethics perspective, this suggests that an individual with a serious substance use disorder may not have the ability to make a free and informed choice to stop using/seek treatment, as they would be experiencing coercion from their addiction. Short-term involuntary care for stabilization purposes is arguably a mechanism to help restore their capacity and therefore, ultimately, a means of respecting their autonomy [71]. It should be noted that while youth with serious substance use disorder may lack decisional capacity in some areas of their care, they may have capacity in relation to other aspects of their care, such as reproductive health, and thus promotion of autonomy requires recognizing that capacity is decision specific. Likewise, infringements on their freedoms should be limited to those necessary to realize the goals of treatment and not extended unnecessarily to other activities. This means that even in the context of stabilization or secure care, youth ought to be supported if they, for example, wish to leave the premises to smoke or take a walk.

Proportionality is also an important consideration and requires that any involuntary intervention must be proportional in terms of the anticipated benefits and risks of harm. While desperate situations may justify significant intrusions on freedoms, these same interventions may not be ethically permissible in situations where consequences were perhaps less severe or where the benefits were less likely to accrue. Moreover, it would be ethically problematic to design a system in which youth were routinely involuntarily placed in secure care when less restrictive approaches would likely be effective. This highlights the importance of providing a continuum of care to ensure access to the least intrusive services.

Intervention Does Not Cause Greater Harm Than It Seeks to Prevent (Non-maleficence)

While there is a duty to respect the youth's evolving autonomy, there is also a recognized societal duty to protect youth from harm (as outlined, for example, in child protection legislation). In the context of minors engaged in high-risk substance use, the duty to protect would reasonably seem to include taking steps to protect those youth from the significant risks of harm and death associated with that drug use. However, this does not translate into a license to involuntarily treat all youth who use substances. Although the anticipated benefits of involuntary interventions—for example, detoxification, assessment, stabilization (including improved decisional capacity), and connection with additional resources and supports—may be compelling, they must still be weighed against the risks associated with such interventions, including the risks associated with overriding the youth's evolving autonomy and preferences. Adolescence has been described as a "developmental stage when trust of adults comes grudgingly, must be earned, and can be lost at first betrayal." [72] In addition to the physical harms associated with treatment (e.g., withdrawal symptoms), erosion or loss of trust in the healthcare team and healthcare institutions and the implications this loss of trust has for the willingness and ability of the youth to seek medical care and form therapeutic relationships must also be considered when reflecting on harms associated with involuntary treatment. Similarly, the loss of freedom and restricted choice as well as the stigma associated with being labeled as an addict and involuntarily treated would need to be considered.

To summarize, in considering this element, it is important to acknowledge that our obligation to protect does not negate or reduce the significance of infringing a person's autonomy/right to self-determination. While some youth may later appreciate this approach and continue to engage in treatment, consideration must also be given to the outcomes of those who stop engaging with care or who never present for care, for fear that mandated treatment may be imposed on them.

Social Context and the Principle of Justice

On a related note, we must also consider the long-term implications of infringing on autonomy, particularly in the social contexts of past harms perpetuated by medical system on certain groups (e.g., indigenous; transgender population), and take steps to ensure that in striving to protect these youth, we are not replicating past harms or perpetuating trauma. Adopting a trauma-informed approach to care in this context would likely be helpful.

The last two criteria outlined below are rooted in the principle of justice. Justice includes, for example, our responsibilities to ensure that all people have equitable access to healthcare services and to fairly distribute resources. This also includes consideration of procedural justice, which involves, for example, transparency in decision-making and ensuring access to a fair appeal process.

Intervention Is Nondiscriminatory (Justice)

Where involuntary interventions are implemented, justice requires that the criteria on which such treatment would be based are clear, as this helps ensure that those who are being treated involuntarily are not being held to a higher standard than others who are similarly situated—or otherwise stated that "like cases are treated alike."

On a related note, justice considerations may be raised both in support of involuntary interventions for youth with serious substance use disorders and in terms of caution around concerns to be addressed if such an approach is implemented. For example, if substance use disorders disproportionately impact marginalized populations (e.g., indigenous people, those who are socioeconomically disadvantaged), then by failing to assertively intervene and treat these youth, are we neglecting our obligations or discriminating against these populations by not offering adequate care because of stigma or devaluation? Conversely, concerns may be raised that secure care may be used disproportionately with marginalized populations as a form of social control.

Intervention Is Fair (Justice)

The kinds of targeted interventions being considered in this chapter may form part of a response to the significant risks of harm to youth with serious substance use disorders. However, justice requires that these discussions take place within a broader effort to address the social determinants of health which are widely recognized as leading to health inequities in general and as also often being at the root of problematic substance use specifically. For example, personal and environmental risk factors that are known to increase likelihood of problematic substance use include (among others) exposure to problematic substance use in the home or peer networks, exposure to abuse or trauma, adverse childhood experiences, lack of parental support/supervision, poor academic performance, uncertain employment/loss of employment, early initiation of substance use, and experiences of racism and discrimination [73]. Tackling the profound health inequities in our society by addressing such broad social, environmental, and personal risk factors is undeniably complex and requires strong leadership, as well as coordinated and sustained efforts from all sectors of society.

Procedural justice is also relevant here. For example, explicit criteria should be established for treatment duration and discharge and clear processes put in place for individuals to appeal involuntary admission. More generally, the concerns outlined above help to highlight the importance of meaningful and effective consultation with stakeholders as part of the exploration and development of policy and procedures around involuntary treatment for youth with serious substance use disorders. Relevant stakeholders include, but are not limited to, youth with substance use disorders, parents of youth with substance use disorders, healthcare providers working with this population, risk management, and ethics. Representation of youth and parents with a variety of experiences with accessing substance use treatment services would be important in this process. Moreover, working in close partnership with key stakeholder groups at a broader system level to ensure any involuntary interventions are designed and implemented in a way that is nondiscriminatory and culturally competent is strongly recommended.

Conclusion

Given the rapidly rising incidence of opiate exposure and overdose among adolescents and the sum of the evidence regarding risk of subsequent overdose death and impaired cognition, there is a compelling need to adopt effective approaches to interrupting adolescent exposure to opiates. Youth experience persistent negative effect on cognition and judgment following exposure to opiates. Many youth who are exposed to opiates are homeless and disconnected from healthy adult relationships and will return immediately after resuscitation to the very high-risk environment from which he or she came if immediately discharged after resuscitation. This warrants new approaches to assertive management of youth who present with an opioid overdose. Unless there are compelling reasons not to, in most circumstances notification and engagement of the youth's parent or legal guardian is advisable, with admission to hospital for stabilization, involuntarily if necessary, is the most responsible first step in keeping the youth safe while allowing time to craft a care plan. Such a plan includes a thorough evaluation of mental health status, evaluation of associated medical or infectious complications, identification and optimization of community supports, discussion of substance use intervention treatment options, and implementation of a harm reduction strategy. When available, many adolescents who have engaged in opiate abuse or other life-endangering substance use may benefit from secure engagement in inpatient care. As with any involuntary engagement, significant ethical questions arise, which must be balanced against the real threat to the youth's life.

References

1. BC Coroners Service. Fentanyl-detected illicit drug overdose deaths, January 1, 2012, to March 31, 2019. Available at https://www2.gov.bc.ca/assets/gov/birth-adoption-death-marriage-and-divorce/deaths/coroners-service/statistical/fentanyl-detected-overdose.pdf. Viewed on 6/2/2019.
2. BC Coroners Service. Child mortality in British Columbia, 2016. Prepared by the Child death Review Unit of the British Columbia Coroners Service. Released May 2018. Available at https://www2.gov.bc.ca/assets/gov/birth-adoption-death-marriage-and-divorce/deaths/coroners-service/child-death-review-unit/reports-publications/child-mortality-2016.pdf. Viewed 6/2/2019.
3. Hedegaard H, Miniño AM, Warner M. Drug overdose deaths in the United States, 1999–2017. NCHS data brief no. 329. 2018. https://www.cdc.gov/nchs/products/databriefs/db329.htm.
4. Fentanyl contamination of other drugs is increasing overdose risk; content source: Centers for Disease Control and Prevention, National Center for Injury Prevention and Control, Division of Unintentional Injury Prevention. 2018, https://www.cdc.gov/drugoverdose/data/otherdrugs.html
5. Lankenau SE, Teti M, Silva K, Jackson Bloom J, et al. Initiation into prescription opioid misuse amongst young injection drug users. Int J Drug Policy. 2012;23(1):37–44.

6. Pradip K. Muhuri, Joseph C. Gfroerer, M. Christine Davies. Center for Behavioral Health Statistics and Quality (SBHSQ), Substance Abuse and Mental Health Administration (SAMHSA), Associations of Nonmedical Pain Reliever Use and Initiation of Heroin Use in the United States, August 2013. https://www.samhsa.gov/data/sites/default/files/DR006/DR006/nonmedical-pain-reliever-use-2013.htm.
7. Jordan CJ, Andersen SL. Sensitive periods of substance abuse: early risk for the transition to dependence. Dev Cogn Neurosci. 2017;25:33.
8. Santa Maria DM, Narendorf SC, Cross MB. Prevalence and correlates of substance use in homeless youth and young adults. J Addict Nurs. 2018;29(1):23–31.
9. Special Advisory Committee on the Epidemic of Opioid Overdoses. National report: apparent opioid-related deaths in Canada (January 2016 to March 2018) web-based report. Ottawa: Public Health Agency of Canada; 2018.
10. MMWR. Drug and opioid-involved overdose deaths – United States, 2013–2017. 2019. https://www.cdc.gov/mmwr/volumes/67/wr/mm675152e1.htm?s_cid=mm675152e1_w.
11. Caudarella A, Dong H, Milloy MJ, Kerr T, et al. Non-fatal overdose as a risk factor for subsequent fatal overdose among people who inject drugs. Drug Alcohol Depend. 2016;162:51–5.
12. Weiner SG, Baker O, Bernson D, Schuur JD. One-year mortality of opioid overdose victims who received Naloxone by Emergency Medical Services. Ann Emerg Med. 2017;70(4S)
13. Christenson J, Etherington J, Grafstein E, et al. Early discharge of patients with presumed opioid overdose: development of a clinical prediction rule. Acad Emerg Med. 2000;7:1110–8.
14. Rudolph MD, Miranda-Dominguez O, Cohen AO, Breiner K, Steinberg L, Bonnie RJ, et al. At risk of being risky: the relationship between "brain age" under emotional states and risk preference. Dev Cogn Neurosci. 2017;24:93–106.
15. Richer I, Bertrand K, Vandermeerschen J, Roy E. A prospective cohort study of non-fatal accidental overdose among street youth: the link with suicidal ideation. Drug Alcohol Rev. 2013;32:398–404.
16. Apfelbaum JL, Silverstein JH, Chung FF, Connis RT, Fillmore RB, Hunt SE, Nickinovich DG, Schreiner MS, Silverstein JH, Apfelbaum JL, Barlow JC, Chung FF, Connis RT, Fillmore RB, Hunt SE, Joas TA, Nickinovich DG, Schreiner MS; American Society of Anesthesiologists Task Force on Postanesthetic Care. Practice guidelines for postanesthetic care, an updated report by the American Society of Anesthesiologists Task Force on Postanesthetic Care. Anesthesiology, V 118 • No. 2. 2013.
17. Alderson P. Competent children? Minors' consent to health care treatment and research. Soc Sci Med. 2007;65(11):2272–83.
18. Weithorn L, Campbell S. The competency of children and adolescents to make informed treatment decisions. Child Dev. 1982;53:1589–98.
19. Etchells E, Sharpe G, Elliott C, Singer PA. Bioethics for clinicians: 3. Capacity. Can Med Assoc J. 1996;155(6)
20. Coughlin K. Medical decision-making in paediatrics: infancy to adolescence. Paediatr Child Health. 2018:138–46.
21. Johnson SB, Blum RW, Giedd JN. Adolescent maturity and the brain: the promise and pitfalls of neuroscience research in adolescent health policy. J Adolesc Health. 2009;45(3):216–21. https://www.ncbi.nlm.nih.gov/pmc/articles/PMC2892678/.
22. Blakemore S, Robbins T. Decision-making in the adolescent brain. Nat Neurosci. 2012;15(9):1184.
23. Peper JS, Dahl RE. Surging hormones: brain-behaviour interactions during puberty. Curr Dir Psychol Sci. 2013;22(2):134–9.
24. Blakemore S, Choudhury S. Development of the adolescent brain: implications for executive function and social cognition. J Child Psychol Psychiatry. 2006;47(3):296–312.
25. Goddings AL, et al. The influence of puberty on subcortical brain development. NeuroImage. 2014;88:242–51.
26. Fuhrmann D, Knoll LJ, Blakemore SJ. Adolescence as a sensitive period of brain development. Trends Cogn Sci. 2015;19(10):563.

27. Conrod PJ. Personality-targeted interventions for substance use and misuse. Curr Addict Rep. 2016;3:427.
28. Gould TJ. Addiction and cognition. Addict Sci Clin Pract. 2010;5(2):4–14.
29. Kerensky T, Walley AY. Opioid overdose prevention and naloxone rescue kits: what we know and what we don't know. Addict Sci Clin Pract. 2017;12(4):4.
30. Barash JA, Ganetsky M, Boyle K, Raman V, et al. Acute amnestic syndrome associated with fentanyl overdose. NEJM. 2018;378(12):1157–8.
31. O'Brien P, Todd J. Hypoxic brain injury following heroin overdose. Brain Impairment. 2009;10(2):169–79. https://doi.org/10.1375/brim.10.2.169.
32. Rapeli P, Kivisaari R, Autti T, Kahkonen S, Puskari V, Jokela O, et al. Cognitive function during early abstinence from opioid dependence: a comparison to age, gender and verbal intelligence matched controls. BMC Psychiatry. 2006;6:9.
33. Biernacki K, McLennan S, TerrettIzelle G, Labuschagne P. Decision-making ability in current and past users of opiates: a meta-analysis. Neurosci Biobehav Rev. 2016;71:342–51.
34. Arias F, Arnsten JH, Cunningham C, Coulehan K, et al. Neurocognitive, psychiatric, and substance use characteristics in opioid dependent adults. Addict Behav. 2016;60:137–43.
35. Kuntsi J, et al. Separation of cognitive impairments in attention deficit hyperactivity disorder into two familial factors. Arch Gen Psychiatry. 2010;67(11):1159–67.
36. Castenada AE, et al. A review on cognitive impairments in depressive and anxiety disorders with a focus on young adults. J Affect Disord. 2008;106(1–2):1–27.
37. A meta-analysis of depression severity and cognitive function. J Affect Disord. 2009;119(1–3):1–8.
38. Treatment of opioid use disorder for youth, guideline supplement. BC Center on Substance Use. Published June 13, 2018. p. 25. Available at http:/www.bccsu.ca/care-guidance-publications/.
39. Webster L. Risk factors for opioid-use disorder and overdose. Anesth Analg. 2017;125(5):1741–1748(8).
40. American Psychiatric Association. Diagnostic and statistical manual of mental disorders (DSM). 5th ed. Arlington: American Psychiatric Publishing; 2013.
41. U.S. Department of Health and Human Services (HHS), Office of the Surgeon General. Facing addiction in America: the surgeon General's report on alcohol, drugs, and health. Washington, DC: HHS; 2016. p. 3-1.
42. Volkow ND, et al. Neurobiologic advances from the brain disease model of addiction. NEJM. 2016;374(4):363–4.
43. Carter A, Hall W. Informed consent to opioid agonist maintenance treatment: recommended ethical guidelines. Int J Drug Policy. 2008;19:85.
44. Clinical practice guidelines for the BC Eating Disorders Continuum of Services. http://mh.providencehealthcare.org/sites/default/files/BC%20Eating%20Disorders%20Clinical%20Practice%20Guidelines.pdf. Accessed 28 Apr 2019.
45. Arcelus J, Mitchell AJ, Wales J, et al. Mortality rates in patients with anorexia nervosa and other eating disorders a meta-analysis of 36 studies. Arch Gen Psychiatry. 2011;68(7):724–31. https://doi.org/10.1001/archgenpsychiatry.2011.74.
46. Rafful C, Orozco R, Rangel G, Davidson P, et al. Increased non-fatal overdose risk associated with involuntary drug treatment in a longitudinal study with people who inject drugs. Addiction. 2018;113:1056–63.
47. Strang J, McCambridge J, Best D, Beswick T, et al. Loss of tolerance and overdose mortality after inpatient opiate detoxification: follow up study. BMJ. 2003;326:959–60.
48. BC Coroners Service. A review of overdose deaths in youth and young adults 2009–2013. A report to the Chief Coroner of British Columbia. January 2016. Accessed at https://www2.gov.bc.ca/assets/gov/birth-adoption-death-marriage-and-divorce/deaths/coroners-service/child-death-review-unit/reports-publications/overdose-death-youth-young-adult.pdf, on 4 June 2019.
49. Pritchard E, Mugavin J, Swan A. Compulsory treatment in Australia: a discussion paper on the compulsory treatment of individuals dependent on alcohol and/or other drugs; 2007. p. 170.

50. Werb D, Kamarulzaman A, Meacham MC, Rafful C, Fischer B, Strathdee SA, et al. The effectiveness of compulsory drug treatment: a systematic review. Int J Drug Policy. Elsevier BV. 2016;28:1–9. Available from https://doi.org/10.1016/j.drugpo.2015.12.005.
51. Wild TC, Roberts B, Cooper EL. Compulsory substance abuse treatment: an overview of recent findings and issues. European Addiction Research, 2002;8(2):84–93.
52. Broadstock M, Brinson D, Weston A. The effectiveness of compulsory, residential treatment of chronic alcohol or drug addiction in non-offenders: Health Services Assessment Collaboration (HSAC); 2008. p. 88.
53. Werb D, Kamarulzaman A, Meacham MC, Rafful C, Fischer B, Strathdee SA, et al. The effectiveness of compulsory drug treatment: a systematic review. Int J Drug Policy. Elsevier B.V. 2016;28:1–9. Available from https://doi.org/10.1016/j.drugpo.2015.12.005.
54. Lindahl ML, Öjehagen A, Berglund M. Commitment to coercive care in relation to substance abuse reports to the social services. A 2-year follow-up. Nord J Psychiatry. 2010;64(6):372–6.
55. Padyab M, Grahn R, Lundgren L. Drop-out from the Swedish addiction compulsory care system. Eval Program Plann. Elsevier Ltd. 2015;49:178–184. Available from https://doi.org/10.1016/j.evalprogplan.2014.12.016.
56. Pasareanu AR, Opsal A, Vederhus JK, Kristensen Ø, Clausen T. Quality of life improved following in-patient substance use disorder treatment. Health Qual Life Outcomes. 2015;13(1):1–8.
57. Dore G, Sinclair B, Murray R. Treatment resistant and resistant to treatment? Evaluation of 40 alcohol dependent patients admitted for involuntary treatment. Alcohol Alcohol. 2016;51(3):291–5.
58. Pasareanu AR, Vederhus JK, Opsal A, Kristensen Ø, Clausen T. Improved drug-use patterns at 6 months post-discharge from inpatient substance use disorder treatment: results from compulsorily and voluntarily admitted patients. BMC Health Serv Res. 2016;16(1):1–8.
59. Lundgren L, Blom B, Chassler D, Sullivan LM. Using register data to examine patterns of compulsory addiction treatment care in Sweden: program planning and methodological implications. Eval Program Plann. 2015;49:149–52.
60. Ekendahl M. Aftercare and compulsory substance abuse treatment: a venture with potential? Contemp Drug Probl An Interdiscip Q. 2007;34(1):137–62. Available from http://ovidsp.ovid.com/ovidweb.cgi?T=JS&PAGE=reference&D=psyc5&NEWS=N&AN=2011-14660-007.
61. Pasareanu AR, et al. Improved drug-use patterns at 6 months post-discharge from inpatient substance use disorder treatment: results from compulsorily and voluntarily admitted patients. BMC Health Serv Res. 2016;16:291.
62. Slopen N, Goodman E, Koenen K, Kubzansky L. Socioeconomic and other social stressors and biomarkers of cardiometabolic risk in youth: a systematic review of less studied risk factors. PLoS One. 2013;8(5)
63. Stewart E, Manion I, Davidson S, Cloutier P. Suicidal children and adolescents with first emergency room presentations: predictors of six-month outcome. J Am Acad Child Adolescent Psychiatry. 2001;40(5):580–7.
64. Sinha R. Chronic stress, drug use, and vulnerability to addiction. Ann N Y Acad Sci. 2008;1141:105–30.
65. Representative for Children and Youth. Paige's story: abuse, indifference and a Young life discarded. Victoria: Representative for Children and Youth; 2015.
66. Clark BA, Preto N, Everett B, Young JM, Virani A. An ethical perspective on the use of secure care for youth with severe substance use. CMAJ Can Med Assoc J. 2019;191(7):E195–6. https://doi.org/10.1503/cmaj.71504.
67. Beauchamp T, Childress J. Principles of biomedical ethics. 7thÂ ed. New York: Oxford University Press; 2013.
68. Hall W, Farrell M, Carter A. Compulsory treatment of addiction in the patient's best interests: more rigorous evaluations are essential. Drug Alcohol Rev. 2014;33:268–71. (Australia)
69. Volkow ND, Koob GF, McLellan AT. Neurobiologic advances from the brain disease model of addiction. N Engl J Med. 2016;374(4):363–71.

70. Caplan AL. Ethical issues surrounding forced, mandated, or coerced treatment. J Subst Abus Treat. 2006;31(2):117–20.
71. Caplan AL. Denying autonomy in order to create it: the paradox of forcing treatment upon addicts. Addiction. 2008;103(12):1919–21.
72. Kelley M. Refusals of treatment in adolescents and young adults. In: Diekema DS, Mercurio MR, Adam MB, editors. Clinical ethics in pediatrics: a case-based textbook: Cambridge University Press; 2011. p. 23–7, at 25.
73. Health Canada. Background document. public consultation on strengthening Canada's approach to substance use issues. Ottawa; 2018. Available at https://www.canada.ca/content/dam/hc-sc/documents/services/substance-use/canadian-drugs-substances-strategy/strengthening-canada-approach-substance-use-issue/strengthening-canada-approach-substance-use-issue.pdf.

Chapter 10
Providing Clinical Care to Youth Experiencing Homelessness

Eva Moore and Curren Warf

Introduction

Youth's Barriers to Accessing Care

Homeless youth commonly face significant challenges in addition to their lack of stable housing. Many LGBTQ youth have felt rejected by their family of origin[1]; immigrant, migrant, and refugee youth live in fear of apprehension and deportation; African American youth may have faced harassment by law enforcement officers; youth who have left multiple placements in foster care may feel that they will never be accepted.

Additionally, while literally homeless, young people are most vulnerable to escalating substance use, including injection drug use, as well as to exposure to sexually transmitted infections, skin problems, flair-ups of chronic disease (asthma, allergies, and other chronic medical problems), and other acute medical problems (injuries, infections, etc.).

Accessing medical care, in addition to meeting preventive, acute, and chronic medical needs, can provide a unique opportunity for linkage to other services. Connections with youth workers or outreach workers can introduce youth to

[1] A Practitioner's Resource Guide: Helping Families to Support Their LGBT Children; SAMHSA (Substance Abuse and Mental Health Services Administration), https://www.aap.org/en-us/advocacy-and-policy/aap-health-initiatives/Pages/LGBT-Resources.aspx (Accessed November 5, 2019)

E. Moore
Division of Adolescent Health and Medicine, Department of Pediatrics, University of British Columbia, Vancouver, BC, Canada
e-mail: eva.moore@cw.bc.ca

C. Warf (✉)
Department of Pediatrics (Retired), Division of Adolescent Health and Medicine, British Columbia Children's Hospital, University of British Columbia, Vancouver, BC, Canada

C. Warf, G. Charles (eds.), *Clinical Care for Homeless, Runaway and Refugee Youth*, https://doi.org/10.1007/978-3-030-40675-2_10

lower-risk environments and move youth toward engagement in school and stability of housing.

It is essential that those engaged in working with youth reject stereotyping or generalizations and get to know each unique individual. Clinic staff should maintain a posture of *nonjudgmental positive regard* when working with homeless youth including in cases when youth have not adhered to care plans.

Homeless youth may be more distrustful than other young people, more fearful of system involvement, and may come with a history of prior negative experiences that are transferred to the provider. Nonetheless, they are entitled to the same level of respect and confidentiality as other youth [1].

Circumstances of Homeless Youth and Opportunities for Intervention

Youth experiencing homelessness vary in their living environment and include youth who are literally homeless on the streets as well as those who are couch surfing from place to place, have insecure housing, or are staying in shelters. Some youth are members of homeless families. Some are "doubled up" with other families. Conditions for individual youth can be very fluid and shift between living on the streets, in parks, in abandoned buildings, in shelters, and with friends. All of these conditions make it challenging for youth to engage in many of the activities of housed youth including attending school (though many continue to do so), accessing medical care in traditional settings, or adhering to medical treatment.

Access to medical care is generally episodic and initiated only when there is an acute need. Youth may access care in emergency rooms, acute care centers, or walk-in clinics, utilizing a variety of services and locations leading to fragmented care. Adhering to treatment regimens which require regularly taking medications or engaging in other follow-up care can be highly challenging. Access to showers, laundry, clean clothing, and nutrition is problematic and can impact provider recommendations for how to care for oneself while sick or infectious. The most challenging group of youth who have the hardest time accessing health services are those who are literally homeless or "street living" youth [2]. By definition, they lack the stable and predictable environments and the consistent relationship and supervision of caring adults that young people need and deserve.

The longer youth remain on the street, the more likely they are to acculturate and the more barriers that will stand in their way. Their concrete health concerns, whether for major or minor problems, may be a critical link that can bring them into contact with a broader range of supportive and stabilizing services. Low barrier medical services that are linked to targeted social services can play a pivotal role in engaging these youth in services and taking initial steps to stabilization. Having positive experiences with clinical care and other services can create greater potential to address chronic health problems including accessing substance use and mental health services.

Given the complex needs of homeless youth, it is useful to provide medical care within an interdisciplinary setting, with sensitive and well-trained staff. In a team setting, case managers, youth workers, social workers, or others may be available to help build a relationship with the youth, address their specific needs, and facilitate stabilization. (*See* Chap. 4.)

Developmental Considerations

Youth who are homeless may initially appear to be more independent than similarly aged peers and may be engaged in some behaviors associated with adults, including sexual activity and alcohol and other drug use. However, the reality is that they are extremely vulnerable and poorly prepared for adult life. They may be behind in school, have a history of significantly traumatic experiences with emotional consequences, commonly face the loss or rejection of their families, and continue to struggle with their emerging sense of identity and place in the world. Given the common history of rejection and loss that they have faced, there are frequently initial barriers to developing trust and accepting services. These developmental challenges are more accentuated among youth with cognitive problems [3] (including the legacy of fetal alcohol effects), learning disabilities, and emotional and mental health problems. Through fostering caring relationships with clinicians, youth workers, and outreach and social workers, housing stabilization, and engagement in school or employment, much of this distrust can be overcome.

The Clinical Environment and Encounter

Given the lack of structure in the lives of most homeless youth, it is important that clinical services have available times for walk-in appointments, particularly for new patients who may be hesitant to come to the clinic. Walk-in healthcare appointments can improve accessibility for patients, and extended hours into the early evening encourage continuing engagement in school or employment.

It is important to establish whether the youth has a place to stay and if they will be in a safe environment and have access to regular meals after they leave the clinic. These concerns offer opportunities for engagement. Clinic staff should be notified immediately if youth need referrals to facilitate prompt response and access to a shelter or drop-in center.

Any clinic that offers health services to homeless youth needs to create a welcoming, accepting, and supportive environment for young people of diverse sexual orientations, gender identities and expressions, cultural and religious backgrounds, ethnicities and colors, immigration status, and other backgrounds. Including youth in the design and decorating of the clinical waiting area can be valuable. A welcoming environment can be developed through including posters portraying diverse young people of varied colors, ethnicities, cultures and gender expression, and multilingual educational materials. Similarly, including youth-specific health information and brochures in the examining room and including material for same sex, opposite sex, and gender diverse youth communicates an openness and acceptance of young people who may have had difficulty accessing services in other environments. Rainbow and gender diversity flags or decals on room doors or bulletin boards can indicate openness and acceptance [4].

When feasible, it is preferable to have specific waiting areas for adolescents and young adults. Youth who are homeless, particularly those new to the streets, find waiting areas with homeless adults to be frightening and uncomfortable and may expose youth to individuals with more advanced mental health and substance use problems. On the flip side, adolescents may not feel welcome in a pediatric clinic decorated for young children. Young children and their families may be uncomfortable waiting with adolescents. Youth-specific waiting areas can frequently be created by having designated youth clinic hours and by including educational materials, posters, and other decor that reflect young people's interests.

In some clinics, designating one or more specific examination rooms to meet the health education needs of youth is possible. The examination room should be large enough to accommodate a companion of the youth if they bring someone and the examination table should always be facing away from the room door. Relevant health education materials on hygiene, contraception, STIs, condom use, hotline phone numbers, and local youth drop-in center information, hours and locations should be made available.

Youth may come with a friend, family member, or youth worker, and the youth may want the presence of this supportive person in the room with them at the time of the health visit. A youth's preference for a supportive person present should be prioritized, but the provider may also need to ask them to leave and not assume that confidential and personal issues may be discussed in front of this person. Alternatively, an advocate for the youth may be made available at the clinic to provide emotional support given how overwhelming the healthcare experience may be.

Organizing Care

Many vulnerable youth may not seek primary or preventative care and may only present to the medical system in crisis. Overuse of emergency departments, walk-in clinics, and/or urgent care centers is common for many homeless and at-risk youth reflecting the chaos and uncertainty of their lives. Any contact with the healthcare system should be seen as an opportunity to engage the youth in their healthcare. Immunizations, contraception, STI testing and treatment, and other primary care measures should be offered at each healthcare encounter, even in emergency settings.

While youth should be directed to and educated on the benefits of a medical home and having their own primary care provider, consistent care at one location may not be feasible or seen as valuable to the youth. Youth and their adult allies should be encouraged to take charge of their own healthcare information – such as medication names and dosing, consultant physician names and phone numbers, test results, and follow-up plans – which can be lost between healthcare systems. Youth who have smartphones can use note pages, calendars, and contact pages to organize their medical care (see "Just TRAC it"[2] for ideas). Simple pen and paper or business cards can also be used in this way. Support workers may need to manage this for their youth clients, as many homeless youth will not have the capacity to organize their health information and will not be able to maintain a smartphone and/or paperwork.

Meeting the Youth Experiencing Homelessness: The First Encounter

Homeless youth frequently have poor access to medical care and have differing personal barriers to accepting care; many enter with preconceptions of the clinic and an initial level of distrust, while other youth may have had very positive experiences with physicians, nurses, and other clinical staff and be comfortable and open.

Youth should be met with warmth and a smile and welcomed. One can acknowledge how difficult it may have been to come into the clinic. Youth may be accompanied by a parent or caregiver, social worker, or youth worker, and the youth may want the presence of this supportive person in the room with them at the time of the medical visit.

Keep in mind that the young person is coming to the clinic either to get help for a concrete problem or on the advice of someone who has picked up on their situation. The clinician is there to be a knowledgeable and caring resource. There is no expectation or desire on the part of the youth that the clinician dresses like, speaks like, or behaves like an adolescent.

Communication

(*See* Chap. 3.)

Many of the issues addressed in the medical evaluation and examination are sensitive, and the history taking, examination, counseling, and teaching should be provided in a confidential setting taking care not to convey judgment or blame.

The focus of the clinician's attention should be on the youth; note-taking during the interview should be minimized as this can pose a barrier to the relationship and communication. Appointments with youth should be uninterrupted as much as possible. Frequent interruptions can interfere with understanding and communication.

It is essential to remain focused on what the young person is saying, ask questions that show that you understand his or her concerns, help elaborate on their concerns, and reflect back what you understand. Being dismissive of the youth's

[2] BC Children's Hospital, Just TRAC it, viewed at http://www.bcchildrens.ca/our-services/support-services/transition-to-adult-care/just-trac-it

concerns through tone of voice, body language, or use of words gives a clear message that you don't care about him or her. Empathetic comments that acknowledge their experiences like "I'm sorry you had to go through that…" can enable youth to appreciate that you have listened to them.

Acknowledge and accentuate the authentic positive characteristics that you see in the youth such as their resourcefulness; their willingness to get help; the care they express for their friends, family, or pet; and their artistic creativity, humor, or emotional insight.

Don't lecture them on what they are doing wrong. Hold off on giving advice until you are sure you understand what you are being asked. Make sure to maintain a nonjudgmental tone. Don't express judgments of parents, even if the youth expresses anger at them; emotional connections with parents almost invariably continue to be strong, even for youth who have been maltreated.

Interpreters

Some youth and their parents may not be fluent in English, and an interpreter may need to be used. It is best practice to use professional interpreters if personal information is covered. Do not use children as interpreters beyond answering concrete questions such as locating the restroom.

Hidden Disabilities and Challenges

Be alert for hidden disabilities such as cognitive deficits, educational deficits, and mental health problems. Traumatic histories are common and frequently difficult to talk about and may have shaped much of the young person's life. Cognitive, emotional, and mental health problems, effects of trauma, and insecurity of housing may affect the ability of the young person to understand clinical advice or follow through with recommendations. Youth may struggle to communicate. Many traumatized youth have great difficulty in direct communication, and homeless youth suffer disproportionately from developmental challenges, traumatic brain injuries, and learning difficulties, further impacting communication. The young person's body language should be attended to including eye contact, tearfulness, facial expressions, and posture.

Getting to Know the Young Person

Particularly at the first encounter, when trust has not yet been established, it may be useful to help the youth identify the problem that they would first like to address. Based on the urgency of the medical need and the receptivity of the youth, a thorough history and psychosocial assessment may need to be deferred. The connection that is made with the young person is more important than the thoroughness of the social history that is obtained. Try to address and resolve the concrete problems a youth brings and involve clinic staff and/or an outreach worker as needed. Schedule an early follow-up appointment for ongoing care to build confidence and trust and address medical needs.

Awareness of One's Own Biases

Providers and clinic staff need to be aware of their own biases that can inadvertently create barriers for youth. Homeless young people may come to clinic poorly dressed, unwashed, and disheveled and possibly intoxicated. Their dress style may be a kind of self-expression or statement that is unappreciated by the examiner. Some youth may be withdrawn and uncommunicative. They may be socially isolated and have been ignored and treated badly on the streets. Their social skills may be limited. All of these factors may lead the examiner to form an initial impression at odds with the vulnerability and potential of the young person.

Ethnic Minority Youth

African American and Native American (indigenous) youth are overrepresented among homeless young people and have likely experienced discrimination and bias on the streets or in other settings. Given youths' vulnerability, clinical staff need to establish a warm, welcoming, affirming, and nonjudgmental environment for all homeless young people [5].

Lesbian, Gay, Bisexual, Transgender, and Questioning (LGBTQ) Youth

Gay, lesbian, bisexual, nonbinary, transgender, and questioning (LGBTQ) youth are disproportionately represented among homeless youth and may have had previous negative experiences with services and felt ridiculed, victimized, or excluded. Clinicians should not presume sexual orientation or gender identity. Sexual behaviors do not always correspond to sexual orientation. Many youth who identify as heterosexual have had sexual experiences with the same sex, and many youth who identify as gay or lesbian have had, or continue to have, sexual relations with the opposite gender [4].

Homophobia refers to an irrational fear and resulting hatred of homosexuality and is pervasive in our culture; it is reflected in higher rates of bullying and violence suffered by sexual minority youth and may lead to self-destructive behaviors. Heterosexism is the expectation that heterosexuality is the expected norm and that LGBTQ youth are "abnormal"; heterosexism is more insidious and more damaging, particularly for adolescents' development of their self-image [4].

Clinicians need to have offices that are not only youth friendly but also welcoming to sexual and gender minority youth. Being gay, lesbian, or gender diverse is not in itself a risk factor, and the majority of LGBTQ youth emerge as adults without significant increase in risk behaviors compared to other youth and as adults lead to happy and productive lives [4].

All young people, regardless of sexual or gender identity, need to know how to express their sexuality in healthy ways, avoid STIs, and avoid unwanted pregnancy. Healthcare providers can play an important role in opening these discussions.

Adolescents who are open about their LGBTQ orientation, or even perceived to be LGBTQ, commonly face verbal harassment or physical threats at school, avoid attending school, or drop out of school because of perceived risk of violence. Sometimes assaults on gay or transgender youth result in homicide; in other cases, there are increased risk of mental health disorders and suicide [4] (*See* Chap. 15). Resources for youth who have been bullied or victimized can be found at "It Gets Better."[3]

Given the disproportionate representation of LGBTQ youth among youth experiencing homelessness, it is important that clinicians caring for them convey acceptance and affirm their feelings, including of gender dysphoria when appropriate, and make appropriate referrals when needed. Obtaining a confidential, thorough, developmentally appropriate history allows for the recognition and affirmation of strengths and assets as well as risks [4]. Clinicians can refer to the American Academy of Pediatrics (AAP) materials which include modules on caring for LGBT youth from the National LGBT Health Education Center of the Fenway Institute for Education and Learning.[4,5,6]

If a young person hasn't yet "come out" to friends or family members, they may need support. Parental support for their adolescent children in affirming their sexual orientation and gender identity is an important factor in reducing risk behavior, suicidality, drug use, and depression; negative parental responses are associated with increased risk behaviors [4]. Organizations such as Parents, Families and Friends of Lesbians and Gays can provide valuable resources.[7,8]

Prior or Existing Medical Care

If the youth has an existing source of accessible primary medical care or a medical home, verify that it is still accessible and if he or she would prefer to return to the prior clinic. Common barriers include the lack of health insurance, physical dis-

---

[3] http://www.itgetsbetter.org/

[4] American Academy of Pediatrics, LGBT Resources, https://www.aap.org/en-us/advocacy-and-policy/aap-health-initiatives/Pages/LGBT-Resources.aspx (Accessed November 5, 2019)

[5] National LGBT Health Education Center, Fenway Institute https://www.lgbthealtheducation.org/lgbt-education/learning-modules/ (Accessed November 5, 2019)

[6] Creating a Welcoming and Safe Environment for LGBT People and Families; GLMA Health Professionals Advancing LGBTQ Equality. http://www.glma.org/index.cfm?fuseaction=page.viewPage&pageID=1031&nodeID=1 (Accessed November 5, 2019)

[7] www.pflag.org

[8] Gay Family Support http://www.gayfamilysupport.com

tance or lack of transportation, or inadequate resources at the existing clinic to address their health needs given their current circumstances.

For homeless youth who remain in school, school-based clinics may be available which the young person can utilize. Well-resourced school-based clinics may have access to social workers and nurses and be well-situated to engage parents and extended family members or other supportive adults.

Youth Presenting with Emergent Medical Conditions

Youth who present to the clinic with a life-endangering or other emergent issue must be quickly evaluated and referred to the closest emergency department (ED) by ambulance as indicated.

Common emergent medical and psychiatric issues include acute suicide risk, psychosis, serious acute injuries, recent sexual assault, and opiate overdose.

All clinics serving homeless youth should have naloxone kits on-site with staff trained in their use[9]; all youth with significant opioid overdose should be referred to the closest emergency department after naloxone has been administered. With the current prevalence of fentanyl and other synthetic opioids, potentially lethal overdoses can occur unintentionally with the use of fentanyl-contaminated marijuana, amphetamines, cocaine, or other drugs. Given the high potency of fentanyl, multiple doses of naloxone may need to be administered, and sufficient observation time after administration may be required, depending on the dose administered for reversal.

Youth who come to clinic after a recent (under 72 to 96 hours) sexual assault should be immediately referred to the appropriate emergency department with capacity for forensic evaluation and evidence collection.

(*See* Chaps. 14 and 15.)

Consent, Confidentiality, and Reporting of Child Maltreatment

All health professionals, including physicians, nurses, and social workers, have a legal responsibility to contact child protective services or the police if there is disclosure by a minor or significant suspicion of child abuse or severe neglect. If available, a social worker should be involved when reporting disclosures of child maltreatment and when interacting with child protective services. Many youth

[9] Reference to BC CDC http://www.bccdc.ca/resource-gallery/Documents/Guidelines%20and%20Forms/Guidelines%20and%20Manuals/Epid/Other/BC%20Overdose%20Prevention%20Services%20Guide_Jan2019_Final.pdf and CDC protocols https://www.cdc.gov/drugoverdose/prevention/reverse-od.html

experiencing homelessness have a history of involvement with child protective services and may have an existing social worker.

The clinician should be clear with the patient about both their right to confidentiality and the limits of confidentiality and communicate requirements for mandatory reporting regarding concerns for safety. This can be a very difficult conversation with the youth; it is important to be transparent regarding one's legal responsibilities and explicit about the goal of assuring their safety.

Minors have rights to confidentiality regarding consensual sexual relations, substance use, and other sensitive matters, though there are limitations related to age discrepancy of sexual partners and disclosure of intrafamilial sexual abuse. Laws governing mandated reporting requirements in the United States vary state by state. These issues are frequently difficult to negotiate and the youth may be angry and/or need support.

Victims of Sexual Exploitation and Sex Trafficking

Youth who are surviving on the streets without a means of support are at very high risk for involvement in "survival sex" and commercial sexual exploitation. Sexual exploitation affects both males and females; LGBTQ youth are at highest risk for involvement among youth experiencing homelessness.

Studies indicate that the age of entry into sex trafficking and commercial sexual exploitation may be as young as 12 to 16 years when youth are most vulnerable to manipulation and have limited life experience [6]. There is some dispute regarding age of entry, with more recent studies indicating that the median age for entry into commercial sexual exploitation was 18 years [7]; variation may be ascribed to differences in samples.

Commercial sexual exploitation is "any sex act in which anything of value is given or received by any person" [7]. Commercial sexual exploitation of a minor includes "crimes of a sexual nature committed against juvenile victims for financial or other economic reasons…include trafficking for sexual purposes, prostitution, sex tourism, pornography, stripping and performing in sexual venues" [6]. In the United States, adolescents under age 18 involved in commercial sexual exploitation do not need to have been subject to force, fraud, deception, or coercion to legally be considered a victim of a crime. As a caution, though commercial sexual exploitation of a minor is an offense under federal law, in some states, youth who have been engaged in commercial sex, or survival sex, are evaluated as being "prostitutes" and treated more as criminals than victims, reducing the likelihood that they will receive the services they need and resulting in reentry into sex trafficking and escalating risk behaviors [8].

Sexual exploitation and sex trafficking expose young people to emotional trauma, potential for assault, exposure to sexually transmitted infections, and high risk for involvement in serious substance use.

In the clinical setting, the patient should be told that he or she is not required to answer any questions, helping give them a sense of control of the interview process. The youth should be interviewed away from those accompanying him or her and must be listened to carefully for concerns about safety. Patients who have been victims of commercial sexual exploitation may present medically for treatment of sexual assault or other physical injury, drug overdose, or other complication, for reproductive health, or to meet other needs. The youth may have been told to lie about his or her circumstances [6]. The clinician needs to be aware of the sensitivity surrounding these issues and the vulnerability the youth may feel, as well as the real danger youth may be in, proceed carefully through the interview process, and ensure that they know the resources youth may need when issues are disclosed. Physicians should become familiar with state-specific laws governing child sexual exploitation [9]. The Institute of Medicine has issued a report on ethical issues related to reporting commercial sexual exploitation of children [6, 8].

Setting the Stage for Medical Evaluation and Management

Interviewing the Patient and Obtaining a Medical History

A thorough social and medical history may or may not be possible or reasonable on the first encounter because of time considerations, reservations of the youth, and his or her tolerance for a long interview. A good place to start is to identify the principal concern of the youth that has brought him or her to clinic, such as a concern about STIs, a need for contraception, an acute injury, or a specific symptom.

Safety concerns should always be prioritized and reviewed, in particular, whether the youth has a safe place to sleep and is interested in locating a drop-in center or shelter.

The HEADSS or SHADDES interview models provide a reasonably time-efficient approach to conducting a “psychosocial biopsy” and identifying key stabilization issues to be addressed. (*See* Chap. 3.)

Acknowledging Patient Strengths

It is important to ask about, and acknowledge, patient strengths as part of the assessment (close relationships; attendance in school; interests in sports, arts, etc.); if the youth cannot identify any, the interviewer can acknowledge their courage in coming to the clinic, their resourcefulness in addressing the challenges they have confronted while homeless, or specific and concrete items that came up during the interview. The acknowledgement of strengths allows one to help build youth’s confidence, encourage continuity of care, and end with a positive and hopeful component in what is commonly a stressful experience for the youth. (*See* Chap. 3.)

Chaperones

Institutions have different policies regarding use of chaperones; it is important that clinicians follow institutional guidelines, respecting patients' comfort, privacy, and perception of safety [10], while being attentive to their own professional concerns regarding potential vulnerability. It is recommended that male and female examiners have chaperones for all breast, pelvic, and genital exams. The chaperone may need to be introduced to the patient as a reassuring person who can assist or provide support if the patient wishes. The name of the chaperone should be recorded in the medical chart. Chaperones, with the exception of those assisting the exam, should always be positioned at the head of the bed. Peers or adult allies of the youth from outside the clinic should never be used as chaperones.

Physical Examination

The examination may need to be problem-focused. It is important to appreciate and respect patient modesty, and it may not be possible or necessary to complete a breast or genital exam. In conducting the examination, it is reassuring to provide the reasons for examining various parts of the body and to make reassuring comments about the normalcy of findings.

Accommodation to modesty can be made by focusing on the elements of the examination most pertinent to the complaint, examining parts of the body serially and not asking the young patient to unclothe completely. A drape can be provided so that the youth can be partially covered during the examination. There may be additional sensitivities for youth who have experienced sexual assault or abuse.

Signs of personal neglect and lack of access to routine healthcare are common and include poor dental hygiene, untreated caries, and other oral problems reflecting poor access to dental care. In addition, youth need vision screening and funding and referral for corrective lenses if visual acuity is poor.

Dermatological exam may show presence of various infections related to neglect, lack of hygiene, trauma, use of drugs, or other more routine problems such as acne.

There may be signs of poorly managed or untreated chronic medical problems such as asthma or diabetes.

Genital and Gynecologic Exam

The genital exam is an important part of the physical exam. It can identify findings of STIs and other infections and evaluate for pelvic inflammatory disease, as well as the potential for testicular tumors in biologic males. For some youth, genital exams can be embarrassing; for youth who have experienced sexual assault, genital examinations may trigger traumatic memories. Youth with gender diversity may feel shame or severe dysphoria with parts of the exam. If the patient expresses a desire for a specific gender examiner, that preference should be respected when possible; if not, the exam may need to be rescheduled.

During a genital examination, the clinician should always explain the reason for the exam, provide verbal reassurance about the normalcy of findings, and approach the examination in a neutral, efficient matter-of-fact way. Be aware of judgmental language, such as "everything looks good," and instead say "everything looks normal." Conduct the examination efficiently, without delays, and discontinue the examination if the patient indicates that they want to stop.

Consider using gender-neutral terms for body parts, especially for youth with gender diversity, for example, internal genitalia instead of vagina, chest instead of breast, and external genitalia instead of penis or labia.

The rectal exam can usually be omitted unless specifically indicated. Youth engaging in anal sex may have physical finding suggestive of infection which often requires more intensive treatment regimens and indicates different risk stratification. Youth can self-collect samples if clinician examination is declined by the patient.

If there has been a recent sexual assault (generally recognized to be within 72 to 96 hours depending on local guidelines), the patient should not be examined at the outpatient clinic but referred for a forensic examination to the local qualified specialty clinic commonly located in a specified emergency department. Gynecologic examination can interfere with evidence collection [11]. Biologic females who have been sexually assaulted should be provided emergency contraception. (*See* Chap. 14.)

The US Centers for Disease Control and Prevention (CDC) has issued guidelines for testing and treatment of sexually transmitted infections in cases of acute sexual assault [12]. These include testing for *Chlamydia trachomatis*, *Neisseria gonorrhoeae*, syphilis, *Trichomonas vaginalis*, HIV, and hepatitis B and hepatitis C as well as a pregnancy test for females. Presumptively treat chlamydia, gonorrhea, and trichomonas (if pregnancy test is negative) and provide postexposure prophylaxis for HIV when indicated. Vaccines for hepatitis B and HPV should be considered. If the youth has not had hepatitis B vaccine, hepatitis B immune globulin may be considered. (*See* Chap. 12.)

Clinical Management Considerations

Clinical management guidelines for homeless youth are fundamentally the same as for those youth who are housed. However, multiple factors can interfere with the ability to prioritize medical problems and adhere to treatment recommendations including the absence of shelter or instability of living arrangements, lack of adult supervision, a history of trauma and loss, presence of mental health or substance use problems, and dealing with the social threats of discrimination and hostility [3].

Medical problems can be managed following standard recommendations. Keep prescriptions, recommendations, and scheduling as simple as possible while retaining efficacy, and when possible use single-dose observed treatments; if not possible, use the least frequent dosage for the shortest period feasible and schedule a prompt follow-up appointment.

Contraception

Contraception, including emergency contraception, should be offered and dispensed at no cost. In particular, emergency contraceptive pills should be available on-site. Contraceptive counseling to assess youths' knowledge and provide information about options should be provided to help youth select the most acceptable method. As with all sexually active females, long-acting reversible contraceptives (LARC) should be promoted, and efforts should be made to provide LARC on-site. Information about contraceptive options should be offered in a straightforward, nonjudgmental manner; pregnancy counseling should be provided when needed and youth should be referred for pregnancy support services or safe and legal termination. Clinicians need to know their local laws and resources. *Contraceptive technology*[10] is an excellent clinical reference book for current contraceptive methods. (*See* Chap. 11.)

Condoms (both external and internal) should be distributed and made readily available in the waiting room and exam rooms. Youth should see a health worker or health educator, if available at the clinic, to review the use of condoms and address any specific questions.

Sexually Transmitted Infections

Urine and serological screening for STIs should be provided for all youth who have been sexually active; treatment and management should follow applicable guidelines (e.g., protocols from the US CDC[11] or British Columbia CDC[12]). Single-dose treatments are preferable and partner treatment is recommended; if there are multiple partners, an appropriate number of doses of medications should be dispensed for partner treatment, and an attempt should be made to encourage the partners to come to the clinic.

Complications of STIs, in particular pelvic inflammatory disease (PID), are not uncommon in young homeless women and can have life-altering complications of

[10] http://www.contraceptivetechnology.org/the-book/

[11] CDC Centers for Disease Control and Prevention, Sexually Transmitted Infections; https://www.cdc.gov/std/default.htm Accessed June 23, 2019

[12] British Columbia Centre for Disease Control, Sexually Transmitted Infections; http://www.bccdc.ca/health-professionals/clinical-resources/communicable-disease-control-manual/sexually-transmitted-infections. Accessed June 23, 2019

impaired fertility and/or ectopic pregnancy. Low clinical threshold for diagnosis and treatment of PID is important in high-risk populations. Clinical suspicion of PID needs to be treated with a completed course of appropriate antibiotics, including dispensing antibiotics for partner treatment when consistent with guidelines. Inpatient treatment should be considered for all adolescents with PID, given the risk of infertility, to assure adequate adherence and completion of treatment. If outpatient treatment is provided, it is advisable to ask the youth to identify someone who can help remind her to take the scheduled medications and assure that treatment is complete with prompt medical follow-up. (*See* Chap. 12.)

HIV

Frequency of HIV testing depends on risk status and exposure. All youth who are at high risk for HIV infection related to sexual or drug use practices should be tested every 3–6 months according to CDC guidelines[13] and encouraged to use pre-exposure prophylaxis (PreP).[14] Those youth who have a risk of exposure to HIV in the previous 72 hours should be given postexposure prophylaxis (PEP).[15] (*See* Chap. 13.)

Youth who are positive for HIV should be referred to an appropriate clinic with the resources to manage and monitor their status over time.

Hepatitis C

Youth who have multiple sexual partners, who are engaged in survival sex, or who have a history of injection drug use are at increased risk for hepatitis C. Risk increases with time, so that a young person who has begun injection drug use has cumulative increased risk if he or she continues and shares needles.[16]

Dermatologic Concerns

Dermatologic complaints are common including acne, minor infections, injuries, and infestations (including lice and scabies). Supplies for treatment should be dispensed on-site when possible with sufficient supplies provided for partners. Youth should be referred for showers and laundry for clothing and bedding to prevent reinfection (*See* Chap. 16).

[13] CDC HIV Testing in Clinical Settings; https://www.cdc.gov/hiv/testing/clinical/index.html Accessed Oct 7 2019

[14] USCDC, https://www.cdc.gov/hiv/basics/prep.html (Accessed Oct.3, 2019)

[15] USCDC, https://www.cdc.gov/hiv/basics/pep.html (Accessed Oct 3, 2019)

[16] CDC Viral Hepatitis, Professional Resources https://www.cdc.gov/hepatitis/hcv/profresourcesc.htm Accessed November 10, 2019

Dermatological findings can indicate systemic disease including syphilis. Be up to date on local syphilis epidemics, as youth, sex workers, men who have sex with men, and transgender females are especially vulnerable in syphilis epidemics. The threshold for suspicion should be very low, and youth need to be screened, particularly those with multiple sexual partners or engaged in survival sex.

Signs of battery and of self-injury can also be found with the dermatological examination and can raise concerns about the safety of the young person. For minors, reporting mandates to child protective services or the police may be triggered if there is a suspicion of interpersonal violence or sexual abuse. If signs suspicious of battery are found, it is important to thoroughly document findings, including photographing lesions, particularly of minors, in the event of a forensic evaluation. All victims of battery should be given a high priority for immediate shelter.

Injection Drug Use

Some youth may present with needle tracks raising concern regarding the use of injection drugs. Injection drug users commonly have complications of cellulitis and abscesses and are at very high risk for endocarditis, sepsis, and systemic infections. While these youth may benefit from engaging in substance use treatment programs, you need to assess their readiness and refer when appropriate. Youth continuing to use injection drugs should be referred to safe injection sites and needle exchange programs if available. Youth who are engaged in opiate use can be offered opioid agonist treatment. Suboxone is considered first line for youth with moderate to severe opioid use disorder. Other opioid agonist treatment, such as methadone, long-acting morphine, injectable buprenorphine, and/or injectable full opioid agonists, may alternatively be indicated, where available.[17] Providers treating youth with opioid dependency should complete buprenorphine training, available free,[18] to be able to serve the needs of their patient population (*See* Chaps. 8 and 9).

Immunizations

Youth who have been on the streets and out of school, as well as refugee and migrant youth, may be behind in their vaccinations. It is important to provide immunizations on-site or refer to an appropriate clinic so that all youth are up to date with immunizations for hepatitis B, hepatitis A,[19] HPV, DPT, MMR, varicella, meningococcal,

---

[17] See BC Centre for Substance Use Clinical Care Guidance, at https://www.bccsu.ca/clinical-care-guidance/ and SAMHSA's FInd Treatment Resources page https://www.samhsa.gov/find-treatment

[18] Free training and provider resources available at Providers Clinical Support System, at https://pcssnow.org/

[19] Grading of Recommendations, Assessment, Development, and Evaluation (GRADE) for Hepatitis A Vaccine for Persons Experiencing Homelessness, CDC https://www.cdc.gov/vaccines/

pneumococcal[20] vaccine, and polio. Homeless youth should receive annual influenza vaccines. Youth usually need documentation of immunization status for school enrollment, and immunizations may need to be duplicated if documentation is not readily available.

The US CDC[21] and the BCCDC[22] are excellent references for vaccine recommendations.

Tuberculosis Screening

Homeless persons are at high risk for infection with tuberculosis. Homeless youth need to have a written record of PPD status. Many shelters require documentation of negative status, or history of treatment, to accept youth. This can be difficult to arrange given that there is a minimum of 48 hours waiting period to read the results of the test. Many agencies recommend testing every 6 months for literally homeless people.

Some migrants from high prevalence areas may have a history of BCG vaccine which commonly results in a positive skin test to PPD and leaves ambiguity of evidence of TB. Though there is some evidence of efficacy, the CDC recommends that all patients with positive PPD receive treatment regardless of a history of BCG.[23] Management guidelines continue to evolve, and the CDC website should be checked for current recommendations.

Management of Chronic Medical Conditions

Youth with chronic medical conditions including insulin-dependent diabetes or asthma may benefit from referral to an accessible specialty clinic; however, many homeless youth have difficulty negotiating the processes of complex medical systems and need to be treated in the local clinic with specialty consultation as available. These conditions are very challenging for youth to manage under the best of circumstances and much more so in the event of unstable housing and lack of adult supervision. When homeless, medications may be lost or stolen and need to be replenished. Arrangements may be made to keep them at a youth drop-in center or

acip/recs/grade/hav-homeless.html

[20] Standing Orders for Administering Pneumococcal Polysaccharide Vaccine to Children and Teens Purpose, https://www.immunize.org/catg.d/p3075a.pdf (Accessed Oct 4, 2019)

[21] CDC Immunizaton Schedule https://www.cdc.gov/vaccines/schedules/hcp/imz/child-adolescent.html

[22] BC CDC Immunization schedule http://www.bccdc.ca/resource-gallery/Documents/Guidelines%20and%20Forms/Guidelines%20and%20Manuals/Epid/CD%20Manual/Chapter%202%20-%20Imms/Part_1_Schedules.pdf

[23] https://www.cdc.gov/tb/topic/basics/vaccines.htm

youth shelter. These youth need frequent follow-up, access to medical supplies, and active case management with persistent attempts to stabilize housing.

In the United States, all youth, in particular those with chronic medical conditions, should be referred to, and assisted with, enrollment in Medicaid or other public health insurance, in accordance with state-specific eligibility requirements.

Management of Mental Health Problems

Youth who are homeless have very commonly experienced significant trauma and loss and at presentation to the new clinician may seem depressed, incommunicative, anxious, or distrustful. In addition, youth on the street are at very high risk for continuing trauma as long as their living situation remains unsafe and unstable. The single most important intervention in most cases is to stabilize housing and provide safety and security. Many drop-in centers, shelters, and transitional housing programs can provide access to experienced mental health practitioners and help with referrals to other supportive services.

When feasible, youth should be linked with evidence-based interventions for mental health treatment and provided with short-term, problem-focused interventions to support healing. Trauma-informed approaches recognize the role trauma plays in the lives of youth and shift the clinical perspective from "what's wrong with you" to "what happened to you" by recognizing and accepting difficult behaviors as strategies developed to cope with childhood trauma. A trauma-informed approach focuses on creating safe, accepting, and respectful environments to help youth heal from the effects of trauma and teaches youth skills to improve coping; manage emotions; connect with others; and find hope, purpose, and meaning.[24]

Starting Psychotropic Medications

Psychotropic medications should only be introduced when there is a clarity of diagnosis; identified targeted symptoms; ability to clinically follow the patient by the prescriber, social worker, or caseworker; informed consent regarding potential benefits and adverse responses; and certainty that the benefits outweigh the risks. Psychotropic medications are not a substitute for stabilization and safety nor a replacement for clinical services and trauma-informed care.

[24] SAMHSA - Center for Integrated Care Solutions https://www.integration.samhsa.gov/clinical-practice/trauma-informed

Positive Reinforcement, Follow-Up, and Adherence

It is important to provide recognition and positive feedback for each small step that a young person makes in adhering to treatment, following up with referrals and keeping appointments. Positive recognition for small and large steps can play a significant role in sustaining engagement and adherence.

Young people are commonly late for or miss medical appointments. Clinics and practitioners need to adjust to this unpredictability and avoid setting up unrealistic barriers to follow-up care.

Schedule prompt and frequent follow-up visits as needed to monitor and promote adherence, preferably with a consistent clinician. Prescribe medications on as simple a regimen as possible such as single-dose treatment or a single daily dose if possible. Only the amount of medication needed for a short course should be dispensed as youth may have no safe place to store medications.

Basic needs such as food, shelter, and clothing can feel higher in priority than medical interventions to homeless youth. It may be difficult, even unrealistic, to expect youth to follow through with medical recommendations if their need for shelter and access to food are not addressed.

Engagement with a youth worker or case manager can be important in promoting adherence.[25] Holding medications in a drop-in center or shelter may be needed to secure reliable access to medications and other supplies.

Frequent, even weekly follow-up visits, may be a way to help manage medication storage and replenish lost supplies.

Concrete Health Needs and Common Referrals

Dental care: Homeless adolescents and young adults have commonly not had access for dental care. In the United States, all adolescents and children to age 21 should be enrolled for Medicaid benefits. Medicaid provides funding for limited-scope dental care.[26] It is helpful if the clinic has prearranged referral sources for youth. These can sometimes be found in collaborating dental schools. Clinics should also provide toothbrushes, floss, and other items to maintain dental hygiene.

Nutrition: Homeless youth commonly lack regular access to healthy food. Identifying and referring to accessible youth drop-in centers, food programs, shel-

[25] National Health Care for the Homeless Network, General Recommendations for the Care of Homeless Patients: Summary of Recommended Practice Adaptations.https://nhchc.org/wp-content/uploads/2019/08/General-Recommendations-for-Homeless-Patients.pdf Accessed November 10, 2019

[26] Keep Kids Smiling: Promoting Oral Health Through the Medicaid Benefit for Children & Adolescents https://www.medicaid.gov/medicaid/benefits/downloads/keep-kids-smiling.pdf (Accessed Nov 10, 2019)

ters, or other agencies is an important step in assuring adequate nutrition for youth as well as a step toward stabilization.

Feminine hygiene supplies: Homeless girls and young women often suffer from lack of access to these items and may have to choose between food and feminine hygiene products, shoplift, or use inadequate solutions like rags and toilet paper. Provision of tampons, sanitary pads, menstrual cups, and underwear is essential, and young women should be linked with drop-in centers, shelters, and transitional living programs.

Transportation: Many homeless youth have no access to transportation which can be a significant barrier to clinical care and accessing services. When feasible, it is useful for case managers, youth workers, clinicians, and others to have bus tokens or vouchers available to help youth utilize public transportation. This an important measure not only to improve healthcare access but to enable school attendance and access to shelter, drop-in centers, housing, and other services.

Linking Youth to Additional Services

Staff of the clinic should be knowledgeable about the locations of drop-in centers, emergency shelters, housing programs, adolescent substance abuse programs, mental health resources, schools, and other community resources and refer youth as appropriate. If a youth expresses an interest in accessing services, it is important to promptly facilitate linkage. You can contact the staff of the agency, who may be able to come to the clinic personally and engage with the youth, or there may be a resource navigator available in your community who can help the youth access services. (*See* Chap. 4.)

When working in an interdisciplinary setting, the clinician should notify case management staff as soon as a need for shelter or housing is identified as it generally takes time to contact agencies and make referral arrangements. If deferred to the end of the visit, the moment may be lost. Clinicians who work in a setting without case management staff are limited in the support they can provide for service linkage and access to care.

The Medical Home for Youth Experiencing Homelessness

While the clinical care of youth experiencing homelessness is often episodic and driven by an acute problem, their need for consistently available care reinforces the importance of the concept of a "medical home." This model of care is organized around improving access, continuity, and preventive care, recognizing that, while maintaining the relationship with each patient is central, clinicians need to develop relationships with families and with community institutions to fully address their patients' needs.

The concept of the medical home recognizes that developmentally appropriate, quality care for adolescents and young adults includes helping them develop autonomy, responsibility, and adult identity and notes that longer appointment times may be necessary to facilitate the transition of youth with chronic medical problems into adult care [13]. The developmentally appropriate orientation of the medical home model can help utilize opportunities to engage youth with supportive community and public agencies, drop-in centers, shelters, and schools and, when appropriate, contribute to family stability and/or reunification.

The National Academy of Medicine Report on Inequities and Addressing Adolescent and Young Adult Health Services [14]
Principles that guide the design and delivery of adolescent and young adult health services

- **Equitable:** *all young people, not just selected groups, are able to obtain the health services, and services do not discriminate against any sector of youth on grounds of gender, ethnicity, religion, disability, social status, sexual orientation, or any other reason.*
- **Reach out to the most vulnerable of those who lack services:** *geographically and financially accessible, easily identifiable, and easy-to-access services both by appointment and walk-in.*
- **Integration of primary and behavioral healthcare services:** *screen and refer for sexual and reproductive health issues, substance use, and mental health concerns.*
- **Confidential and obtaining informed consent from young people themselves:** *separate waiting room for youth; guarantee confidentiality and adolescent minors' rights to consent to sexual and reproductive healthcare; informational, social, psychological, and physical privacy.*
- **Developmentally tailored and appropriate:** *age-appropriate approach and health education materials by adolescent and young adult-friendly providers.*
- **Relationship based:** *mentorship of youth by providers, recognition of the importance of relationships with providers on youth development, availability of providers who spend enough time with the youth.*
- **Sensitive, trained, and reflective staff:** *staff receive training and support regarding working with adolescents; services are effective because they are delivered by trained and motivated healthcare providers; care provided by adolescent specialists; adolescent health resources and mechanisms for providers, including subspecialty sources of care and reference*

materials, provider collaboration; efficient division of responsibility (care delivered by most appropriate providers); staff sensitivity to young people; compensation for providers; build staff capacity to serve adolescent patients.

- **Safe space and approach that is nonjudgmental and without stigma**: *welcoming with visual teaching aids; youth-friendly environment that signals diversity and the competence of the service to listen to and help with any concern or question, no matter what.*
- **Respectful:** *providers who take youth seriously, listen, do not scold them; providers support youth in making their own decisions; exams are done with maximum respect for youth's dignity.*
- **Culturally competent:** *culturally appropriate health education materials, celebrating diversity.*

From: *Perspectives on Health Equity and Social Determinants of Health*, US National Academy of Medicine, 2017 [14].

Conclusion

Clinicians providing care to youth experiencing homelessness provide vital services to address acute and chronic healthcare needs and build trusting relationships with young people that can be a bridge to a fuller system of care. During a clinical visit, youth can be linked with drop-in centers, shelters, and transitional living programs that provide further support and stabilization. Clinical environments need to be welcoming, accepting, and supportive of youth with diverse sexual orientations, gender expressions and identities, ethnicities, national origins, and cultural and religious backgrounds. If healthcare is delivered with attention and thoughtfulness, providers have the potential to make a significant difference in the lives of these young people.

References

1. Bogard K, Murry V, Alexander C, editors. Perspectives on health equity and social determinants of health. Washington, DC: National Academy of Medicine; 2017. p. 15–6.
2. Slesnick N, Prestopnik JL, Meyers RJ, Glassman M. Treatment outcome for street-living, homeless youth. Addict Behav. 2007;32:1237–51. https://doi.org/10.1016/j.addbeh.2006.08.010. Accessed 12 Nov 2019.
3. Bonin E, Brehove T, Carlson C, Downing M, Hoeft J, Kalinowski A, Solomon-Bame J, Post P. Adapting your practice: general recommendations for the care of homeless patients. Nashville: Health Care for the Homeless Clinicians' Network, National Health Care for the Homeless Council, Inc.; 2010. p. 50. https://docs.google.com/document/d/1hjhFjKwufsGIb0NGWU8-do3NArmNvT2OIxVWwr8F988/edit. Accessed 10 Nov 2019.

4. Levine DA, Committee on Adolescence. Office-based care for lesbian, gay, bisexual, transgender, and questioning youth. Pediatrics. 2013;132(1):e297–313. https://doi.org/10.1542/peds.2013-1283.
5. US Interagency Council on Homelessness. Preventing and ending youth homelessness, a coordinated community response. p. 3. https://www.usich.gov/resources/uploads/asset_library/Youth_Homelessness_Coordinated_Response.pdf. Accessed 14 June 2019.
6. Greenbaum J, Crawford-Jakubiak JE, Committee on Child Abuse and Neglect. Child sex trafficking and commercial sexual exploitation: health care needs of victims. Pediatrics. 2015;135(3):566–74. https://doi.org/10.1542/peds.2014-4138.
7. Murphy LT. Labor and sex trafficking among homeless youth: a ten-city study full report. Modern Slavery Research Project Loyola University New Orleans; 2016.
8. Institute of Medicine and National Research Council. Confronting commercial sexual exploitation and sex trafficking of minors in the United States. Washington, DC: The National Academies Press; 2013.
9. Shared Hope International. Protected innocence challenge: state report cards on the legal framework of protection for the nation's children. Vancouver: Shared Hope International (SHI); 2013. Available at: http://sharedhope.org/wp-content/uploads/2014/02/2013-Protected-Innocence-Challenge-Report.pdf.
10. Use of chaperones during the physical examination of the Pediatric patient, Committee on Practice and Ambulatory Medicine; Pediatrics, 2011, 1275; American Academy of Pediatrics, Policy Statement https://pediatrics.aappublications.org/content/127/5/991. Accessed 3 Oct 2019.
11. Jenny C, Crawford-Jakubiak JE, Committee on Child Abuse and Neglect, American Academy of Pediatrics. The evaluation of children in the primary care setting when sexual abuse is suspected. Pediatrics. 2013;132(2). Available at: www.pediatrics.org/cgi/content/full/132/2/e558. pmid:23897912.
12. Workowski KA, Berman S, Centers for Disease Control and Prevention (CDC). Sexually transmitted diseases treatment guidelines, 2010. MMWR Recomm Rep. 2010;59(RR-12):1–110. pmid:21160459.
13. Committee on Adolescence, American Academy of Pediatrics. Policy statement: achieving quality health services for adolescents. Pediatrics. 2016;138(2):e20161347. https://doi.org/10.1542/peds.2016-1347.
14. Bogard K, Murry V, Alexander C, editors. Perspectives on health equity and social determinants of health. Washington, DC: National Academy of Medicine; 2017. p. 134–5. https://nam.edu/perspectives-on-health-equity-and-social-determinants-of-health/. Accessed 11 June 2019.

Resources

SAMHSA (Substance Abuse and Mental Health Services Administration). A practitioner's resource guide: helping families to support their LGBT children. https://www.aap.org/en-us/advocacy-and-policy/aap-health-initiatives/Pages/LGBT-Resources.aspx. Accessed 5 Nov 2019.

Chapter 11
Contraception

Meera Beharry and Celia Neavel

Contraception is considered one of the top 10 public health developments of the twentieth century [1]. In addition to allowing people to plan for pregnancy and child-rearing, there are non-contraceptive benefits. Condoms can reduce the risk of sexually transmitted infections. Hormonal methods can be used to treat dysmenorrhea, menorrhagia, polycystic ovarian syndrome, iron deficiency anaemia and premenstrual dysphoric disorder [2]. Many hormonal methods can be used for menstrual suppression and in reducing the frequency of menses which may be beneficial for women with limited access to menstrual hygiene products [3]. Hormonal birth control can decrease the risk of pelvic inflammatory disease (PID), ectopic pregnancy, seizures and some migraine headaches [2].

Reproductive Health Issues

There are many issues facing women who are pregnant while homeless. Preventing pregnancy can reduce these risks. Women experiencing homelessness also are likely to be victims of rape, human trafficking or survival sex [4, 5]. Having access to contraception, including emergency contraception, can reduce harm and abortions [6]. Abstinence and periodic abstinence are not options for those forced into sexual activity. However, this may be an option for some youth and should be encouraged when it is feasible. Ensign [7] noted that homeless youth who were using abstinence have been offended that providers assumed that they were sexually active. It is also

M. Beharry (✉)
Adolescent Medicine, McLane Children's Medical Center Specialty Clinic, Temple, TX, USA
e-mail: Meera.Beharry@BSWHealth.org

C. Neavel
Center for Adolescent Health, People's Community Clinic, Austin, TX, USA
e-mail: celian@austinpcc.org

C. Warf, G. Charles (eds.), *Clinical Care for Homeless, Runaway and Refugee Youth*, https://doi.org/10.1007/978-3-030-40675-2_11

important to remember that providers need to treat the patient based on their practices, preferences and biology. Transgender males who still have their female reproductive organs can get pregnant. Additionally, sexual minority women have higher risks of unintended pregnancy [8].

Contraceptive use rates among men and women experiencing homelessness are not well known. Of the studies that were done, male condoms are the most commonly used method followed by birth control pill [9, 10]. Male and female condoms are available over the counter, and almost all women can start non-intrauterine hormonal contraception without the need for a pelvic exam [11]. A visit to discuss, start or continue contraception provides an opportunity to assess for abuse, human trafficking and safety concerns [12]. We recommend taking a thorough menstrual history for natal females and using the 5 Ps assessment tool with all patients to help with contraceptive decision-making [13] (Table 11.1).

In this chapter, we will review hormonal and non-hormonal contraceptive options, including risks, benefits and the advantages of the different methods in a variety of situations. While sterilization is highly effective for contraception, it is not a method that is recommended for use with teenagers and young adults since their desire to have a family may change over time. Safe and legal abortions should be available to

Table 11.1 The 5 Ps

The 5 Ps of sexual history taking	
First, set the stage and let the patient know that these are questions you ask of all your patients. Explain confidentiality. Ask questions in a non-judgmental and matter of fact manner. Adapt language to improve understanding. Clarify terms as needed	
Partners	**Ask:** "Are you currently sexually active?" or **Ask:** "Are you currently having sex?" **If no, ask** "Have you ever had sex?" **If no**, ask about history of sexual abuse which they may not count as sexual activity. Ask about future plans. Encourage safe practices and inform about availability of contraception, if needed in the future **If yes, ask:** "How many sex partners have you had in the past 3 months?" "How many sex partners have you had in the past 12 months?" "How many sex partners have you had in your life?" "Have you had sex with men, women or both?"
Practices	**State:** "I am going to be more explicit here about the kind of sex you've had over the last 12 months to better understand if you are at risk for STDs." **Ask:** "What kind of sexual contact do you have or have you had? Genital (i.e. penis in the vagina)? Anal (penis in the anus)? Oral (mouth on penis, vagina or anus)?" **Ask:** "Has anyone forced you to have sex?" **If yes**, assess for safety and offer resources as needed **Ask:** "Have you ever exchanged sex for food, clothing, money or shelter?" (survival sex)

Table 11.1 (continued)

The 5 Ps of sexual history taking	
First, set the stage and let the patient know that these are questions you ask of all your patients. Explain confidentiality. Ask questions in a non-judgmental and matter of fact manner. Adapt language to improve understanding. Clarify terms as needed	
Prevention of STDs	**Ask:** "Do you and your partner(s) use any protection against STDs?" **For survival sex or forced sex, you may need to ask specifically about partners by choice* versus *others. You may miss information about health risk if you ask about "partners".* **If not, ask** "Could you tell me the reason?" **If yes, ask** "What kind of protection do you use?" How often do you use this protection? If "sometimes", ask "In what situations or with whom do you use protection?" **Ask:** "Are you able to use protection in all situations or are there times when you don't have a choice?" *Encourage appropriate use when it is reported* **Ask:** "Do you have any other questions, or are there other forms of protection from STDs that you would like to discuss today?"
Past history of STDs	**Ask:** "Have you ever been diagnosed with an STD?" If yes, "When? How were you treated?" **Ask:** "Have you had any recurring symptoms (discharge, pain with sex, pain with urination) or diagnoses?" **Ask:** "Have you ever been tested for HIV or other STDs? Would you like to be tested?" **Ask:** "Has your current partner or any former partners ever been diagnosed or treated for an STD?" If yes, "Were you tested for the same STD(s)?" **If yes**, "When were you tested? What was the diagnosis? How was it treated?"
Prevention of pregnancy	**Ask:** "Are you currently trying to conceive or father a child?" **Ask:** "Are you concerned about getting pregnant or getting your partner pregnant?" **Ask:** "Are you using contraception or practicing any form of birth control?" "Do you need any information on birth control?" or **Ask:** "Would you like any information on birth control?"

Adapted from "A Guide to Taking a Sexual History" from the Center for Disease Control. Accessible at: https://www.cdc.gov/std/treatment/sexualhistory.pdf [13]

all women including homeless youth. When women are denied quick access to safe abortions, they may resort to dangerous actions which can result in severe injury, infection or death [7]. All providers caring for women should maintain accurate and up-to-date lists of providers and facilities who can provide prenatal care and abortions if they are unable to provide these services in their setting. It is also imperative to maintain a continuously updated awareness of the local and federal laws pertaining to reproductive rights and access to abortion. In the USA, the Center for Adolescent Health and the Law (https://www.cahl.org/) keeps up-to-date information about laws affecting adolescents. The Guttmacher Institute (https://www.guttmacher.org/) compiles information on reproductive health statistics and policies internationally.

Issues of consent and confidentiality in general are important for all young people, especially those experiencing homelessness and those seeking reproductive healthcare. All providers should be familiar with the legal issues related to providing reproductive healthcare to unaccompanied minors. The Society for Adolescent Health and Medicine, the Canadian Pediatric Society, the American College of Obstetrics and Gynecology, the Society of Obstetricians and Gynaecologists of Canada, the American Medical Association, the American Academy of Pediatrics and the American Academy of Family Practice have statements supporting the provision of confidential reproductive healthcare to minors [11, 12, 14]. Policies that limit access to confidential care lead to delayed care, increased morbidity and mortality and, in the case of contraception, unplanned pregnancy with late prenatal care or later-term abortions [6]. Many young people and adults may not know their rights to confidential care [7]. Care providers, including case managers, social workers and shelter staff, can help increase awareness of patient rights. In addition to written resources about consent, confidentiality and patient rights, facilities may wish to develop standard verbal or recorded messages for youth with limited literacy skills. The Adolescent Health Initiative [15] has specific trainings on minor consent and confidentiality which can be accessed at http://www.umhs-adolescenthealth.org/improving-care/confidentiality/.

Contraceptive Options

We divide contraceptive options into hormonal or non-hormonal methods. Non-hormonal methods include the copper intrauterine device, the fertility awareness method, withdrawal and barrier methods, such as male and female condoms. Hormonal methods work primarily by preventing ovulation. Most can also thicken cervical mucus making it harder for sperm to reach an egg in the event of ovulation. Hormonal methods are further subdivided into progesterone-only or combined hormonal methods that contain ethinyl estradiol and a progestin. The most effective methods for contraception are referred to as LARC, long-acting reversible contraception or HERC (highly effective reversible contraception). Intrauterine contraceptive devices (IUDs) and the contraceptive implants are LARC methods. They are as effective as sterilization at pregnancy prevention but are completely reversible [2, 11].

Long-Acting Reversible Contraception

There are intrauterine devices (IUDs) which contain the hormone levonorgestrel and the non-hormonal option of the copper IUD. These methods are over 99% effective at preventing pregnancy. For the copper IUD, the main side effects of concern are worsening cramps and heavier menstrual bleeding in the first few months of use. The copper IUD has the advantage of being effective for use as emergency contraception if inserted within 5 days of unprotected sex. It can be used for 10 years [2, 11, 16].

IUD

The hormonal IUDs can be used for 3 or 5 years depending on the product chosen. The progesterone hormone in these methods usually helps decrease menstrual bleeding and can be beneficial for women who have dysmenorrhea. However, as with all progesterone-only methods, bleeding can be unpredictable. Women need to be prepared for this as it may be problematic if hygiene supplies aren't always available. Occasionally bleeding can be heavier. The hormone may also cause some physical side effects, such as breast tenderness or weight gain, headache, hair loss and change in mood. The hormonal IUDs come in varying sizes, duration of use and hormonal level. The IUD which contains 52 mg of levonorgestrel and is marketed under the name Mirena® has indication for heavy menstrual bleeding and dysmenorrhea [2, 11, 16]. Some providers have placed it in women solely for this benefit.

Uterine perforation is exceedingly rare with IUD use (less than 0.1%) but is more likely to occur in lactating women. Another potential problem with the IUD is expulsion or migration. Though uncommon (~4%), this would decrease the efficacy of the device. In the case of migration, surgical intervention will be needed to remove the IUD. Condoms should be used if the patient is unsure if the device is in place.

Contraindications for use of IUDs are few. The most likely condition that an adolescent would have would be infection. Uterine anomalies may be a contraindication to insertion or may require placement with ultrasound guidance. If there is a high suspicion for infection, the patient should be treated prior to insertion. Current pelvic inflammatory disease is a contraindication to insertion of the IUD; however, past pelvic inflammatory disease is not. If a woman acquires infection after IUD placement, the IUD does not need to be removed. The initial step would be to treat infection and reassess clinically [17–19] (see Table 11.2).

Myths about IUDs abound. Misunderstandings about LARC can result in underutilization of these generally safe methods [20]. When talking to youth, it is critical to ask about and dispel any erroneous information they may have heard. IUDs do not cause infertility and migration within the body is rare. Due to issues with previous IUDs, even medical providers may propagate these myths, such as taking out previously placed IUDs when there is a sexually transmitted infection [18, 19]. Also, the young person is not required to perform string checks. In a study of homeless young women in Pittsburgh, Dasari and colleagues [21] found that women would prefer to know that they can discontinue use of the implant or IUD early if desired and to have more complete information about methods and side effects from their provider. They also voiced a preference for having a visual guide, such as the CDC's Effectiveness of Family Planning Methods (Fig. 11.1) or those available at bedsider.org, to help guide their decision.

Many women are worried about pain with insertion. Young people tend to be more sensitive to their body experiences. Pre-treating with high-dose ibuprofen or naproxen may decrease the likelihood of cramping. Some providers use cervical blocks, whereas others introduce lidocaine to the uterus to decrease pain and cramping [22]. Close follow-up of patients who are likely to experience pain is recommended.

Summary Chart of U.S. Medical Eligibility Criteria for Contraceptive Use

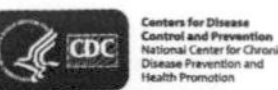

Condition	Sub-Condition	Cu-IUD I	Cu-IUD C	LNG-IUD I	LNG-IUD C	Implant I	Implant C	DMPA I	DMPA C	POP I	POP C	CHC I	CHC C
Age		Menarche to <20 yrs:**2**		Menarche to <20 yrs:**2**		Menarche to <18 yrs:**1**		Menarche to <18 yrs:**2**		Menarche to <18 yrs:**1**		Menarche to <40 yrs:**1**	
		≥20 yrs:**1**		≥20 yrs:**1**		18-45 yrs:**1**		18-45 yrs:**1**		18-45 yrs:**1**		≥40 yrs:**2**	
						>45 yrs:**1**		>45 yrs:**2**		>45 yrs:**1**			
Anatomical abnormalities	a) Distorted uterine cavity	4		4									
	b) Other abnormalities	2		2									
Anemias	a) Thalassemia	2		1		1		1		1		1	
	b) Sickle cell disease[‡]	2		1		1		1		1		2	
	c) Iron-deficiency anemia	2		1		1		1		1		1	
Benign ovarian tumors	(*including cysts*)	1		1		1		1		1		1	
Breast disease	a) Undiagnosed mass	1		2		2*		2*		2*		2*	
	b) Benign breast disease	1		1		1		1		1		1	
	c) Family history of cancer	1		1		1		1		1		1	
	d) Breast cancer[‡]												
	i) Current	1		4		4		4		4		4	
	ii) Past and no evidence of current disease for 5 years	1		3		3		3		3		3	
Breastfeeding	a) <21 days postpartum					2*		2*		2*		4*	
	b) 21 to <30 days postpartum												
	i) With other risk factors for VTE					2*		2*		2*		3*	
	ii) Without other risk factors for VTE					2*		2*		2*		3*	
	c) 30-42 days postpartum												
	i) With other risk factors for VTE					1*		1*		1*		3*	
	ii) Without other risk factors for VTE					1*		1*		1*		2*	
	d) >42 days postpartum					1*		1*		1*		2*	
Cervical cancer	Awaiting treatment	4	2	4	2	2		2		1		2	
Cervical ectropion		1		1		1		1		1		1	
Cervical intraepithelial neoplasia		1		2		2		2		1		2	
Cirrhosis	a) Mild (*compensated*)	1		1		1		1		1		1	
	b) Severe[‡] (*decompensated*)	1		3		3		3		3		4	
Cystic fibrosis[‡]		1*		1*		1*		2*		1*		1*	
Deep venous thrombosis (DVT)/Pulmonary embolism (PE)	a) History of DVT/PE, not receiving anticoagulant therapy												
	i) Higher risk for recurrent DVT/PE	1		2		2		2		2		4	
	ii) Lower risk for recurrent DVT/PE	1		2		2		2		2		3	
	b) Acute DVT/PE	2		2		2		2		2		4	
	c) DVT/PE and established anticoagulant therapy for at least 3 months												
	i) Higher risk for recurrent DVT/PE	2		2		2		2		2		4*	
	ii) Lower risk for recurrent DVT/PE	2		2		2		2		2		3*	
	d) Family history (*first-degree relatives*)	1		1		1		1		1		2	
	e) Major surgery												
	i) With prolonged immobilization	1		2		2		2		2		4	
	ii) Without prolonged immobilization	1		1		1		1		1		2	
	f) Minor surgery without immobilization	1		1		1		1		1		1	
Depressive disorders		1*		1*		1*		1*		1*		1*	

Key:	
1 No restriction (method can be used)	3 Theoretical or proven risks usually outweigh the advantages
2 Advantages generally outweigh theoretical or proven risks	4 Unacceptable health risk (method not to be used)

Table 11.2 Rating of risk for prescribed contraceptives in specific medical conditions. (From Centers for Disease Control and Prevention (CDC), Division of Reproductive Health, National Center for Chronic Disease Prevention and Health Promotions. United States Medical Eligibility Criteriea (USMEC) for Contraceptive Use, 2010. Summary Chart of US Medical Eligibility Critera for Contraceptive Use. Updated 2017. https://www.cdc.gov/reproductivehealth/contraception/mmwr/mec/summary.html)

Summary Chart of U.S. Medical Eligibility Criteria for Contraceptive Use

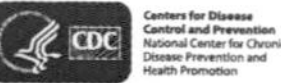

Condition	Sub-Condition	Cu-IUD I	Cu-IUD C	LNG-IUD I	LNG-IUD C	Implant I	Implant C	DMPA I	DMPA C	POP I	POP C	CHC I	CHC C
Diabetes	a) History of gestational disease	1		1		1		1		1		1	
	b) Nonvascular disease												
	i) Non-insulin dependent	1		2		2		2		2		2	
	ii) Insulin dependent	1		2		2		2		2		2	
	c) Nephropathy/retinopathy/neuropathy‡	1		2		2		3		2		3/4*	
	d) Other vascular disease or diabetes of >20 years' duration‡	1		2		2		3		2		3/4*	
Dysmenorrhea	Severe	2		1		1		1		1		1	
Endometrial cancer‡		4	2	4	2	1		1		1		1	
Endometrial hyperplasia		1		1		1		1		1		1	
Endometriosis		2		1		1		1		1		1	
Epilepsy‡	(*see also Drug Interactions*)	1		1		1*		1*		1*		1*	
Gallbladder disease	a) Symptomatic												
	i) Treated by cholecystectomy	1		2		2		2		2		2	
	ii) Medically treated	1		2		2		2		2		3	
	iii) Current	1		2		2		2		2		3	
	b) Asymptomatic	1		2		2		2		2		2	
Gestational trophoblastic disease‡	a) Suspected GTD (immediate postevacuation)												
	i) Uterine size first trimester	1*		1*		1*		1*		1*		1*	
	ii) Uterine size second trimester	2*		2*		1*		1*		1*		1*	
	b) Confirmed GTD												
	i) Undetectable/non-pregnant ß-hCG levels	1*	1*	1*	1*	1*		1*		1*		1*	
	ii) Decreasing ß-hCG levels	2*	1*	2*	1*	1*		1*		1*		1*	
	iii) Persistently elevated ß-hCG levels or malignant disease, with no evidence or suspicion of intrauterine disease	2*	1*	2*	1*	1*		1*		1*		1*	
	iv) Persistently elevated ß-hCG levels or malignant disease, with evidence or suspicion of intrauterine disease	4*	2*	4*	2*	1*		1*		1*		1*	
Headaches	a) Nonmigraine (mild or severe)	1		1		1		1		1		1*	
	b) Migraine												
	i) Without aura (includes menstrual migraine)	1		1		1		1		1		2*	
	ii) With aura	1		1		1		1		1		4*	
History of bariatric surgery‡	a) Restrictive procedures	1		1		1		1		1		1	
	b) Malabsorptive procedures	1		1		1		1		3		COCs: 3 P/R: 1	
History of cholestasis	a) Pregnancy related	1		1		1		1		1		2	
	b) Past COC related	1		2		2		2		2		3	
History of high blood pressure during pregnancy		1		1		1		1		1		2	
History of Pelvic surgery		1		1		1		1		1		1	
HIV	a) High risk for HIV	2	2	2	2	1		2*		1		1	
	b) HIV infection					1*		1*		1*		1*	
	i) Clinically well receiving ARV therapy	1	1	1	1	If on treatment, see Drug Interactions							
	ii) Not clinically well or not receiving ARV therapy‡	2	1	2	1	If on treatment, see Drug Interactions							

Abbreviations: C=continuation of contraceptive method; CHC=combined hormonal contraception (pill, patch, and, ring); COC=combined oral contraceptive; Cu-IUD=copper-containing intrauterine device; DMPA = depot medroxyprogesterone acetate; I=initiation of contraceptive method; LNG-IUD=levonorgestrel-releasing intrauterine device; NA=not applicable; POP=progestin-only pill; P/R=patch/ring ‡ Condition that exposes a woman to increased risk as a result of pregnancy. *Please see the complete guidance for a clarification to this classification: www.cdc.gov/reproductivehealth/unintendedpregnancy/USMEC.htm.

Tab. 11.2 (continued)

Summary Chart of U.S. Medical Eligibility Criteria for Contraceptive Use

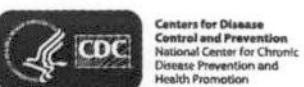

Condition	Sub-Condition	Cu-IUD	LNG-IUD	Implant	DMPA	POP	CHC
		I / C	I / C	I / C	I / C	I / C	I / C
Hypertension	a) Adequately controlled hypertension	1*	1*	1*	2*	1*	3*
	b) Elevated blood pressure levels (*properly taken measurements*)						
	i) Systolic 140-159 or diastolic 90-99	1*	1*	1*	2*	1*	3*
	ii) Systolic ≥160 or diastolic ≥100‡	1*	2*	2*	3*	2*	4*
	c) Vascular disease	1*	2*	2*	3*	2*	4*
Inflammatory bowel disease	(*Ulcerative colitis, Crohn's disease*)	1	1	1	2	2	2/3*
Ischemic heart disease‡	Current and history of	1	I: 2 / C: 3	I: 2 / C: 3	3	I: 2 / C: 3	4
Known thrombogenic mutations‡		1*	2*	2*	2*	2*	4*
Liver tumors	a) Benign						
	i) Focal nodular hyperplasia	1	2	2	2	2	2
	ii) Hepatocellular adenoma‡	1	3	3	3	3	4
	b) Malignant‡ (hepatoma)	1	3	3	3	3	4
Malaria		1	1	1	1	1	1
Multiple risk factors for atherosclerotic cardiovascular disease	(e.g., older age, smoking, diabetes, hypertension, low HDL, high LDL, or high triglyceride levels)	1	2	2*	3*	2*	3/4*
Multiple sclerosis	a) With prolonged immobility	1	1	1	2	1	3
	b) Without prolonged immobility	1	1	1	2	1	1
Obesity	a) Body mass index (BMI) ≥30 kg/m²	1	1	1	1	1	2
	b) Menarche to <18 years and BMI ≥ 30 kg/m²	1	1	1	2	1	2
Ovarian cancer‡		1	1	1	1	1	1
Parity	a) Nulliparous	2	2	1	1	1	1
	b) Parous	1	1	1	1	1	1
Past ectopic pregnancy		1	1	1	1	2	1
Pelvic inflammatory disease	a) Past						
	i) With subsequent pregnancy	I: 1 / C: 1	I: 1 / C: 1	1	1	1	1
	ii) Without subsequent pregnancy	I: 2 / C: 2	I: 2 / C: 2	1	1	1	1
	b) Current	I: 4 / C: 2*	I: 4 / C: 2*	1	1	1	1
Peripartum cardiomyopathy‡	a) Normal or mildly impaired cardiac function						
	i) <6 months	2	2	1	1	1	4
	ii) ≥6 months	2	2	1	1	1	3
	b) Moderately or severely impaired cardiac function	2	2	2	2	2	4
Postabortion	a) First trimester	1*	1*	1*	1*	1*	1*
	b) Second trimester	2*	2*	1*	1*	1*	1*
	c) Immediate postseptic abortion	4	4	1*	1*	1*	1*
Postpartum (*nonbreastfeeding women*)	a) <21 days			1	1	1	4
	b) 21 days to 42 days						
	i) With other risk factors for VTE			1	1	1	3*
	ii) Without other risk factors for VTE			1	1	1	2
	c) >42 days			1	1	1	1
Postpartum (*in breastfeeding or non-breastfeeding women, including cesarean delivery*)	a) <10 minutes after delivery of the placenta						
	i) Breastfeeding	1*	2*				
	ii) Nonbreastfeeding	1*	1*				
	b) 10 minutes after delivery of the placenta to <4 weeks	2*	2*				
	c) ≥4 weeks	1*	1*				
	d) Postpartum sepsis	4	4				

Tab. 11.2 (continued)

Summary Chart of U.S. Medical Eligibility Criteria for Contraceptive Use

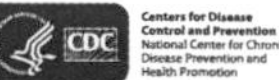

Condition	Sub-Condition	Cu-IUD I	Cu-IUD C	LNG-IUD I	LNG-IUD C	Implant I	Implant C	DMPA I	DMPA C	POP I	POP C	CHC I	CHC C
Pregnancy		4*		4*		NA*		NA*		NA*		NA*	
Rheumatoid arthritis	a) On immunosuppressive therapy	2	1	2	1	1		2/3*		1		2	
	b) Not on immunosuppressive therapy	1		1		1		2		1		2	
Schistosomiasis	a) Uncomplicated	1		1		1		1		1		1	
	b) Fibrosis of the liver†	1		1		1		1		1		1	
Sexually transmitted diseases (STDs)	a) Current purulent cervicitis or chlamydial infection or gonococcal infection	4	2*	4	2*	1		1		1		1	
	b) Vaginitis (*including trichomonas vaginalis and bacterial vaginosis*)	2	2	2	2	1		1		1		1	
	c) Other factors relating to STDs	2*	2	2*	2	1		1		1		1	
Smoking	a) Age <35	1		1		1		1		1		2	
	b) Age ≥35, <15 cigarettes/day	1		1		1		1		1		3	
	c) Age ≥35, ≥15 cigarettes/day	1		1		1		1		1		4	
Solid organ transplantation‡	a) Complicated	3	2	3	2	2		2		2		4	
	b) Uncomplicated	2		2		2		2		2		2*	
Stroke‡	History of cerebrovascular accident	1		2		2	3	3		2	3	4	
Superficial venous disorders	a) Varicose veins	1		1		1		1		1		1	
	b) Superficial venous thrombosis (acute or history)	1		1		1		1		1		3*	
Systemic lupus erythematosus‡	a) Positive (or unknown) antiphospholipid antibodies	1*	1*	3*		3*		3*	3*	3*		4*	
	b) Severe thrombocytopenia	3*	2*	2*		2*		3*	2*	2*		2*	
	c) Immunosuppressive therapy	2*	1*	2*		2*		2*	2*	2*		2*	
	d) None of the above	1*	1*	2*		2*		2*	2*	2*		2*	
Thyroid disorders	Simple goiter/ hyperthyroid/hypothyroid	1		1		1		1		1		1	
Tuberculosis‡ (*see also Drug Interactions*)	a) Nonpelvic	1	1	1	1	1*		1*		1*		1*	
	b) Pelvic	4	3	4	3	1*		1*		1*		1*	
Unexplained vaginal bleeding	(suspicious for serious condition) before evaluation	4*	2*	4*	2*	3*		3*		2*		2*	
Uterine fibroids		2		2		1		1		1		1	
Valvular heart disease	a) Uncomplicated	1		1		1		1		1		2	
	b) Complicated‡	1		1		1		1		1		4	
Vaginal bleeding patterns	a) Irregular pattern without heavy bleeding	1		1	1	2		2		2		1	
	b) Heavy or prolonged bleeding	2*		1*	2*	2*		2*		2*		1*	
Viral hepatitis	a) Acute or flare	1		1		1		1		1		3/4*	2
	b) Carrier/Chronic	1		1		1		1		1		1	1
Drug Interactions													
Antiretroviral therapy All other ARV's are 1 or 2 for all methods.	Fosamprenavir (FPV)	1/2*	1*	1/2*	1*	2*		2*		2*		3*	
Anticonvulsant therapy	a) Certain anticonvulsants (phenytoin, carbamazepine, barbiturates, primidone, topiramate, oxcarbazepine)	1		1		2*		1*		3*		3*	
	b) Lamotrigine	1		1		1		1		1		3*	
Antimicrobial therapy	a) Broad spectrum antibiotics	1		1		1		1		1		1	
	b) Antifungals	1		1		1		1		1		1	
	c) Antiparasitics	1		1		1		1		1		1	
	d) Rifampin or rifabutin therapy	1		1		2*		1*		3*		3*	
SSRIs		1		1		1		1		1		1	
St. John's wort		1		1		2		1		2		2	

Updated in 2017. This summary sheet only contains a subset of the recommendations from the U.S. MEC. For complete guidance, see: http://www.cdc.gov/reproductivehealth/unintendedpregnancy/USMEC.htm. Most contraceptive methods do not protect against sexually transmitted diseases (STDs). Consistent and correct use of the male latex condom reduces the risk of STDs and HIV.

CS266008-A

Tab. 11.2 (continued)

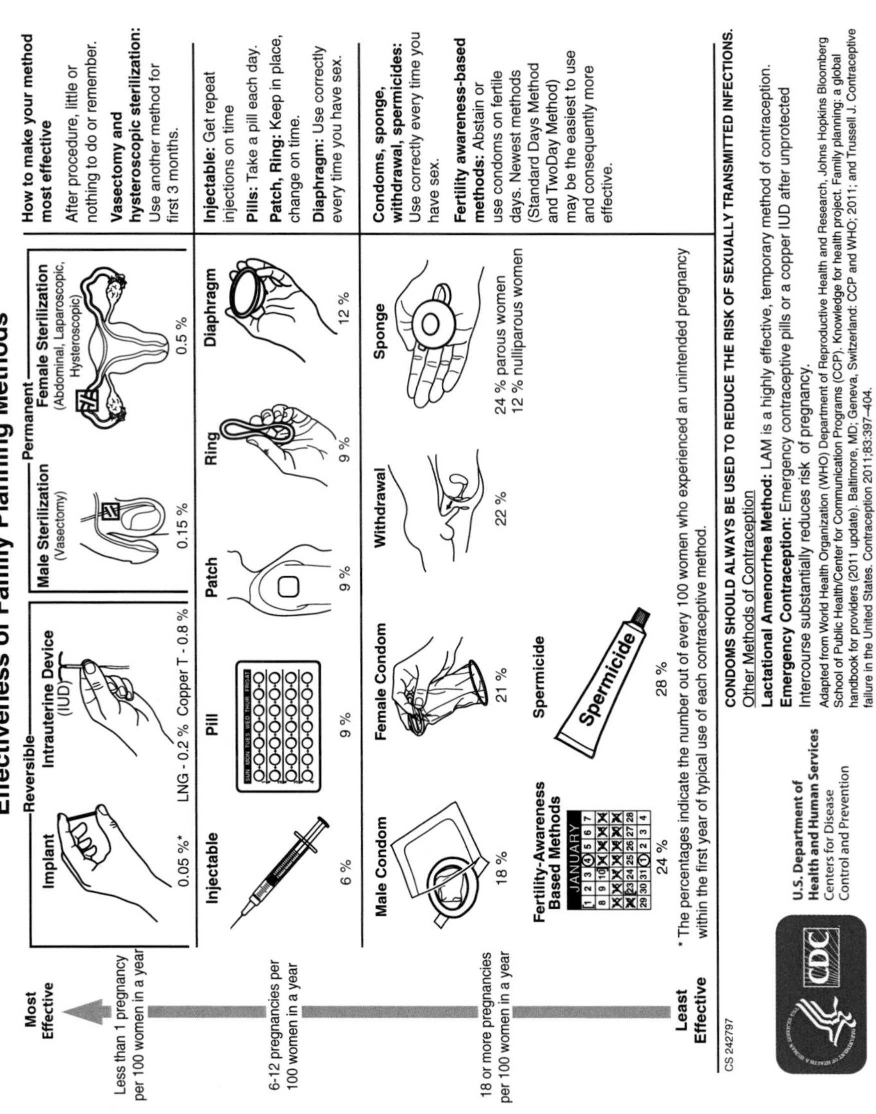

Fig. 11.1 Visual guide for youth of most to least effective contraception based on typical use. Available at https://www.cdc.gov/reproductivehealth/contraception/mmwr/mec/intro.html and https://www.cdc.gov/reproductivehealth/unintendedpregnancy/pdf/contraceptive_methods_508.pdf [17]

Implant

The contraceptive implant that is available for use in North America is the etonogestrel implant. It is inserted in the upper arm just under the skin and lasts for at least 3 years. The most common side effect that is bothersome to adolescents is irregular bleeding. According to package insert, more frequent or heavier menstrual bleeding occurs for about one-third of patients. Another one-third will have no menstrual bleeding or have just occasional spotting throughout the 3 years of implant use. Some women experience weight gain or mood changes which are bothersome enough to have the implant removed [2, 16].

Some youth are uncomfortable with the idea of having a foreign body in their arm or are worried that their partner or abuser may feel the implant. As with other methods, myths abound. Some are worried that the implant will cause them to be infertile. Others are worried that it will move within their body, be painful or limit their participation in physical activity. For women living on the street or engaged in sex trafficking, unpredictable menstrual bleeding may be a significant barrier to the use of this method [23].

Another potential barrier to the use of the LARC methods is the ability to access providers trained in placing them. For the IUD, a pelvic exam is required. This is not needed for implant placement.

Major medical organizations and research support LARC as the first-line and most effective forms of pregnancy prevention for adolescents and young adults. Progesterone-containing LARC may be an option for youth who are transgender men or gender non-conforming. Transmen, even if on testosterone, still need to think about birth control if they are having intercourse with natal male partners. Progesterone-containing LARC also can help ameliorate menstrual bleeding.

Injection and Progestin-Only Pill

A key advantage of progesterone-only methods is that they can be used immediately post-partum or in other conditions when the use of oestrogen as in combined hormonal contraception is contraindicated (see Table 11.2) [17]. A progesterone-only method may be a consideration for a transgender male who needs contraception or menstrual suppression.

Injection

Depot-medroxyprogesterone acetate (DMPA) is an injection that is given every 12–13 weeks into a deep muscle, usually the gluteus. Side effects include irregular menstrual bleeding and may include weight gain and mood changes [2]. Women who experience weight gain can have significant increases which can be very distressing. Many women do not have these side effects and enjoy using this method.

According to the package insert, 55% of those who use DMPA for more than a year will achieve amenorrhea. Women who use DMPA for more than 2 years may have decreased bone mineral density [11]. If a woman is planning on using this contraceptive method for more than 2 years, she should be advised to consider one of the LARC options noted above. If a woman chooses to use DMPA, engaging in weight-bearing exercise and taking calcium and vitamin D supplements can help decrease adverse effects on the bone [11]. One key advantage for the use of DMPA is that it is the only completely invisible method. The primary disadvantages are the need to return regularly for injections and the unpredictable bleeding pattern.

There are almost no contraindications to Depo Provera, making it a useful option when there is limited medical history or other health concerns [17].

Progestin-Only Pills

Like DMPA, progestin-only pills have few contraindications. To effectively suppress ovulation, progestin-only pills must be taken at the exact same time every day. Failure of consistency with this method can result in pregnancy and/or breakthrough bleeding. This may be a challenge for youth without a watch, phone or clock to help them keep track of time. Carrying the pills can also be a challenge, especially for those who travel a lot. The efficacy of progestin only pills is similar to other user dependent methods [11].

Combined Hormonal Contraception

Combined hormonal contraception is the term that refers to the products that contain ethinyl estradiol and a progestin. These include the combination birth control pill, the patch and the vaginal ring. They work by suppressing ovulation through the administration of hormones similar to what women have in early pregnancy. Therefore, many of the potential side effects of these methods are similar to what women may experience in pregnancy and include breast tenderness, weight gain, mood changes, nausea and headaches. Many of the side effects resolve after a few months. Women who have migraines with aura should be advised to consider another option for contraception as they may be at increased risk of stroke with the use of combined hormonal contraception [2, 11, 21, 24]. There are also risks of venous thromboembolism which can be fatal. Any woman with a personal history of a venous thromboembolism or increased risk of blood clot formation due to an underlying medical condition should use another method. A complete list of contraindications can be found in the World Health Organization's Medial Eligibility Criteria [24] for contraceptive use. In the USA, the Centers for Disease Control and Prevention have adapted this guideline to reflect additional conditions and medications commonly used in this country [21]. Some providers may not be aware of these references and could be providing inaccurate information about which methods are safe and which are contraindicated for use. Both of the references are in the public domain and can be accessed by patients or those who are not medically trained. We have included the summary pages of the USMEC as part of this chapter in Table 11.2. There also is an app that can be downloaded which helps health professionals in decision-making around contraceptive recommendations.

It is important to remember and counsel women and transmen that any birth control is safer than pregnancy unless there are contraindications. There are significant medical risks, including the risk of blood clots, in pregnancy. This is true whether or not the pregnancy is wanted or planned.

The use of ethinyl estradiol in combined hormonal methods can allow women to have a "withdrawal bleed" which mimics the normal menstrual period if desired. Overall, combined hormonal contraception allows for more control over menstrual bleeding. The ethinyl estradiol can provide non-contraceptive benefits including improvement in acne, reduction in menstrual cramps and reduction in menstrual flow [2, 3].

Combined Oral Contraceptive Pill

The combined oral contraceptive (COC) pill remains the most commonly used hormonal birth control method. The formulations have changed to include a variety of doses and different types of progestin. The traditional packet of pills contains 21 active pills and 7 days of placebo pills. The week of placebo pills induces the week of the "withdrawal bleed" to mimic a menstrual period. Some manufacturers have opted to shorten this by including 24 active pills and 4 placebo pills. Others include the placebo pills every 3 months which can allow the woman to have menses only four times a year. While packaging pills in this way makes it more convenient to use, these methods of menstrual manipulation can be used with any packet of pills [3]. It is not medically necessary to have a withdrawal bleed while using the COC [13]. It can also be advantageous to suppress menses in a variety of conditions, including anaemia, dysmenorrhea, menstrual migraine, ovarian cysts, premenstrual syndrome and endometriosis [3, 25]. Additionally, pills may be more effective if they are used without the hormone-free interval every 4 weeks [25]. It is important to explain this to patients as many women are taught that if they do not have a period, there is something wrong with them. We recommend giving patients a handout on how to use OCPs, including for continuous cycling and reviewing what to do if they miss pills. An example of such a handout is included in Fig. 11.2 [26].

A primary advantage of COC is the ability for a woman to control when or if she wants to bleed. Generally, there is no significant change in weight. Other advantages include decreasing anaemia, protecting against ovarian and uterine cancer and treating acne, polycystic ovarian syndrome, hirsutism and bleeding disorders [2]. While COCs can have interactions with other medications such as some of those used for as mood stabilizers or for seizure disorders, most antibiotics do not interfere with use [21, 24].

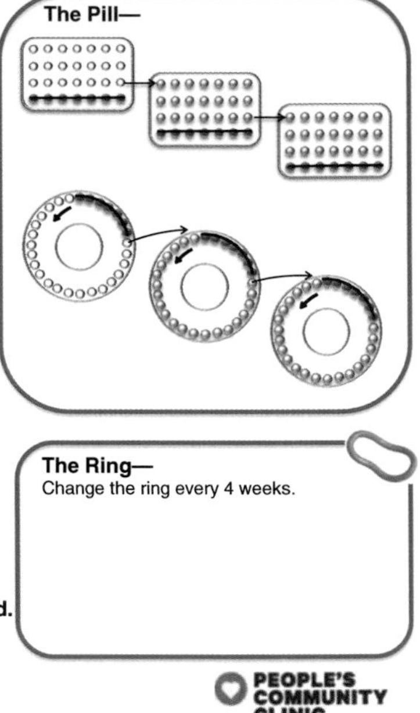

Fig. 11.2 Example handout on using traditional OCP packs or the vaginal contraceptive ring for continous hormonal cycling. Developed by People's Community Clinic, Austin, Texas, US, and used with permission [26]

However, it can be difficult to consistently use COC when living on the streets or travelling. The packets of pills could be stolen. Ideally, COC pills should be taken around the same time every day. While newer formulations of the pill allow increased efficacy if there is one missed pill and the woman takes two pills the next day, patients will be at risk of pregnancy if they miss pills very often. Therefore, this may not be the best method for those who are not keeping track of days, do not have a calendar or are not staying sober. Since all pills come in a packet, this may be difficult method to keep secret.

For those who choose to use the pill, they can usually start it immediately if there is a negative pregnancy test. If they have engaged in unprotected sex in the past 5 days, emergency contraception with levonorgestrel or the Yuzpe method can be given prior to initiation. Previously, women were advised to start COC pills on the first Sunday after their last menstrual period. There is no medical reason to do this, but some providers and pharmacists still dispense this advice. If a woman chooses to do this "quick start" (see Table 11.3), it is recommended that she have a repeat pregnancy test in 2 weeks after starting or if she does not have a withdrawal bleed when expected [2, 11]. There is no known risk to the woman, the course of the pregnancy or the fetus if hormonal contraception is started [17]. However, failure to recognize or diagnose an early pregnancy can lead to delayed pre-natal care or later term abortions.

Table 11.3 Quick start and backup recommendations

Method	When to start (if provider is reasonably certain that the woman is not pregnant)[a]	Additional contraception (i.e. backup) needed	Examinations or tests needed before initiation
Copper-containing IUD	Anytime	Not needed	Bimanual examination and cervical inspection
Levonorgestrel-releasing IUD	Anytime	If >7 days after menses started, use backup method or abstain for 7 days	Bimanual examination and cervical inspection
Implant	Anytime	If >5 days after menses started, use backup method or abstain for 7 days	None
Injectable	Anytime	If >7 days after menses started, use backup method or abstain for 7 days	None
Combined hormonal contraception	Anytime	If >5 days after menses started, use backup method or abstain for 7 days	Blood pressure measurement
Progestin-only pill	Anytime	If >5 days after menses started, use backup method or abstain for 2 days	None

[a]A healthcare provider can be reasonably certain that a woman is not pregnant if she has a negative pregnancy test, no symptoms or signs of pregnancy and meets *any one* of the following criteria:

Is ≤7 days after the start of normal menses.

Has not had sexual intercourse since the start of last normal menses.

Has been correctly and consistently using a reliable method of contraception.

Is ≤7 days after spontaneous or induced abortion.

Is within 4 weeks post-partum.

Is fully or nearly fully breastfeeding (exclusively breastfeeding or the vast majority (≥85%) of feeds are breastfeeds), amenorrhoeic and <6 months post-partum [17].

Lower-dose pills with only 20 μg of ethinyl estradiol have been marketed as less likely to cause adverse side effects; however, they are more likely to cause breakthrough bleeding or contraceptive failure if doses are missed. Many providers use the 30–35 μg pills to reduce the likelihood of these problems [11]. Higher doses, 50 μg of ethinyl estradiol, are used rarely when a woman has breakthrough bleeding on lower-dose pills or uses medications which decrease efficacy of the pills, such as certain anti-epileptic medications and HIV medications. We generally prefer monophasic COCs for young people. "Monophasic pills" refers to packs in which the hormonal dose stays the same throughout the pack and can be less confusing than pills that change hormone levels and have multiple colours of pills. Monophasic pills may be easier for continuous cycling or when needing to double up due to a missed pill or needing to treat abnormal uterine bleeding.

Providers may choose to use different brands because of personal preference or because of the type of progestin. Newer progestins are less likely to cause breakthrough bleeding with missed pills. They are also less likely to have androgenic effects and adverse effects on lipids. Drospirenone has anti-androgenic effects, which may be beneficial to women with polycystic ovarian syndrome. However, there is some conflicting data about whether the newer progestins increase the risk of thromboembolic events [2, 11]. Women should be counselled about the possibility of the thromboembolic events so that they can seek care in the unlikely event that these occur. As when discussing potential side effects from birth control, the authors remind professionals and the youth themselves that pregnancy also can have serious negative health consequences.

Transdermal Patch

The contraceptive patch delivers hormone transdermally. The daily dose is 150 μg of the progestin norelgestromin and 35 μg of the ethinyl estradiol. The patch contains slightly more than 7 days' worth of hormones and therefore should be changed once a week. The patch should be applied to clean dry skin, and the old patch should be removed before placing a new one. The area of patch placement should change from week to week to avoid adverse effects on the skin. This is done for three consecutive weeks with a fourth patch-free week to induce a withdrawal bleed [2].

The patch is not recommended for use in women who weigh more than 90 kg as it may not be effective. There is also some data supporting increased risk of thromboembolic events compared to other methods [11]. Some teens do not like the idea of having something stuck to their skin. Others prefer this. Some teens have a sensitivity to the adhesive making it contraindicated for use. The need to change it only once a week makes it more convenient for some patients to use. This method can be visible to others.

Vaginal Ring

The vaginal ring is another combined hormonal contraceptive option which delivers 120 μg etonogestrel and 15 μg of ethinyl estradiol a day through contact with the vaginal mucosa. The ring is heat activated and should be kept at room temperature or lower until it is ready for use. It should not be used if it has been exposed to temperatures higher than 30 °C. According to the prescribing information, the ring contains enough hormone for 4 weeks of contraception. It can be used cyclically with removal and a ring-free period of 7 days to induce withdrawal bleed or continuously with replacement every 4 weeks for menstrual suppression (Fig. 11.2). It can be removed for up to 3 hours and reinserted if the woman or the person she is having sex with feels uncomfortable having it in place during sex. Most males and females do not feel the ring during sex and should be encouraged to keep the ring in place during sex to decrease the likelihood of forgetting to replace it after sex [27].

In addition to the typical side effects associated with combined hormonal contraception such as venous thromboembolism, breast tenderness and nausea, some women have side effects related to the intravaginal placement of the device, such as development of vaginal irritation, yeast infections or bacterial vaginosis [27]. Another potential problem with using the ring is storage of the device if they receive it more than 1 month at a time. Monthly trips to a pharmacy to pick up the ring will eliminate the problem of storage but adds the hindrance of frequent pharmacy visits.

For all prescribed methods, the more user responsibility required, the potentially less effective the method. The authors recommend offering as many packs or boxes as feasible or appropriate for pills, the ring and the patch so that accessing refills is less of an issue. When starting any method, we recommend a 2-week follow-up, as possible, to recheck a pregnancy test and to ensure that the young person remains comfortable with the method. This is another opportunity to dispel any myths around the contraceptive and review potential side effects and expected changes.

Barrier Methods

Condoms

Condoms are the most commonly used and easily available barrier method. When used correctly, they can be effective at reducing the risks of contracting STDs in addition to preventing pregnancy. However, typical use results in 18 women out of 100 getting pregnant [11]. This is usually due to incorrect use. The primary challenge with use of barrier methods is that they must be obtained in advance and then used at the time of sexual activity. Discomfort during sex is often cited as a reason why people do not use condoms. The main contraindication is allergy to latex, which is the most common material used for male condoms. Female condoms, also known as “internal condoms”, and non-latex condoms are available but are more expensive. An advantage of the female condom is that the woman can insert it herself and have more control in preventing sexual infections and pregnancy. Female condoms are also significantly larger than the male condom and eliminate concerns about the fit of the condom and some of the discomfort with use.

Anyone counselling youth about contraception should be able to counsel about how to use condoms. Condom use with all sexual encounters needs to be part of the discussion, even if an effective hormonal method is being used. Studies with homeless youth have demonstrated increased use of condoms when they are taught how to use condoms and provided condoms [28]. It is important not to assume that anyone knows how to correctly use condoms. Many people are not aware that condoms have expiry dates, can be more likely to break if they have been exposed to extreme temperatures or can have small tears if they are placed by someone with long fingernails or rings. Both males and females should be familiar with correct condom use. Figure 11.3 includes some information from the CDC about the importance of condom use [29]. This can be given to patients to help increase correct use of condoms. A sex positive approach, if that is appro-

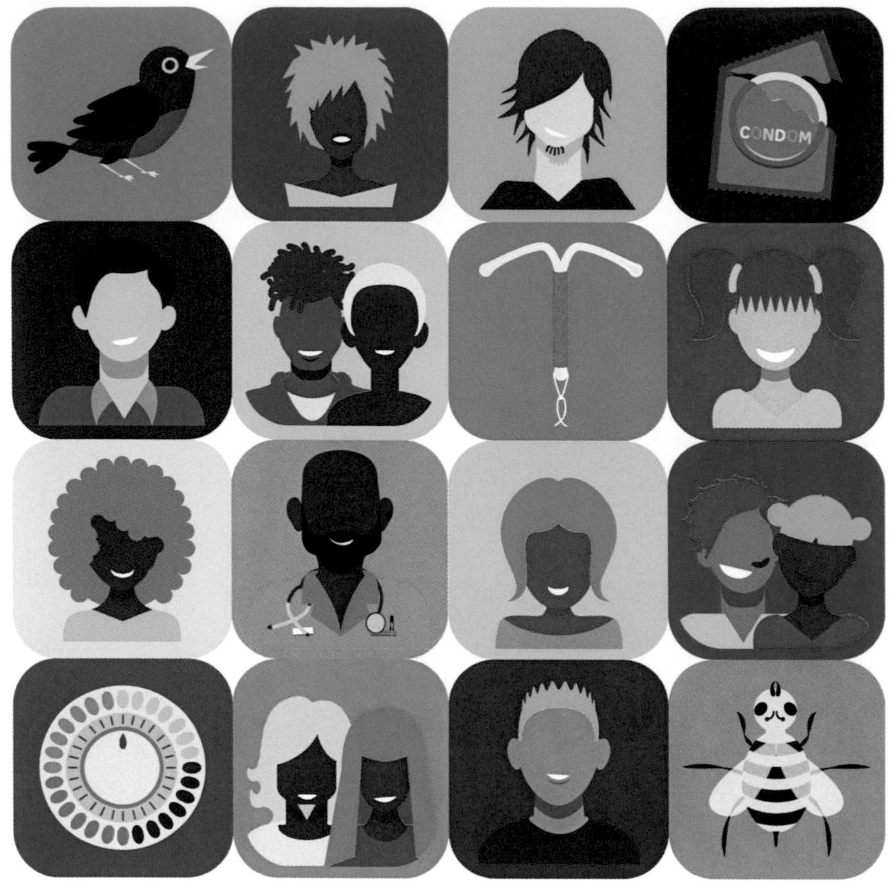

Fig. 11.3 Example Handout from the CDC on condom use [29]

If you are sexually active and are not ready to become a parent, it is important to use birth control to protect yourself from pregnancy.

It is also important to reduce your risk of getting sexually transmitted diseases (STDs), including HIV.

Condoms are the only birth control that reduces your risk of both pregnancy and STDs, including HIV. But, in order to work, condoms must be used correctly and must be used every time you have sex. It's important to know, however, that they cannot completely protect you and your partner from some STDs, like herpes, syphilis, or human papillomavirus (HPV), the virus that causes genital warts and cervical cancer. Also, condoms can break, slip, or leak, especially if they are not put on and taken off properly.

The only sure way to prevent pregnancy and STDs is NOT to have sex.

If you do have sex, use DUAL PROTECTION.

Even if you or your partner is using another type of birth control, agree to use a condom every time you have sex, to reduce the risk to both of you for HIV and most other STDs.

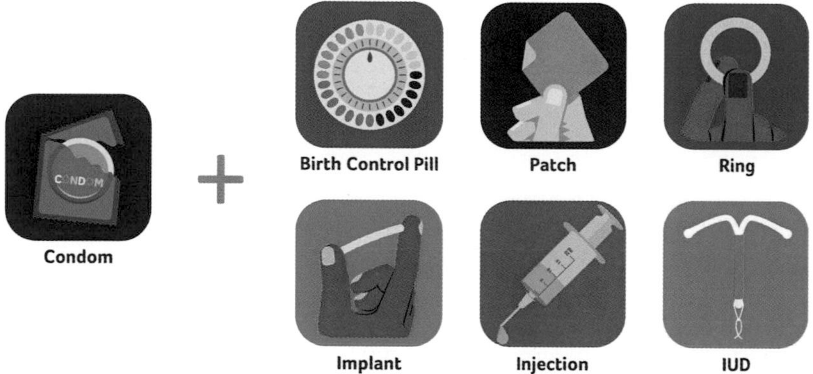

Remember!

- Use a condom and birth control.
- Condoms must be used correctly and used every time you have sex.
- Sometimes you or your partner might not know if one of you has an STD.

Fig. 11.3 (continued)

Know how to use a condom the right way, every time.

How do you put a condom on correctly?

The condom should be put on before any genital contact. Sperm may come out of the penis before the male ejaculates, so put the condom on before any skin-to-skin contact begins. You should also know that some STDs can be transmitted without intercourse, through genital (skin-to-skin) contact. To reduce the risk of pregnancy and STDs (including HIV), males need to wear a condom the entire time from the beginning to the end of genital contact, each and every time.

1 When you are opening the package, gently tear it on the side. Do not use your teeth or scissors because you might rip the condom that's inside. Pull the condom out of the package slowly so that it doesn't tear.

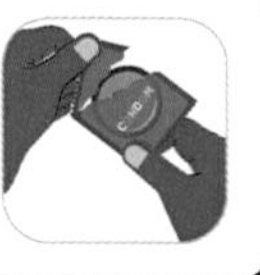

2 Put the rolled up condom over the head of the penis when it is hard.

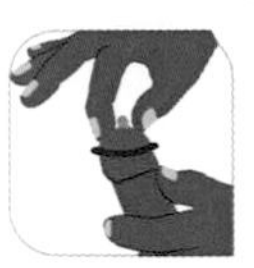

3 Pinch the tip of the condom enough to leave a half-inch space for semen to collect.

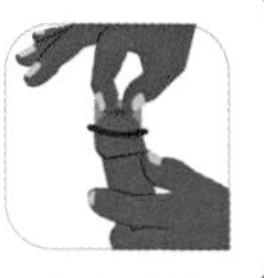

4 Holding the tip of the condom, unroll it all the way down to the base of the penis.

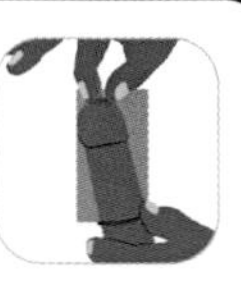

When the condom is on, it should feel snug enough so that it won't fall off during sex, but not too tight.

- If you accidentally put on a condom inside-out, throw it away and get a new one. You can tell a condom is inside-out if it won't roll down the length of the penis easily.
- If the condom ever tears or rips when you are putting it on or when it's being used, throw it away and use a new one.

How do you take off a condom correctly?

The most common mistake is not using condoms from the beginning of sexual contact to the very end, after ejaculation. Immediately after ejaculation, hold the bottom of the condom so it stays on and semen cannot spill out. Then, carefully withdraw the penis while it is still hard. Once the penis is out, you can remove the condom, wrap it in tissue, and throw it in the trash. Do not flush it down the toilet because it might clog.

What if the condom breaks?

If you feel the condom break at any point before or during sex:

Stop immediately! **Withdraw.** **Carefully remove the broken condom and put on a new one.**

If the condom breaks, pregnancy can be prevented with emergency contraception. Emergency contraception (the "Morning-After Pill") works best when it's started as soon as possible after sex, but can be started up to 5 days after sex.

Remember: Emergency contraception helps prevent pregnancy, but it does NOT protect against STDs.

Fig. 11.3 (continued)

Know your CONDOM DOs & DON'Ts

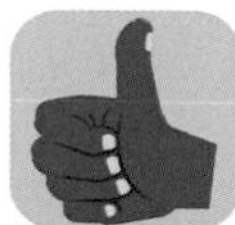

DO

- Read all the information on the package. Know what you are using.
- Check the expiration date on the package. If it is expired, get a new package of condoms and throw away the old ones.
- Use only condoms that are made of latex or polyurethane (plastic). Latex condoms and polyurethane condoms are the best types of condoms to use to help prevent pregnancy, STDs, and HIV.
- Use a pre-lubricated condom to help prevent it from tearing. If you only have a non-lubricated condom, put a little bit of water-based lubricant ("lube") inside and outside the condom.
- Condoms come in different sizes, colors, textures, and thicknesses. Talk with your partner and choose condoms both of you like.

DON'T

- Do not use two condoms at once.
- Do not use condoms made of animal skin, sometimes called "natural" condoms. Animal skin condoms can help prevent pregnancy but don't work as well as latex or polyurethane condoms to prevent STDs, including HIV.
- Do not keep condoms in a place that can get very hot, like in a car. If you keep a condom in your wallet or purse, be sure you replace it with a new one regularly.
- Do not use any kind of oil-based lubricants (like petroleum jellies, lotions, mineral oil, or vegetable oils). These can negatively affect the latex, making it more likely to rip or tear.
- Do not reuse condoms.
- Do not use condoms that are torn or outdated.

www.cdc.gov/teenpregnancy/Teens.html

National Center for Chronic Disease Prevention and Health Promotion
Division of Reproductive Health

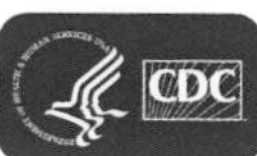

Fig. 11.3 (continued)

priate to the young person's situation, can be used in discussing condom placement as part of foreplay. Water-based lubricants can be recommended to help make condoms more comfortable. Making lubricants that feel, smell and/or taste good available or encouraging purchase through most drug and grocery stores may increase proper use.

Reviewing condom use with males is a good opportunity to discuss their reproductive life plan and when or if they may want children. A guideline for these discussions is available at https://www.cdc.gov/preconception/men.html. Males who are sexually involved with a regular female partner and do not want the responsibility of fathering children right now should be encouraged further to use condoms correctly every time and to discuss with their partners if they are on an effective birth control method. Males may want to encourage their female partners to seek care to review and access effective birth control options.

Condom use may not be possible for youth who are in coercive or abusive situations or being trafficked.

Sponge

The contraceptive sponge is a disposable spermicide-filled device that will release spermicide for up to 24 hours once activated. It is available without a prescription. The primary advantage of this method is that it can be inserted prior to intercourse and is effective for multiple sexual acts if they occur in the 24-hour time period. However, this device offers no protection against sexually transmitted infections and diseases.

Diaphragm and Cervical Cap

The diaphragm and cervical cap are both barrier methods that can be inserted prior to intercourse. They are more effective if used with spermicide. If used correctly, they can be 94% effective at preventing pregnancy [11]. They do not protect against sexually transmitted infections. They are available only with prescription, and a pelvic exam is required for proper fitting which will limit access and ease of use.

Natural Methods

As noted by Gelberg [23], challenges with storing methods, lack of awareness of methods and concerns about birth control being "unnatural" are barriers to use. Though they are not as effective at pregnancy prevention as any other method mentioned above, natural methods can be appealing to many youth. They are most useful for those in committed relationships with good communication between partners.

Periodic Abstinence

Periodic abstinence, fertility awareness or the "rhythm method" can be up to 75% effective at preventing pregnancy if the woman has regular menstrual cycles and uses it correctly [17]. This method is best used by women with regular menstrual cycles who can control when they have unprotected sex. Cycle beads or use of menstrual calendars on paper or as apps can be used to help make this method more effective. However, adolescents and those with hormonal or other disorders may have irregular menstrual cycles making this method less effective. As well, youth who are experiencing homelessness can be at risk for forced sex and sexual assault which would be a barrier to using this method. This method requires careful teaching.

An advantage of the rhythm method is that it has no side effects and can be used without the need for supplies. This may be preferred by youth who wish to stay hormone-free.

Withdrawal

Withdrawal or "pulling out" can be 78% effective at preventing pregnancy [11, 17]. It is the least effective of the methods studied but can reduce risk of pregnancy. This method is dependent on the male partner having control and removing his penis from his partner's vagina prior to ejaculation. It has the advantage of being free with no ahead of time preparation.

Emergency Contraception

Emergency contraception can prevent pregnancy in the case of rape, unprotected sex or contraceptive failure if used in the recommended time period. Ulipristal acetate and the copper IUD are highly effective at preventing pregnancy if prescribed within 5 days of unprotected intercourse [30–33]. Oral ulipristal acetate can be prescribed without a need for an exam. Ulipristal acetate is an antiprogestin. Taking ulipristal at the same time as a quick start hormonal birth control may decrease ulipristal's efficacy in preventing ovulation [32, 33]. A barrier method or abstinence could be used until the hormonal method is started 5 days after use of ulipristal [33]. However, each person's situation should be taken into account and allow for provider flexibility if there are concerns about follow-up and high risk for future pregnancy. Women may have misinformation that emergency contraceptive pills are abortifacient; they will benefit from professionals reviewing that this is not the case [33]. Training is required for IUD placement. Levonorgestrel pills can be used for emergency contraception and are available over the counter in Canada and the USA [34]. The levonorgestrel pills may be less effective for women with higher weights [30].

We recommend giving emergency contraceptive pills as an advanced prescription [30, 31] for women or men only relying on barrier methods, rhythm method and withdrawal ("pulling out") or who aren't using another hormonal method effectively. As appropriate, oral emergency contraception can be given to males for them to give to their partners in the event of contraceptive failure.

The Yuzpe method allows providers to use typical packets of birth control for emergency contraception. Taking two doses of COC with a 100 μg of ethinyl estradiol and 500 μg of levonorgestrel or its equivalent per dose 12 hours apart and within 3 days of unprotected sex can reduce the risk of pregnancy. The efficacy of this method is higher closer to the time of unprotected sex. If taken within the first 24 hours, 77% of pregnancies can be prevented. This wanes to 31% by 72 hours [35]. The emergency contraception website is an excellent resource for up-to-date information about emergency contraception https://ec.princeton.edu/questions/dose.html [36], including options for how to get it. It also includes information about how to make a dose of emergency contraception for the Yuzpe method from different brands of pills.

The use of oral emergency contraception may affect the next menstrual cycle. A repeat pregnancy test should be done 2 weeks after use of all emergency contraception to assess efficacy.

Clinical Issues

Psychosocial issues greatly influence the choice of contraception for all people. For youth experiencing homelessness there are many factors to consider. The HEADSS assessment is a psychosocial screening tool that was developed through work with high risk youth and is now part of routine adolescent health care [37, 38]. Using the modified HEEADSSS format, we have highlighted some issues which may influence the choice of contraception in Table 11.4. All staff members who are working with homeless youth can help medical providers offer the best advice by gathering information for a full medical history including current and past medication use. Using proper anatomic terminology, a respectful tone and science-based information and checking in for frequent understanding will help providers guide decision-making in a way that is useful for the young person. It may be appropriate to use humour at times. In the end, the choice of which method to use should be left to the adolescent or young adult. A method can always be changed to another. If appropriate, the partner or support person can join in the visit. Frequent follow-up can help to build rapport and ensure that the method is being used correctly [35, 39]. Motivational interviewing techniques are useful for assisting youth who are unsure of which option to choose or are uncertain about using contraception at all.

Table 11.4 Adapting the HEADSSS assessment for guiding contraceptive decision-making

HEEADSSS area	Questions	Effect on contraceptive choice
Home	Stable?	If yes, can choose from a variety of methods
	Couch surfing? On the streets?	If yes, they may have difficulty keeping track of methods like the pill, patch or contraceptive ring Also, the ring needs to be kept in a cool dry place before use May need access to free condoms on regular basis
	Foster care?	May wish to keep choice of method private from guardians or other foster children May need help in planning contraceptive coverage if returns to family of origin
	Travelling?	May not be able to make it to appointments to follow up on birth control refills or for the DMPA shots May lose pills, patch or ring while travelling
Education/employment	Native language Literacy level Cognitive impairment	They may not be able to understand information or instructions provided
	Engaged in sex work	May prefer method with predictable bleeding pattern or no bleeding and/or methods that are not visible to others and condoms to prevent STI's
	Working outdoors	Sweating a lot may affect how well the patch can stick to the skin
	Long-term goals	May prefer most effective pregnancy prevention such as LARC (implant or IUD)
Eating	Regular access to food?	If no, may not want methods that cause nausea
	Worried about overweight?	If yes, methods that may increase weight may not be preferred
	Wanting to gain weight?	May want methods more likely to increase weight
	Vegetarian/vegan	May prefer non-hormonal or natural methods like the rhythm method
Activities	What do they do for fun?	May want to have a method that would not interfere with their activities
		If they are uncertain about using birth control, thinking about how a pregnancy might affect their engagement in activities may help them decide

(continued)

Table 11.4 (continued)

HEEADSSS area	Questions	Effect on contraceptive choice
Drugs	Using drugs or alcohol?	If yes, this may interfere with ability to consistently follow through with user-dependent methods
		Decision making and understanding of risk may be impaired. Substance use may increase risk to fetus if does become pregant
		May need more consistent protection against sexually transmitted infections
Sex	5 Ps (see Table 11.1)	Need to have protection for actual sex practices
	Gender identity	Need to treat biology (if transmale has ovaries and uterus, he can still get pregnant)
	Sex abuse, trafficking or survival sex	May not be able to control access to method. Partner may sabotage method. May want concealed and effective method
	Plan for pregnancy	May be in situation with pressures to get pregnant May be seeking or not wanting to prevent pregnancy Consider offering prenatal vitamins, even if ambiguous about pregnancy
	History of previous birth control use?	Level of satisfaction or dissatisfaction with previous method can help with making a decision at this time
	Enjoyment of sex?	If yes, may be worried about method decreasing satisfaction for partner or themselves If no, using birth control and taking away concern about pregnancy may make sex more enjoyable
	Parties and other practices	If engaging in S&M, sharing parties, etc. will need protection from infection
	Abstinence/renewed abstinence	Have they used it? What worked? What didn't? How can they use it now?
Safety/suicidality	History of depression?	If yes, some methods may make better or worse. They may need closer monitoring
	Are mood symptoms worse with menses?	
Strengths	They are here and thinking about their health	Use motivational interviewing techniques to help with decision-making
	What has worked in the past to prevent pregnancy?	Can help with contraceptive decision-making
	What do you do well?	Reproductive control may allow them to have more time to do these things

Issues Specific to Homeless Youth

In addition to the usual considerations when choosing contraception, providers must think about the particular circumstances for youth experiencing homelessness. For youth who move often, there may be issues with storing and keeping some of the methods, being able to return to the office for administration of the method and check-ups. LARC methods can eliminate these concerns, but they may need medical support if there is prolonged irregular bleeding.

Many youth experience violence while homeless [4, 5]. The contraceptive implant is able to withstand pressure but can break if too much pressure is applied or there is repetitive trauma to the area. There have also been incidents of patients or other people cutting out the implant. This is extremely dangerous as there are many important blood vessels and nerves near the implant insertion site. Additionally, other youth may steal prescribed oral hormones for their own use as a contraceptive or for gender-affirming therapy.

Intrauterine devices are unlikely to be damaged through trauma but can increase the risk of serious infection such as pelvic inflammatory disease if the young woman is raped or is engaging in survival sex close to the time of insertion. Partners or those who are trafficking youth may sabotage the contraceptive method as a form of abuse. For these reasons, we recommend that all patients use condoms with hormonal contraception. We also recommend that youth receive treatment if there is any concern for infection or concern that they will not be able to return for treatment or results.

Similar to housed youth, youth experiencing homelessness may have other health conditions. However, they are less likely to have access to regular care. Youth should be encouraged to disclose any health conditions to their providers to guide the choice of contraception. The World Health Organization has complied Guidelines for Contraceptive Use in variety of health conditions. This should be referenced for any young woman with medical conditions who is seeking prescribed contraception. We have included the US version of this document in this chapter to help guide contraceptive decision-making. It is reprinted as Table 11.2.

Clinical Vignettes

Angela

Angela is a 17-year-old young woman who just came into the shelter where you work and plans to stay for at least 30 days. She has engaged in survival sex. Her last sexual encounter was yesterday. She did not use a condom. She is worried because she cannot feel the strings of her IUD. She also is complaining of a yellow discharge from her vagina.

Recommendations:

- Encourage getting a pregnancy test.
- If the pregnancy test is negative, provide emergency contraception as soon as possible.
- Help her access a healthcare provider who can assess and treat for sexually transmitted infections and assess location of the IUD. If the IUD is visible and in place, then this method can be continued. Angela can be treated for gonorrhoea, chlamydia and/or trichomoniasis as appropriate, and the IUD does not need to be removed.
- If the provider cannot feel or visualize the IUD strings either, then a pelvic ultrasound is recommended to assess for device migration. If the IUD is not visible, Angela can start another method or have the device replaced.

Toni

Toni is 16-year-old transmale. He identifies as bisexual. He has been using the DMPA injection for menstrual suppression and pregnancy prevention. He is worried about the weight gain he has had with this method. He would like to use something hormone-free. The provider who is trained in IUD insertion is not available in clinic until next month. Toni is due for his DMPA injection today.

Recommendations:

- Use "bridging"—use of another method of contraception until the IUD can be placed.
- Using a progesterone-only method will help Toni avoid potentially undesirable effects from oestrogen.
- He also could opt to use condoms or abstinence with a backup of emergency contraception until IUD placement.
- If he chooses to engage in sexual activity, condoms should be used to avoid infection prior to the IUD insertion.
- Offer Toni STI testing (oral, urine/vaginal or rectal as appropriate).

Serena

Serena is an 18-year-old woman who is travelling. She comes into your drop-in centre to get some food. While talking to staff, she lets them know that her bag was stolen last night. She has lost her ID and her packets of birth control. She has not had sex with a male in the past 2 months.

Recommendations:

- Assist her with getting her ID as that may be needed to access medical care.

- Assess how she was taking her pills and if she had missed any pills before having them stolen. Offer a pregnancy test if she had missed pills or is concerned.
- Counsel about availability of LARC which may be easier to deal with while travelling.
- If she wishes to continue COC, help her problem-solve if having them stolen or losing them can be prevented in the future.
- Help her obtain condoms and emergency contraception if desired.
- Provide feminine hygiene products if she is having periods with her COC or if you are unable to help her restart them as she may have withdrawal bleeding.

Resources

Web-based

(i) For adolescents and young adults:

1. Sex and U (from the Society of Obstetricians and Gynaecologists: https://www.sexandu.ca/
2. Bedsider.org (contraceptive information): https://www.bedsider.org/
3. Center for Young Women's Health: https://youngwomenshealth.org/
4. Young Men's Health: https://youngmenshealthsite.org/
5. American College of Obstetrics and Gynecology: https://www.acog.org/Patients
6. Society of Obstetricians and Gynaecologists of Canada: https://sogc.org/womens-health-programs/index.html
7. Emergency Contraception reference and clinic finder: https://ec.princeton.edu/
8. Clinic locator US: https://opa-fpclinicdb.hhs.gov/

(ii) For healthcare providers:

1. Family Planning: A Global Handbook for Providers: http://apps.who.int/iris/bitstream/handle/10665/260156/9780999203705-eng.pdf?sequence=1
2. Training Resource Package for Family Planning: https://www.fptraining.org/
3. Society of Obstetricians and Gynaecologists of Canada: https://sogc.org/womens-health-programs/index.html
4. Society for Adolescent Health and Medicine: https://www.adolescenthealth.org/Home.aspx
5. American College of Obstetrics and Gynecology: https://www.acog.org/
6. Center for Adolescent Health and the Law: https://www.cahl.org/
7. Guttmacher Institute: https://www.guttmacher.org/
8. Adolescent Health Initiative: http://www.umhs-adolescenthealth.org/improving-care/confidentiality/

9. Association for Reproductive Health Professionals: https://www.arhp.org/professional-education
10. Physicians for Reproductive Health: https://prh.org/medical-education

(iii) Information handouts for providers to give out:

1. https://www.acog.org/-/media/For-Patients/faq112.pdf?dmc=1&ts=20180909T1700538200
2. https://www.cdc.gov/reproductivehealth/contraception/unintendedpregnancy/pdf/Contraceptive_methods_508.pdf
3. https://www.cdc.gov/teenpregnancy/pdf/Teen-Condom-Fact_Sheet-English-March-2016.pdf
4. https://www.cdc.gov/preconception/men.html

References

1. Centers for Disease Control and Prevention. Ten great public health achievements—United States, 1900-1999. MMWR Wkly. 1999;48(12):241–3.
2. Tracy EE. Contraception: menarche to menopause. Obstet Gynecol Clin. 2017;44(2):143–58.
3. Sulak PJ. Continuous oral contraception: changing times. Best Pract Res Clin Obstet Gynaecol. 2008;22(2):355–74.
4. Elliott AS, Canadian Paediatric Society, Adolescent Health Committee. Meeting the health care needs of street involved youth. Paediatr Child Health. 2013;18(6):317–21.
5. Rickert V, Etter D, Chacko M. Sexual assualt and victimization. In: Neinstein LS, et al., editors. Neinstein's adolescent and young adult health care: a practical guide. 6th ed. Philadelphia: Wolters Kluwer; 2016. p. 610–8.
6. American Academy of Pediatrics Committee on Adolescence. The adolescent's right to confidential care when considering abortion. Pediatrics. 2017;139(2):e20163861.
7. Ensign J. Reproductive health of homeless adolescent women in Seattle, Washington, USA. Women Health. 2000;31(2–3):133–51.
8. Klein DA, et al. Providing Quality Family Planning Services to LGBTQIA individuals: a systemic review. Contraception. 2018;97(5):378–91.
9. Gelberg L, et al. Homeless women: who is really at risk for unintended pregnancy. Matern Child Health J. 2008;12:52–60.
10. Winetrobe H, et al. Pregnancy attitudes, contraceptive service utilization, and other factors associated with Los Angeles homeless youths' use of effective contraception and withdrawal. J Pediatr Adolesc Gynecol. 2013;26(6):314–22.
11. Di Meglio G, Crowther C, Simms J, Canadian Paediatric Society, Adolescent Health Committee. Contraceptive care for Canadian youth. Paediatr Child Health. 2018;23(4):271–7.
12. Society for Adolescent Health and Medicine. Protecting adolescents: ensuring access to care and reporting sexual activity and abuse. J Adolesc Health. 2004;35(5):420–3.
13. US Department of Health and Human Services Centers for Disease Control and Prevention. A guide to taking a sexual history. Available at: https://www.cdc.gov/std/treatment/sexualhistory.pdf. Accessed 10 Oct 2018.
14. American Medical Association. Code of medical ethics opinion. 2.2.2 "Confidential health care for minors." 2016.
15. Adolescent Health Initiative. Confidentiality. Available at: http://www.umhs-adolescenthealth.org/improving-care/confidentiality/. Accessed 20 Oct 2018.

16. Francis JKR, Gold MA. Long-acting reversible contraception for adolescents: a review. JAMA Pediatr. 2017;171(7):694–701.
17. Curtis KM, Tepper NK, Jatlaoui TC, et al. U.S. Medical Eligibility Criteria for Contraceptive Use, 2016. MMWR Recomm Rep 2016;65(No. RR-3):1–104. https://doi.org/10.15585/mmwr.rr6503.
18. Jatlaou TC, et al. The safety of intrauterine devices among young women: a systematic review. Contraception. 2017;95(1):17–39.
19. Grimes DA. Intrauterine device and upper-genital-tract infection. Lancet. 2000;356(9234): 1013–9.
20. Wu JP, Moniz MH, Ursu AN. Long-acting reversible contraception-highly efficacious, safe, and underutilized. JAMA. 2018;320(4):397–8.
21. Dasari M, et al. Barriers to long-acting reversible contraceptive uptake among homeless young women. J Pediatr Adolesc Gynecol. 2016;29:104–10.
22. Anthoulakis C, et al. Pain perception during levonorgestrel-releasing intrauterine device insertion in nulliparous women: a systematic review. J Pediatr Adolesc Gyneco. 2018;31(6):549–56.
23. Gelberg L, et al. Chronically homeless women's perceived deterrents to contraception. Perspect Sex Reprod Health. 2002;34(6):278–85.
24. World Health Organization. Medical eligibility criteria for contraceptive use. 5th ed. Geneva: World Health Organization; 2015. p. 111–33.
25. Wright KP, Johnson JV. Evaluation of extended and continuous use oral contraceptives. Ther Clin Risk Manag. 2008;4(5):905–11.
26. People's Community Clinic. Continuous cycling for the pill and the ring. 2014.
27. Veres S, Miller L, Burington B. A comparison between the vaginal ring and oral contraceptives. Obstet Gynecol. 2004;104(3):555–63.
28. Haignere CS, et al. High-risk adolescents and female condoms: knowledge, attitudes, and use patterns. J Adolesc Health. 2000;26(6):392–8.
29. Centers for Disease Control and Prevention (CDC). It's your future. You can protect it. Created 2 June 2016. Available at: https://www.cdc.gov/condomeffectiveness/index.html. Accessed 30 Oct 2018.
30. Society for Adolescent Health and Medicine. Emergency contraception for adolescents and young adults: guidance for health care professionals. J Adolesc Health. 2016;58(2):245–8.
31. Gold MA, Sucato GS, Conard LE, Hillard P, et al. Provision of emergency contraception to adolescents. J Adolesc Health. 2004;35(1):66–70.
32. Kelly C, Elizabeth GR, Elizabeth W, James T. Emergency Contraception Review. Clinical Obstetrics and Gynecology 57(4):741-750.
33. Trussell, James; Raymond, Elizabeth G; Cleland, Kelly "Emergency Contraception: A Last Chance to Prevent Unintended Pregnancy" January 2019. Accessible at: https://ec.princeton.edu/questions/ec-review.pdf.
34. Fisher WA, Black A. Contraception in Canada: a review of method choices, characteristics, adherence and approaches to counselling. CMAJ. 2007;176(7):953–61.
35. Dunn S, Guilbert E. Society of Obstetrics and Gynecology of Canada. Clinical practice guidelines No. 131. Aug 2003.
36. The Emergency Contraception Website. https://ec.princeton.edu/questions/dose.html. Accessed 13 Oct 2018.
37. Cohen E, et al. HEADSS, a psychosocial risk assessment instrument: implications for designing effective intervention programs for runaway youth. J Adolesc Health. 1991;12(7):539–44.
38. Goldenring JM, Cohen E. Getting into adolescent heads. Contemp Pediatr. 1988; 5:75-82.
39. American College of Obstetrics and Gynecology. Committee opinion no. 710: counseling adolescents about contraception. Obstet Gynecol. 2017;130(2):E74–80.

Chapter 12
Sexually Transmitted Infections and Sexual Healthcare of Homeless and Street-Involved Youth

Troy Grennan, Joshua Edward, and Sarah Chown

> Adolescence is a time of opportunity, but also one of risk.
> –World Health Organization, *Making Health Services Adolescent Friendly*, 2012

Introduction

This quote is emblematic of the challenging paradox presented by the provision of sexual health services to adolescents and young adults (herein, AYA; 'AYA' and 'youth' will be used interchangeably). On the one hand, AYA have among the highest rates of sexually transmitted infections (STIs) of any population [1], and these risks can be exacerbated by some of the experiences of simply being young. On the other hand, though healthcare providers often approach sex among AYA in terms of risk or potential harm, it is critical to remember that sexuality and sexual behaviour are normal parts of healthy development. Thus, providing appropriate, comprehensive and sensitive sexual healthcare to AYA requires a recognition of these oft-competing priorities. Specific resources and treatment guidelines for STIs and other sexual health-related issues in AYA are essential, as AYA not only carry a disproportionate burden of STI diagnoses but may also face structural barriers (e.g. inadequate sexual health education) and other unique considerations (e.g. parental notification of receipt of sexual health services) related to STI testing, diagnosis and successful treatment [2, 3]. In 1995, the World Health Organization (WHO), along

T. Grennan (✉)
BC Centre for Disease Control, Vancouver, BC, Canada
e-mail: troy.grennan@bccdc.ca

J. Edward
Dalhousie University, Halifax, NS, Canada
e-mail: joshua.edward@dal.ca

S. Chown
YouthCO, Vancouver, BC, Canada
e-mail: sarahc@youthco.org

C. Warf, G. Charles (eds.), *Clinical Care for Homeless, Runaway and Refugee Youth*, https://doi.org/10.1007/978-3-030-40675-2_12

with the United Nations Children's Fund (UNICEF) and the United Nations Population Fund (UNFPA), put forth a *Common Agenda for Action* aimed at adolescent health [4]. This document takes a two-pronged approach: first, to acknowledge and support healthy adolescent development, and, second, to prevent and address health issues when they arise. This type of complementary approach must be taken into account in the development of any effective AYA sexual health program and arguably is one of the only ways to resolve the abovementioned paradox.

AYA already face many challenges relating to STIs and sexual healthcare: lack of access to services and appropriate education, embarrassment, fear (real or perceived) of stigma and concern that their confidentiality will be compromised – and these are the proverbial tip of the iceberg. Homelessness worsens all of these and is not a rare problem among AYA. In the United States (USA), homelessness is estimated to impact 1.6 million AYA annually, with the majority being in 18–24-year-old age group [5]. Homelessness alone is an important risk factor for STI and HIV acquisition [6], so it follows that in the context of the many other challenges and barriers experienced by AYA as they struggle to understand emerging issues of sexual health, the impact of these interconnected issues on the health of AYA would be additive and detrimental.

This chapter will provide an overview of the sexual health and STI care of AYA in four parts. The first section will provide two different frameworks offering critical elements in understanding – and ultimately providing care to – AYA experiencing STI and sexual health-related issues. The second section will put forth the context within which AYA – particularly those who are homeless or otherwise marginalized – experience their sexual lives. The third section will provide a practical overview of STI and sexual health clinical care provision, focusing on specific STIs of importance in AYA. The final section will present several priorities for future research.

Fundamental Frameworks for Understanding the Sexual Lives of Adolescents and Young Adults

When considering the care and management of STIs in AYA, with the exception of some subtle differences, issues relating to the diagnosis, clinical manifestations, treatment and prevention are not dissimilar from STI care in adults. Where the significant differences occur and where the provider must pay special attention are in two specific domains: first, how health services are set up for – and accessed by – AYA patients, particularly those experiencing marginalization such as homelessness, and, second, what special circumstances AYA face in experiencing STIs and other issues relating to sexual health. These two areas are best understood through an examination of different theoretical frameworks addressing them. These frameworks set the tone for the following section's discussion on communication, respecting diversity and recognizing the importance of autonomy by presenting several of these ideas in a formalized manner. They provide a foundation for the provision of appropriate STI and sexual health services to AYA, in a way that is acceptable to them and which takes into consideration the unique circumstances and contexts within which they live.

Ensuring STI and Sexual Healthcare Is AYA-Friendly

The first theoretical framework is based on the WHO's 'Quality of Care' document [7] and puts forth a number of criteria required to overcome the most significant barriers experienced by AYA in accessing healthcare services. Though not specific to STIs or sexual health, these are arguably more important for sexual health services than they are for many other health-related issues, given the complex social network within which these are accessed. This WHO framework highlights the following five quality components required in order for services to be considered 'adolescent-friendly':

- *Equitable*: Providing healthcare or services that are *equitable* requires that all AYA are able to obtain such services with no restrictions (e.g. on the basis of age, gender, ethnicity, sexual orientation) and that those providing the services deliver them with equal care and respect to all.
- *Accessible*: The concept of *accessible* services requires that AYA are able to get the services they require, with minimal or no barriers, including cost, hours of service and proximity. Additionally, accessibility requires that those obtaining services are informed about the details of the services provided, and that there is community support and awareness of such services and their intended benefits.
- *Acceptable*: Healthcare services are considered *acceptable* if they meet the expectations of AYA. There are multiple components to this, including the following: the assurance of privacy, comprising formalized processes (e.g. policies) and the 'set-up' of the environment where services are provided; having providers who are relatable and non-judgemental and who are able to make provisions to provide services or make necessary referrals within a short time window; and allowing for the meaningful involvement of AYA in the design and delivery of services, so that their preferences are reflected in the services provided.
- *Appropriate*: In order for healthcare services to be *appropriate*, the specific needs of AYA must be met and must not only be limited to the needs of the general population but also tailored to those with specialized needs (e.g. marginalized groups).
- *Effective*: Health services are considered *effective* if they are provided in a way that positively contributes to the health of AYA. Further, those providing the services must be competent, spend the appropriate amount of time and use evidence-informed guidelines and/or interventions to drive their practice. Finally, the location of service delivery must be equipped with the appropriate resources to deliver quality services.

The previously cited WHO document is an excellent resource for providers and staff of healthcare facilities to assess the quality of the services they provide and puts forth a comprehensive set of in-depth questions for AYA patients, as well as their healthcare providers, and clinic managers to assist with this. Additionally, scripts, interview tools and other detailed resources relating to care provision to youth and adolescents are provided [7].

Applying a Syndemic Approach to the Sexual Healthcare of Homeless AYA

The second theoretical framework relevant to a discussion of STIs and healthcare in AYA is based on the concept of syndemics, originally proposed by Merrill Singer in the mid-1990s [8–10]. STIs – and particularly STIs in youth and adolescents – cannot be considered in isolation. The occurrence of STIs in youth and adolescents is intimately linked to the environment in which youth and adolescents live, the unique situations to which they are exposed and, as noted by the US Centers for Disease Control and Prevention, even heightened biological susceptibility to STI transmission and infection. Additionally, homeless AYA have increased vulnerability to sexual assault and other forms of sexual violence and face unique challenges (e.g. an inability to work legally) in order to obtain food, shelter and other necessities. As such, STIs in youth and adolescents are interconnected to other comorbidities and social factors, including mental health issues, substance use, poverty, stigma, discrimination and other medical illnesses [11]. The interconnections and intersections may combine to create a climate in which basic needs are met through survival sex or other actions that increases STI risk even more, as highlighted in a study of survival sex of young women in Los Angeles, where those engaged in survival sex were primarily motivated by desperation to meet basic needs such as shelter and food for themselves and their young children [12]. According to Singer, syndemics are 'the aggregation of two or more diseases or other health conditions in a population in which there is some level of deleterious biological or behaviour interface that exacerbates the negative health effects of any or all of the diseases involved'. Singer further indicates that, '[s]yndemics involve the adverse interaction of diseases of all types … (and) are most likely to emerge under conditions of health inequality caused by poverty, stigmatisation, stress or structural violence because of the role of these factors in diseases clustering and exposure and in increased physical and behavioural vulnerability' [13]. Though initially conceived in relation to the HIV epidemic in men who have sex with men (MSM) [14], the applicability of the syndemic conceptualization to STIs in adolescents – particularly adolescents who are homeless or experiencing other forms of marginalization – is obvious. See Fig. 12.1 for a conceptual representation of how syndemic conditions may synergistically interact to promote adverse outcomes.

Arguably, in most settings, STI prevention and care efforts focus on the individual and emphasize risk reduction while ignoring broader systemic and environmental factors that may impact risk and behaviours [15], like those discussed above. Efforts and interventions addressing and redressing these larger contextual factors affecting AYA at risk for STIs are critical, as are strategies aimed at mitigating the impact of these underlying conditions [16, 17]. As practitioners and researchers interested in the sexual health and the care of STIs in AYA, it is critical that both of the frameworks presented herein be considered and actively applied when addressing issues of sexual health and STIs and when providing care. By doing so,

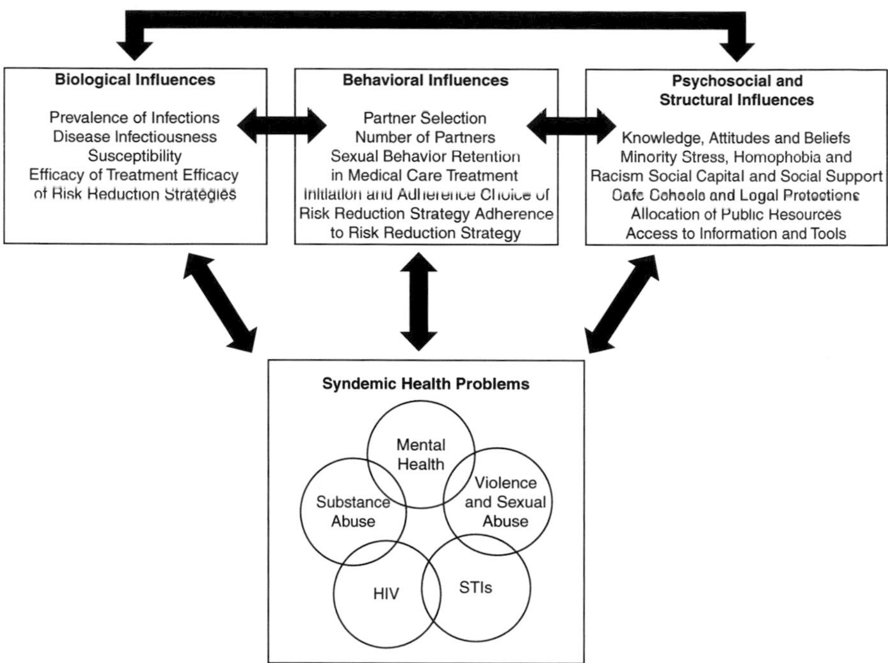

Fig. 12.1 A conceptual representation of how overlapping conditions ('syndemics') can synergistically interact to produce adverse health outcomes. (Reprinted from Halkitis et al. [11])

it will help ensure that practitioners are providing AYA with a safe space for care that is appropriate and acceptable and that a comprehensive understanding of the interacting factors impacting on the sexual health and lives of AYA is taken into consideration.

Contextualizing STIs and Sexual Health in Homeless Adolescents and Young Adults

The Challenges of Homelessness for AYA

Despite increased visibility for lesbian, gay, bisexual, transgender, queer, asexual, pansexual and two-spirit (henceforth, LGBTQ+/2S) AYA in schools, students of all genders and sexualities still struggle to get relevant, reliable, stigma-free information about sexual health in classroom settings [18–20]. Many parents, educators [21], clinicians [22] and foster caregivers are ill-equipped for open conversations about sexual health. For example, these adults may not have up-to-date information about treatment or testing or may not have the language necessary to talk about sex in a way that affirms the gender[1] and sexual identity of the AYA in their lives [20]. Other barriers that can make it difficult for AYA to get relevant sexual health information include the desire on the part of some adults to prevent youth from becoming sexually active and the myth that talking about sex openly encourages young people to become sexually active. Shelters and emergency housing – on which some youth may rely – have varying policies about sex, some of which discourage service providers from sharing sexual health information or supplies such as condoms. In some scenarios, these limitations may mean that providers are unable to speak about abortion services or are prohibited from acknowledging forms of sex that do not lead to procreation. Adults are often especially apprehensive about speaking openly about sexual health with AYA who have physical or developmental disabilities and youth who are being raised with an expectation of abstinence (e.g. in certain immigrant or religious communities).

Street-involved AYA may be navigating sex in the context of poverty and substance use (i.e. survival sex) [23] and often do not have safe, private spaces to experience sexual pleasure. In a study of street-involved youth in 13 municipalities across the Canadian province of British Columbia, 16% of street-involved youth reported unwanted sex as a consequence of substance use in the past year. These circumstances include specific risks that youth with stable housing may not encounter. Notably, youth living on the streets are at greater risk for sexual violence [24].

Policies in many emergency shelters and temporary housing spaces prohibit sexual activity, which can push AYA to have sex in public spaces. These policies are not consistently enforced, sending mixed messages to residents and making it difficult for youth to predict what behaviour is acceptable. For youth who want to engage in sex, this can put them in the precarious or potentially dangerous scenario of being interrupted during sex or facing violence from partners disappointed by an interrupted sexual encounter. AYA who are looking for sexual health information or supplies in these contexts may be unsure if they can speak openly about sex. Having sex in public spaces may limit opportunity to have pleasurable experiences and discourage AYA from taking the time necessary to use condoms and/or other protective measures.

Street-involved AYA may also rely on sex as a source of income, shelter or drugs. These circumstances are known to diminish the capacity that youth have to negotiate healthy sexual relationships and safer sex strategies, including condom use.

[1] Recognizing the broad diversity of sexual identity, sexual orientation and gender identity, we have taken measures in this chapter to ensure the language we use is inclusive and gender-affirming. We have attempted to avoid making assumptions about gender, preferring to use more specific language when appropriate (e.g. person with a cervix rather than female; recognizes that both cisgender females and transgender males may have a cervix). In some situations, particularly when reporting on epidemiologic trends, this was not possible, as most studies use 'male' and 'female' as exclusive gender categories. In these situations, we use the terms as reported. In some situations, for clarity of language, we have used the terms 'biological female' and 'biological male' to refer to individuals who were assigned that particular gender at birth or have the sexual anatomy associated with female or male sex.

Substance use often interacts with sexual decision-making among AYA, especially for street-involved youth, where addiction and concurrent disorders are highly prevalent.

The Sexual Lives of Homeless and Street-Involved AYA

Street-involved AYA disproportionately experience exclusion and rejection, often both as a factor that pushes them into homelessness and as a result of street involvement [23]. These experiences can take the form of bullying at school, being removed from school or family; discrimination when accessing health care (15% of street-involved youth did not access healthcare in the past year due to prior negative experiences [23]), social or public services; or being at the hands of police. Many of these experiences of exclusion and rejection are based in racism, classism, transphobia and homophobia. In response, many AYA become distrustful of the systems intended to offer support [25].

Another message that youth may receive through these experiences is that concealing parts of their identity or experience is a way to protect themselves from harm. For example, youth present as straight and cisgender in order to avoid homophobic and transphobic violence. Youth may also conceal their housing, food or income insecurity, both to avoid judgment from service providers and to prevent involvement of additional systems such as child welfare agencies or police that may return them to housing or a situation that is unsafe for them. The concealment that is required in these unsafe environments often has deleterious impacts on youth mental health, social connection and overall well-being. Within this context, however, it is imperative to recognize that some street-involved AYA, as well as those experiencing homelessness and other forms of housing precarity, may demonstrate poor judgment of their own critical needs – regardless of self-identified gender identity or sexual orientation expressions. Child protective services that are designed to meet the unique needs of street-involved and homeless AYA, including those self-identifying as LGBTQ+/2S, are still best positioned to provide the most readily available stabilizing services. While there may be a legitimate and recognized need for increasing access to interdisciplinary, effective, accepting and compassionate stabilization services that are rooted in evidence and best-practices, there too exists a need to recognize the importance of working with existing public, private and non-profit and other non-governmental agencies and services providing support to street-involved and homeless AYA.

The Importance of Language

There are many tools that clinicians can use to make healthcare more accessible and safer for AYA who are street-involved. Making a conscious choice to use language that avoids assumptions and counters stigma is one such strategy. The language we suggest here also takes a plain language approach to health communication, while also tackling stigma related to STIs and HIV directly, as well as the identities and experiences that are commonly disproportionately associated with these identities and experiences. These language choices may make it easier for AYA to see themselves represented in positive ways, without any action required on their part. Table 12.1 offers some concrete suggestions for clinicians working with AYA in a sexual health context.

STIs, including HIV, are often considered through a public health lens, leading us to use verbs such as infect or spread in conversations, as well as to describe people who are living with STIs as 'infected with'. These words divert attention from the individual patient's needs and instead immediately turn the focus to the public health imperative associated with HIV and STIs. Further, the words 'infect' or 'spread' are associated with a certain degree of malfeasance and overlook evidence that indicates people who are aware of an STI diagnosis often go to great lengths to ensure their partners do not get an STI as well. Alternatives to this language include using the verb 'pass' and stating people with a current STI diagnosis

Table 12.1 Guidance on appropriate language in providing sexual healthcare to AYA

Avoid saying:	Instead, try:
Infect or spread e.g. youth can be infected through sex	Pass e.g. HIV can be passed through unprotected vaginal, anal, or frontal sex
Infected with HIV or suffers from HIV	Living with HIV
Gendered descriptions e.g. female condoms e.g. Pap smears are an important part of healthcare for women	Body parts or actions e.g. insertive condoms e.g. Pap smears are an important part of healthcare for people with a cervix[a]
Prostitution	Sex work
Junkies, addicts, alcoholic	People who use drugs, people experiencing addiction, people with a substance use disorder (this depends on what is being discussed; note, most individuals use drugs, e.g. caffeine, nicotine, over-the-counter medications)
Clean/dirty used to describe equipment or people	To describe people – abstinent, not using/actively using To describe equipment (e.g. needles) – new, unused/used
Normal e.g. normal sex e.g. a normal CD4 cell count is…	More specific language – 'normal' can be othering and exclusive e.g. 'penis in vagina' sex; sex where a mouth is on a bum, vulva e.g. CD4 cell counts above 500 mean our immune system can fight off most infections
Protect e.g. protect against HIV	Prevent e.g. prevent HIV from being passed
Sexually transmitted disease (STD)	Sexually transmitted infection (STI) – infection is more accurate and less stigmatizing

[a]See Footnote [1]

are 'living with [an STI]'. Another word to avoid for these reasons is 'protect' against, with 'prevent' as a possible alternative. Similar considerations also underpin the recommendation to avoid the word 'clean'(to describe people who are HIV-negative, lifestyles, behaviours [e.g. sex work] or new/unused drug paraphernalia) and 'dirty' (to describe people living with an STI, lifestyles or behaviours that pose increased possibility of STI transmission or used drug paraphernalia).

Recognizing Diversity of Identities

There are many relationships that AYA may have to LGBTQ+/2S identities because of continued homophobia, biphobia and transphobia. Many youth – especially those who may have been pushed out of their homes or schools because of their assumed identity as LGBTQ+/2S – may be reluctant to use these labels or share these parts of their identity with care providers. Further, AYA may not have experiences with LGBTQ+/2S people or community and may not connect themselves to these identities now but may in the future. This is clear from studies on sexuality in adolescents, where AYA's uncertainty about their sexual orientation decreases with age: in one study, whereas 26% of 12-year-olds surveyed expressed uncertainty about their sexual orientation, only 5% of 17-year-olds did [26]. Street-involved AYA may be engaged in sexual acts associated with LGBTQ+/2S identities through survival sex work or sexual violence. These scenarios demonstrate circumstances in which AYA either may not have information about an LGBTQ+/2S identity to share with a care provider or choose not to share vulnerable information about themselves.

Much of sexual health education and care has been developed from a cisgender, heterosexual perspective, with this being an underlying assumption. While there have been important shifts to ensure gender affirmation is included in such education, clinics have much more experience providing sexual health to cisgender and heterosexual patients and must be active in meeting needs of LGBTQ+/2S youth. One assumption that still exists in many clinical settings is congruency between sexual identity and sexual behaviour; for example, lesbian women only have sex with other women. These assumptions may sometimes lead to erroneous conclusions or clinical recommendations (e.g. lesbians do not need cervical cancer screening, or they cannot get pregnant). Additionally, these assumptions often erase or ignore transgender people, whether they are the patient or a partner of the patient. In many clinical settings, the onus is on the patient to disclose if they are LGBTQ+/2S or if they are having sex other than the dominant assumption of 'penis-in-vagina' sex. These assumptions can limit the care that is provided to young patients; this may mean patients are not offered contraception, cervical cancer screening, STI testing or information about their sexual health needs that could be right for them. Another potential scenario is clinicians relying on patients to use LGBTQ+/2S language to cue them to use inclusive language or address specific sexual health needs.

Clinicians working in sexual health will benefit from strategies to offer LGBTQ+/2S-inclusive and gender-affirming care without relying on patients to disclose. One such strategy is creating an explicitly LGBTQ+/2S-inclusive clinical setting, by ensuring LGBTQ+/2S people are visible in signage and information that is available and including cues to LGBTQ+/2S-inclusive practice (e.g. sharing pronouns of staff members, asking for patient's pronouns, distinguishing between a person's legal name and the name they prefer to use). AYA are also best served when clinicians avoid substituting gendered descriptions for names of people (e.g. assuming she/her pronouns for a person with developed breasts), sexual acts (e.g. sex between a man and a woman) or names of body parts (e.g. female private parts). These types of gendered descriptions make assumptions that may be untrue for many AYA, including youth who identify as LGBTQ+/2S. Alternatives to gendered descriptions include using a person's name and/or asking for their pronoun, whether in conversation or on an intake form, using names of body parts and their less-gendered equivalents where appropriate. For example, using the term 'insertive condom' rather than female condom is both helpful for people with a vagina who are not females and for reminding people that insertive condoms can be used in the anus as well.

Providing the Opportunity to Exercise Autonomy

Another important strategy for clinicians to use when working with street-involved AYA is to create opportunities for youth to exercise autonomy and make decisions about their own care. Many street-involved AYA typically have limited opportunities in which they are able to exercise autonomy. Street-involved AYA, whether they are couch surfing, staying in shelters or staying in public spaces, do not have a permanent space that they can control. In these scenarios, youth do not have a place to keep things that are important or special to them or the things that may make it easier for them to navigate daily life (e.g. identification such as a health insurance card, extra clothing). Surviving in semipublic spaces means AYA must constantly be aware of their surroundings to keep themselves and their belongings safe, do not have control over their sleeping hours and are subject to regulation by police or shelter workers. Additionally, street-involved AYA may be exposed to specific risks associated with housing precarity and time spent in public and semipublic spaces. Street-involved AYA may be at heightened risk for sexual assault, sexual exploitation and other forms of sexual violence (both by peers and older youth and adults) and may also find themselves exposed to different/more dangerous and addictive drugs than their non-street-involved peers. Offering clinical services that contrast with these experiences can help engage youth.

An illustrative example of how affirming AYA autonomy can be integrated into sexual healthcare is ensuring youth are informed about the confidentiality of their healthcare information, including an assurance that health information will not be shared with caregivers where appropriate and what potential disclosures may occur (e.g. in case of suspected harm). Clinicians may also benefit from providing AYA with information that allows them to make decisions about the types of tests or treatment that may be appropriate, rather than recommending them from the outset. This can also help avoid assumptions about body parts or sexual activity for each individual patient. Other strategies that can help engage LGBTQ+/2S AYA and other street-involved youth include having low-barrier clinic requirements, for instance, not requiring legal identification or follow-up contact information. Other suggestions for low-barrier clinics include offering as many services as possible simultaneously, such as providing harm reduction and safer sex supplies for free on-site or offering treatment ahead of results for suspected STIs as appropriate. Some of these ideas vis-à-vis making services 'low-barrier' and appropriate will be discussed in the next section.

STI Clinical Care in Homeless Adolescent and Young Adult Populations and Communities

Overview

This section will now focus on some of the specific STIs that impact on AYA. In many instances, youth are disproportionately impacted by STIs, with prevalence rates much higher than those seen in adults [27, 28]. Rather than providing an exhaustive review of these infections – which is beyond the scope of this chapter – it will provide guidance for doing an appropriate sexual and STI history, as well as an overview of some of the key infections, with a focus on AYA-specific issues relating to each infection. This section will focus on the following infections: chlamydia, gonorrhoea, syphilis, trichomoniasis, lice, scabies, human papillomavirus and human immunodeficiency virus.

STI Risk Factors

There is tremendous overlap in the risk factors for the various STIs impacting AYA, independent of homelessness and poverty, though these can certainly exacerbate the impact of other risk factors. These risk factors can be broadly divided into behavioural, biological and psychosocial risk factors. *Behavioural* risk factors associated with STI acquisition in AYA include younger age of sexual debut [29–31]; having multiple sexual partners concurrently or partners with multiple partners [32]; having serial, short-lived sexual partnerships [7]; a number of new sexual partners [27, 33], inconsistent use of barrier (e.g. condom) methods [27] and alcohol or drug use [34, 35]. *Biological* risk factors for STI acquisition have not been well studied, and thus there is a paucity of data; the limited data available focuses primarily on biological females. Specifically, one theory postulates that cervical ectopy is responsible for higher susceptibility to STIs in individuals with a cervix [36], though the evidence is conflicting on this [37]. In AYA, the outer surface of the cervix contains columnar cells that are postulated to be more susceptible to certain STIs than squamous cells, which ultimately replace columnar cells once sexual maturity occurs. Other potential biologic mechanisms of STI susceptibility in AYA include lower levels of a specific immunoglobulin level in the cervical mucus [38] and alterations in the composition of the vaginal microbiome [39]. *Psychosocial* risk factors for STIs are typically complex, interrelated and often additive and would include factors such as homelessness or poverty, both of which have been shown to be risk factors for STI acquisition in Canadian and US studies [5, 6]. Concurrent mental illness or mood disorders [7, 40, 41], sex trade work [42], incarceration [7] and substance use [43, 44] have all been shown to be associated with STI acquisition, and many of these are much more likely to co-occur with homelessness and poverty, which then mutually reinforce each other.

The Sexual History

The cornerstone of providing appropriate sexual health and STI care is the sexual history and risk assessment. Eliciting a sexual history in youth and adolescents should be done in a manner that incorporates the abovementioned principles from the WHO in ensuring services are adolescent-friendly [7]; in other words, it should be equitable, accessible, acceptable, appropriate and effective. The history should be done in a non-judgemental manner, in a setting that is comfortable and where confidentiality and privacy can be assured and using language that is understandable and inclusive. See Table 12.2 for a set of questions making up a complete STI history.

Table 12.2 The components of a complete sexual history for AYA

Category	Example questions to guide assessment
General health history	
Medical history	Do you have current or past medical issues? Are you on any medications? Do you have any medication allergies?
Vaccination history	Have you been vaccinated for hepatitis A and/or B and human papillomavirus (HPV)?
Relationships	
Present situation	Do you have a regular sexual partner or partners? If yes, how long have you been with this person?
Identify concerns	Do you have any concerns about your relationship(s)? If yes, what are they (e.g. violence, abuse)?
STI history	
Prior STI screening	Have you ever been tested for an STI or HIV? If so, when was your last test?
Prior STI diagnosis	Have you had an STI in the past? If so, which one and when? Have any of your partners had an STI? Do any of your partners currently have an STI?

Table 12.2 (continued)

Category	Example questions to guide assessment
Current concern	Are you currently having symptoms? If so, what are your symptoms and how long have you been experiencing them? When was your last sexual contact? Have you had any recent sexual encounter that you are concerned about (e.g. the condom broke)?
Sexual activity	
Partners	*Preamble: Many of the following questions are personal. Ensure AYA are told that they do not need to answer any questions that they do not feel comfortable answering. Note: If not immediately pertinent to emerging clinical concerns, questions about sexual activity may create unnecessary barriers to AYA seeking services and may not be appropriate.* Tell me about your partners. Are your partners male, female or both? When did you last have sex? Was it with your regular partner or another partner? How many sexual partners have you had in the last 2 months? In the past year? How many of them could you contact?
Sexual activities	*Preamble: Many of the following questions are personal. Start out by explaining the reason why these questions are important,* e.g. 'In order to better understand your risk for STIs and to know what kind of tests to do, it's important to know what kinds of sex you're having'. Do you perform oral sex (i.e. do you kiss or put your mouth on the genitals or anus of your partner)? Do you receive oral sex? Do you have intercourse (i.e. do you penetrate your partners in the vagina/front or in the anus/bum or do your partners penetrate your vagina/front or anus/bum?)?
Personal risk evaluation	*Preamble: Ensure language used is inclusive and gender-affirming. Can start with a more open-ended question* e.g. 'What do you do to protect yourself from STIs and HIV?' How often do you use a condom for oral, vaginal/frontal or anal sex (sometimes, always, never)? What influences your decision to use a condom or not? How do you meet your sexual partners (e.g. online, on smartphone apps, bathhouse)? If you had to rate your risk for an STI, would you say that you are at no risk, low risk, medium risk or high risk? Why?
Reproductive health history	
Contraception	Do you/your partner(s) use contraception? If yes, frequency and type (e.g. oral contraceptive pill, Depo-Provera, intrauterine device [IUD])?
Reproductive or genitourinary health problems	Have you ever been diagnosed with or told you had a reproductive health issue or a problem with your genitourinary system (e.g. genitals, cervix, uterus, fallopian tubes, testicles, bladder)?
Cervical cancer screening	*Preamble: Given the recent changes to cervical cancer screening guidelines where the age of initiation for cervical cytology has increased, this may not be relevant to many AYA.* Have you ever had cervical cancer screening (either with a Pap test or HPV screening)? If yes, what was the result?
Pregnancy	Have you ever been pregnant? If yes, how many times? What was/were the outcome(s) (number of live births, abortions, miscarriages)?

(continued)

Table 12.2 (continued)

Category	Example questions to guide assessment
Substance use	
Types of substance use	Do you use alcohol? Drugs? If yes, frequency and type? Do you inject drugs? If yes, have you ever shared injecting equipment with someone else? If yes, when was the last time?
Sex under the influence	Have you ever had sex while drunk? If yes, how often? Have you ever had sex while high/under the influence of drugs? If yes, how often? What were the consequences? Do you feel that you need help because of your substance use?
Other percutaneous risk	Do you have tattoos or piercings? If yes, were they done using sterile equipment (i.e. professionally)?
Psychosocial history	
Housing	Do you have a home? If no, where do you sleep? Do you live with anyone?
Sex trade involvement	Have you ever traded sex for money, drugs, shelter or food? Have you ever paid for sex? If yes, how often and when?
Sexual abuse	Have you ever had sex with someone where you felt pressured or forced? If yes, when and by whom?

Adapted from: Canadian STI guidelines [3]

Chlamydia and Gonorrhoea

Chlamydia and gonorrhoea are the two most common bacterial STIs and are caused by the bacteria *Chlamydia trachomatis* and *Neisseria gonorrhoeae*, respectively. In Canada in 2014, the incidence of chlamydia infection – the most common reportable bacterial STI – was 1082 per 100,000 population in the 15–19-year-old age group and 1628 per 100,000 in the 20–24-year-old age group [45]; in the USA in 2016, the chlamydia rates were 1929 per 100,000 in the 15–19 age group and 2644 per 100,000 in the 20–24 age group [46]. In Canada in 2014, the incidence of gonorrhoea was 102 per 100,000 population in the 15–19-year-old age group and 180 per 100,000 in the 20–24 age group [54]; analogous US numbers from 2016 were 380 per 100,000 in the 15–19 age group and 608 per 100,000 in the 20–24 age group [55]. Both infections have been increasing steadily in Canadian and US jurisdictions in the last decade, and AYA (specifically those in the 15–24 age group) are disproportionately impacted, making up 63% of chlamydia cases and 47% of gonorrhoea cases in the USA in 2016 [55].

There is a significant overlap between the clinical presentations of chlamydia and gonorrhoea. Both can cause urethritis, vaginitis, cervicitis, epididymitis, proctitis and pharyngitis [47–50]. In population-based studies, over half of the cases of both chlamydia and gonorrhoea are asymptomatic or present with very mild symptoms [51, 52]. Untreated infection with both *C. trachomatis* and *N. gonorrhoeae* may lead to an ascending infection (from the cervix) causing pelvic

Table 12.3 Treatment recommendations for chlamydia and gonorrhoea

Infection	Recommended regimens	Partner management	Comment
Chlamydia	Azithromycin 1 g orally in a single dose Doxycycline 100 mg orally twice daily for 7 days	All sexual partners within 60 days preceding the diagnosis should be offered testing and treatment	If there are adherence or treatment completion concerns, single-dose therapy is preferred
Gonorrhoea	Ceftriaxone 250 mg intramuscularly in a single dose *If cephalosporin-allergic:* Azithromycin 2 g orally in a single dose		In diagnosed gonorrhoea, co-treatment for chlamydia should be provided

Adapted from: Canadian STI guidelines [3]; US CDC STD guidelines [2]
Note that medication dosages provided are based on adult weight, which should apply to most adolescents and young adults. We recommend consulting with an expert if unsure

inflammatory disease (PID) in biological females, which can lead to scarring and infertility [53]. In biological males, untreated chlamydia and gonorrhoea can lead to epididymitis or epididymo-orchitis, which may also lead to scarring and infertility [54]. This is of particular concern to AYA, who may face multiple barriers to receiving adequate STI screening and may thus go undiagnosed. Management of STIs in AYA should take into account these barriers, and attempts should be made to maximize and support adherence to therapy and the preservation of fertility (e.g. promoting access to a support worker if in a shelter, hospital admission for therapy completion). A recent study of adolescents seen in emergency departments and prescribed antimicrobial therapy for either PID or a diagnosis of chlamydia highlights the importance of this. In this study, fewer than 60% of prescriptions provided to these adolescents were filled, with hospital admission being the only predictor of prescription filling [55].

C. trachomatis or *N. gonorrhoeae* infection is diagnosed via nucleic acid amplification testing (NAAT) of first-catch urine or swabs of the pharynx, vagina, endocervix, rectum, urethra or a lesion. Gonococcal culture can also be performed. The preferred treatments for chlamydia and gonorrhoea are outlined in Table 12.3. Note that this is not an exhaustive resource for the treatment of STIs, and guidance should be sought from local STI experts and from comprehensive guidelines such as those referenced in this chapter [2, 3]. Clinics should take measures to optimize adherence and treatment completion, including on-site availability of medications; when feasible, the option of single-dose, directly observed therapy; and providing therapy for sexual partners. Care should be taken to ensure sexual partners of those diagnosed with chlamydia or gonorrhoea are provided with testing and/or treatment, according to the latest STI guidelines, to prevent onward transmission, delayed diagnoses and possible complications from untreated infection.

Syphilis

Syphilis is a bacterial STI caused by the spirochete *Treponema pallidum* and – like chlamydia and gonorrhoea – has been increasing steadily since the early 2000s in several jurisdictions. In North America and many other parts of the world, the epidemic has been primarily concentrated among gay, bisexual and other men/males who have sex with men/males (MSM) [56, 57]. In Canada in 2014, the incidence of early infectious syphilis (i.e. syphilis acquired within the previous year) was 6.7 per 100,000 population overall, representing a 95% increase from 2005. In the 15–19-year-old age group, the rate was 3 per 100,000 and 11.7 per 100,000 in the 20–24 age group [41]. The overrepresentation of MSM in syphilis rates was noted within these age categories as well: the male rate for 15–19-year-olds was 4 per 100,000 (versus 1.8 per 100,000 for females) and the male rate for 20–24-year-olds was 19.6 per 100,000 (versus 3.4 per 100,000 in females of the same age group). Similar patterns were observed in the USA [42].

The clinical manifestations of syphilis are determined by the stage of the infection. Generally, syphilis is divided into early, or infectious syphilis (diagnosed within 1 year of infection), and late, or non-infectious syphilis (diagnosed greater than 1 year after infection), and the untreated infection progresses stepwise through different stages [58]. Primary syphilis typically occurs within 10–90 days of infection and presents with a localized painless skin lesion called a chancre. Secondary syphilis follows, usually within weeks to several months after initial infection, and represents dissemination of the infection. It may present with a myriad of symptoms, though the hallmark is a systemic illness characterized by a diffuse rash [59]. Other clinical manifestations of secondary syphilis may include (but are not limited to) constitutional symptoms, generalized lymphadenopathy, hepatitis and central nervous system involvement (i.e. neurosyphilis) [43, 44, 60]. Even in the untreated individual, the symptoms of primary and secondary syphilis will usually spontaneously resolve. Additionally, not all individuals with syphilis will be symptomatic. Since a syphilis chancre is painless, it often may go unnoticed. Following the symptomatic stages (if they occur), syphilis enters a latent stage. An asymptomatic infection that is confirmed to have been acquired within the last year is still considered infectious syphilis and would be staged as an early latent infection [3]. An infection acquired more than 1 year previous is a late latent infection. Up to 30% of individuals with untreated late latent infection may develop late or tertiary complications of syphilis, and these may occur up to several decades after the initial infection. These clinical manifestations are variable and may include central nervous system involvement, cardiovascular complications or granulomatous lesions in the skin, bones or organs (called gummatous syphilis) [3]. The preferred treatments for syphilis are outlined in Table 12.4.

Another concerning trend that has been observed recently has been an increase in cases of congenital syphilis. Congenital syphilis occurs when syphilis is transmitted to an infant from an infected mother, typically *in utero* [61], and can have devastating consequences, including death of the infant [62]. In September 2018, the US Centers for Disease Control and Prevention (CDC) issued an advisory that 913

Table 12.4 Treatment recommendations for syphilis

Stage of infection	Recommended regimens	Partner management	Comment
Primary	Benzathine penicillin 2.4 million units intramuscularly in a single dose Alternative regimen: Doxycycline 100 mg orally twice daily for 14 days	Test and treat all sexual partners within 90 days of primary lesion	Doxycycline should not be used in pregnant individuals; penicillin-allergic pregnant individuals should undergo penicillin desensitization
Secondary		Test all partners within 180 days of start of symptoms; treat any partners in the last 90 days	
Early latent (≤1 year)		Test all partners within last year; treat any partners in the last 90 days	
Late latent (>1 year)	Benzathine penicillin 2.4 million units intramuscularly once weekly for 3 weeks *Alternative regimen:* Doxycycline 100 mg orally twice daily for 28 days	Test any long-term partners	

Adapted from: Canadian STI guidelines [3]; US CDC STD guidelines [2]
Note that medication dosages provided are based on adult weight, which should apply to most adolescents and young adults. We recommend consulting with an expert if unsure

babies had been born with congenital syphilis in the USA in 2017, representing an increase of 150% from 2003 and a significant shift from years of sustained reductions in congenital syphilis cases [63]. The increasing recognition of congenital syphilis has particularly concerning implications for AYA, as they may face more barriers than adults in accessing appropriate pregnancy and pre-pregnancy care or counselling, thus putting them at potential higher risk of inadequate care, including prenatal STI screening. This is especially salient given that one of the risk factors for congenital syphilis is either a lack of or inappropriate prenatal care [64, 65].

Human Papillomavirus (HPV)

Though chlamydia and gonorrhoea may be the most common bacterial STIs, the most common STI worldwide is the viral STI human papillomavirus (HPV) [66]. It is estimated that over 80% of sexually active individuals are exposed to HPV at some point in their lifetime, and most HPV infections occur within a decade of sexual debut [67]. There are over 200 genotypes of HPV, with tropism for different tissue types (e.g. cutaneous epithelium, anogenital epithelium), and nearly 50 of these genotypes favour the tissues of the anogenital area [68]. HPV genotypes are further classified according to their potential to cause cancer [69]. The clinical manifestations of HPV are dependent on the location and type of the infection. The most common low-risk types (i.e. those with low or no carcinogenic potential) are HPV-6 and HPV-11, responsible for 90% of the most common HPV-related lesion: condyloma acuminata (or more commonly, genital warts). HPV-16 is the most common high-risk, or oncogenic, type and is postulated to have the highest risk of progression to cancer. It, along with other oncogenic types (e.g. HPV-18, HPV-31, HPV-33, HPV-45, HPV-52, HPV-58), may cause precancerous lesions that can eventually lead to cervical cancer [70], vaginal and vulvar cancers [71], penile cancers [72], anal cancers [73] and some oropharyngeal cancers [74].

HPV infection is of particular relevance to AYA as it is often acquired during this time period, is very common in this population yet is entirely preventable via very effective vaccines. In areas where routine HPV vaccination has been implemented, marked decreases have been noted in the prevalence and incidence of HPV infection, genital warts and other HPV-associated diseases (including precancerous lesions of the cervix and anal canal) [75–78] in both males and females. Both the Canadian National Advisory Committee on Immunization (NACI) [79] and the US Advisory Committee on Immunization Practices (ACIP) [80] recommend the HPV vaccine to all individuals prior to sexual debut (i.e. age 9–14 years) but up to the age of 26 years in those unvaccinated. Both bodies also recommend the use of HPV vaccination in MSM, as well as individuals living with HIV. As of this writing, all Canadian provinces and territories provide HPV vaccination via a gender-neutral school-based program, and some also provide publicly funded vaccinations for others deemed at higher risk for HPV-associated malignancies, including those living with HIV and MSM [81]. Though the data indicates that school-based programs are effective in achieving broad vaccination coverage [82], several studies have demonstrated suboptimal uptake in many areas (despite a clear decrease in HPV-associated disease) [83]. Negative parental attitudes persist towards HPV vaccine, with many parents concerned that their support for HPV vaccination will encourage sexual activity and risky behaviours [84, 85]. A recent adolescent study in the Canadian province of British Columbia (BC) examined the impact of the implementation of public HPV vaccine program on sexual behaviours in adolescent girls. Comparing the period pre- and post-HPV vaccine program implementation, this study found a decrease in the proportion of girls self-reporting ever having had sexual intercourse, a decrease in the proportion self-reporting sexual intercourse before the age of 14, a decrease in substance use before intercourse, a decrease in pregnancy and an increase in condom use [86].

Trichomoniasis, Lice and Scabies

While trichomoniasis, lice and scabies may be less likely to cause serious complications, for AYA (and especially for those facing homelessness, housing insecurity or other forms of housing precarity) these STIs warrant meaningful and effective responses whenever possible. Trichomoniasis is a protozoal infection caused by

Trichomonas vaginalis, most commonly infecting the urogenital tract [87]. Unlike chlamydia, gonorrhoea and syphilis, it is not typically reported to public health authorities, so prevalence is difficult to establish. While some AYA may demonstrate specific symptoms linked to trichomoniasis infection, very few (less than 20%) will present with typical symptoms, which – when present – are usually urethral-type symptoms, including dysuria, discharge, urinary frequency and dyspareunia [88]. For young women, trichomoniasis warrants special concern, as it is associated with a two-to-threefold increase in HIV transmission risk, premature and preterm birth and other pregnancy complications. AYA engaged in survival sex work, those who use illicit drugs and those residing in high-prevalence correctional institutions, shelters and treatment facilities may be considered to be at elevated risk for trichomoniasis and should be screened accordingly [89]. Although the identification of the organism with its characteristic motility on wet mount is diagnostic, this method lacks sensitivity [90]. The diagnostic gold standard for trichomonas infection is the NAAT of urine or urethral/vaginal swab [91]. The only effective drugs for *T. vaginalis* are the 5-nitroimidazoles (i.e. metronidazole and tinidazole) [2, 3].

Lice and scabies are ectoparasitic infections of the skin and/or hair and are largely considered nuisance infections [92]. Neither lice nor scabies are associated with significant or serious, long-term complications, but both *are* associated with institutional settings [93], including those in which AYA may be residing (e.g. treatment centres, youth correctional facilities or AYA shelters), and both can be troublesome and cause discomfort and embarrassment for infected youth. As such, institutional settings serving AYA, and especially AYA facing homelessness and housing precarity, should ensure ready access to scabicides and pediculicides and should provide staff support for successful treatment.

Human Immunodeficiency Virus (HIV)

Human immunodeficiency virus (HIV) infection remains an infection of global significance among AYA, with over 30% of all new infections globally occurring in those aged 15–25 years old [94]. HIV in AYA also presents a complex clinical challenge, as it may result from vertical transmission from a mother living with HIV, in which case it is experienced as a lifelong, chronic illness; or it may be transmitted via sexual and drug use behaviours during youth. This section will focus exclusively on sexually transmitted HIV infection in high-income countries.

Just as there are for all STIs in AYA, there are unique challenges in the care and prevention of HIV in these populations. In Canada in 2016, there was an 11.6% increase in the number of HIV cases diagnosed compared to 2015, after several years of decreases and relative stability. Though the cases in the 20–29-year-old age group remained stable in 2016 (representing nearly 25% of new cases), there has been a steady increase in reported cases in the 15–19-year-old age group for the 5 years prior to 2016, and this age group now represents over 2% of new cases [95]. Similar numbers are observed in the USA, where, in 2009, 7% of new cases were between 13 and

24 years old; in 2010, nearly 25% of new cases were seen in this age group [96]. The concept of syndemics is particularly salient to HIV infection and risk in AYA, as those at highest risk live in environments where multiple, overlapping vulnerabilities exist: heterosexual AYA females, young MSM, youth who inject drugs, youth engaged in sex work and young transgender women having sex with men [97]. Further, minority groups are disproportionately impacted [84], and one model of HIV incidence in young black MSM in the USA predicts that 40% of these individuals will be living with HIV by the age of 30 in the absence of changes to current prevention efforts [98].

One of the most significant developments in biomedical HIV prevention has been the advent of HIV pre-exposure prophylaxis (PrEP), where the HIV medication tenofovir-emtricitabine (TDF-FTC) is taken (usually) daily to prevent HIV acquisition. Despite multiple randomized controlled trials (RCT) demonstrating efficacy of once-daily PrEP in MSM [99] and heterosexual men and women [100, 101], subsequent demonstration studies and pragmatic trials demonstrating feasibility and/or effectiveness [102–104] and one study in MSM showing efficacy of event-driven, intermittent PrEP [105], none of these large seminal studies has examined PrEP use in individuals under the age of 18. Recently, the results of one demonstration project were published, where TDF-FTC was given to 72 MSM aged 15–17 years to examine safety, tolerability, acceptability, adherence and sexual risk behaviour [106]. In this study, 46 (64%) participants completed 48 weeks of follow-up, and three participants acquired HIV infection, for an annualized HIV incidence of 6.4 (95% confidence interval, 1.3–18.7) per 100 person-years. There was no indication of risk compensation in this study, as evidenced by the lack of significant change noted in the number of sexual partners, condomless sex acts and bacterial STI diagnoses over time.

This study on HIV PrEP use in young MSM did highlight one priority area that merits further investigation: medication adherence. Adherence was measured via TDF levels on dried blood spot (DBS) testing, and protective levels were extrapolated from the results of a prior study indicating that a mean of four pills or more per week was sufficient to achieve protective levels of drug in the rectal tissue [90]. At week 4, 54% of participants had TDF levels consistent with protective adherence, and this value decreased throughout the study, reaching 22% by week 48. Common reasons cited by participants for missing drug doses were being away from home, being too busy, forgetting and changes in routine. Participants with suboptimal TDF levels were also more likely to endorse a statement indicating concern about others seeing them take the medication and thinking they were HIV-positive.

STI Screening, Testing, Diagnosis and Treatment Concerns and Considerations in AYA

The approach to screening for bacterial STIs in AYA should be responsive to their needs (e.g. using language that is respectful and understandable, ensuring confidentiality) and sensitive and inclusive to all, including LGBTQ+/2S AYA; specifically, it should be gender-affirming. Thus, instead of discussing chlamydia and gonorrhoea screening in terms of male and female testing, an anatomic site-based approach is preferred. Generally, as discussed previously, screening for chlamydia and gonorrhoea is done using NAAT on urine samples or swabs of specific sites (e.g. vagina, cervix, rectum), though culture for *N. gonorrhoeae* is also often indicated [2, 3]. Screening for syphilis is generally done via serologic testing; in instances where a chancre or other infectious lesion is present, direct tests (e.g. darkfield microscopy, polymerase chain reaction) may also be done [3]. There are no universal, evidence-based recommendations on the frequency of STI screening in any population and no specific recommendations for AYA. Generally, STI treatment guidelines recommend STI screening yearly in those who are sexually active [2, 3] and more frequently if certain situations deemed a higher risk for STI acquisition are present (e.g. new sex partner, multiple sex partners, a sex partner with multiple partners or a sex partner with a known STI) [107].

For street-involved and homeless AYA, barriers to testing, diagnosis and successful treatment may be even more significant. AYA facing homelessness, housing insecurity and other forms of housing precarity may lack the resources (e.g. a transit pass or reliable transportation) necessary to visit sexual health clinics specialising in AYA needs, and complex treatment protocols (e.g. PID or syphilis requiring multiple treatment visits) may present additional challenges to accessing care. Additionally, for AYA facing housing, food and economic insecurity, accessing sexual healthcare, including STI testing, diagnosis and treatment, may simply rank as a lower priority than meeting the more emergent needs of food and a safe, warm and dry place to sleep.

For any clinician, especially male clinicians and trainees, the presence of a legal chaperone or neutral clinical observer is essential when completing any pelvic, genital or breast exam. When possible, AYA should be presented with the option to specify their preferred gender in an attending clinician and should be empowered to play an active role in determining how sensitive examinations proceed, including by whom.

Directions for the Future

STIs are infections of adolescents and young adults, and there are a multitude of reasons why this is so, many of which have been discussed above. By virtue of simply being young, AYA find themselves in a complicated physical, emotional and psychosocial milieu, as they struggle to understand their emerging sexualities and issues relating to their sexual health. The addition of homelessness, poverty or other forms of marginalization further exacerbates this, and evidence indicates that homeless AYA as an already-disadvantaged group experience even worse health outcomes particularly around STIs and HIV than their housed peers. As providers, researchers and policymakers in the field of AYA sexual health, it is our responsibility to shift and broaden the paradigm of AYA sexual health [108] to one focused on sexuality and sexual behaviour as normal, healthy and meaningful, to promote empowerment and resilience in these individuals [109].

With this in mind, there are four priorities to consider in future work and research relating to STIs and sexual health in homeless AYA. The first two priorities cut across all aspects of sexual health and STI care, whereas the latter two recognize the limitations of our current and historic prevention efforts and focus on more novel biomedical prevention tools for two infections with the potential for significant, lifelong health impacts. These priorities include:

1. *Approaching and providing STI and sexual healthcare in a way that is appropriate for all AYA*. This was discussed in detail above and emphasizes the importance of ensuring sexual health and STI services provided to AYA demonstrate a commitment to AYA-friendly care, including confidentiality and privacy, normalization and lack of judgement, respect, avoiding jargon, avoiding assumptions and facilitating opportunities for AYA autonomy. Implicit within this, and arguably one of the most critical elements of this, is an assurance that the care provided is gender-affirming and inclusive of all AYA. Examples of this include the following: avoiding assumptions about the gender of sexual partners based on the person's reported sexual orientation (e.g. an individual identifying as straight male may have male sexual partners), providing site-based testing as opposed to testing based on gender or gender of sexual partners and ensuring the 'healthcare experience' is appropriate and follows the principles of AYA-friendly services, from initial contact (i.e. sign-in desk, reception) to follow-up (e.g. phone call to discuss results).
2. *Incorporating an understanding of syndemics into the care of AYA*. As AYA often face true or perceived barriers to healthcare – and particularly STI and sexual healthcare – any encounter with a healthcare provider must be seen as an opportunity to address ongoing issues. STIs, homelessness and other health issues do not occur in isolation and are intimately connected to other health and social issues that may be co-occurring in AYA: mental health, poverty, substance use and stigma. An understanding of the link and interconnectedness between these often synergistic epidemics is critical to providing appropriate care, and healthcare providers should ensure that they are inquiring about these issues with every healthcare contact.
3. *Exploring and evaluating the role of HPV vaccination in AYA*. Though there is an abundance of data on the use of HPV vaccination in young females, there are several priority areas that require further consideration and study. As a highly effective prevention tool against cervical cancer and other forms of cancer and given that HPV is typically acquired during the early years following sexual debut, efforts must focus on ways in which vaccine uptake can be ameliorated to ensure the highest rates of population-level protection are achieved. Still, uptake of school-based girls' vaccination programs is suboptimal. More recently, school-based HPV vaccination programs have become gender-neutral, making HPV vaccination of school-aged boys a fledgling but under-investigated area of inquiry. Studies on uptake, parental attitude, the feasibility of earlier childhood vaccination and longer-term efficacy are important next steps, particularly as data emerges on the disproportionate

impact of HPV-associated disease and cancers in some male subpopulations (e.g. anal and oral cancers in gbMSM living with HIV).

4. *Examining the use of HIV PrEP in AYA*. Very few studies have investigated the use of HIV PrEP in AYA populations, particularly those under the age of 18 years. Recognizing that AYA living with additional vulnerabilities (e.g. homelessness, racial or gender minorities) are at particularly high risk for HIV and these same subpopulations are historically those with the lowest rates of condom use and are often forced into survival sex, new prevention modalities are critically needed. More studies must be done in these populations, with a particular focus on adherence, as this was seen as one of the most important barriers to PrEP use in the previously cited study of young MSM. Further, access is another important priority. AYA may face stigma (e.g. from families, cultural communities) by self-identifying as MSM, thus preventing them from accessing services. The issues of access and adherence were highlighted in a recent position statement on PrEP in AYA by the Society for Adolescent Health and Medicine, which highlighted the need for youth-focused PrEP research, the incorporation of PrEP into youth sexual health education and the development of AYA-appropriate PrEP services [95].

References

1. Weinstock H, Berman S, Cates W. Sexually transmitted diseases among American youth: incidence and prevalence estimates, 2000. Perspect Sex Reprod Health. 2004;36:6.
2. United States Centers for Disease Control and Prevention. 2015 Sexually transmitted diseases treatment guidelines. 2015. Available at: https://www.cdc.gov/std/tg2015/specialpops.htm#adol. Accessed 26 Mar 2019.
3. Public Health Agency of Canada. Canadian guidelines on sexually transmitted infections. 2019. Available at: https://www.canada.ca/en/public-health/services/infectious-diseases/sexual-health-sexually-transmitted-infections/canadian-guidelines/sexually-transmitted-infections.html#toc. Accessed 26 Mar 2019.
4. World Health Organization. Adolescent-friendly health services: an agenda for change. 2004. Available at: www.who.int/child_adolescent_health/documents/fch_cah_02_14/en/index.html. Accessed 15 Aug 2018.
5. Caccamo A, Kachur R, Williams SP. Narrative review: sexually transmitted diseases and homeless youth – what do we know about sexually transmitted disease prevalence and risk. Sex Transm Dis. 2017;44:466.
6. Marshall BD, Kerr T, Shoveller JA, Patterson TL, Buxton JA, Wood E. Homelessness and unstable housing associated with an increased risk of HIV and STI transmission among street-involved youth. Health Place. 2009;15(3):753.
7. Quality of Care. A process for making strategic choices in health systems. Geneva, World Health Organization; 2006; Quality Assessment Guidebook. A guide to assessing health services for adolescent clients. Geneva, World Health Organization; 2009.
8. Singer M. A dose of drugs, a touch of violence, a case of AIDS: conceptualizing the SAVA epidemic. Free Inq Creat Sociol. 1996;24:99.
9. Singer M. Introduction to syndemics: a systems approach to public and community health. San Francisco: Jossey-Bass; 2009.
10. Singer M, Bulled N, Ostrach B, Mendenhall E. Syndemic and the biosocial conception of health. Lancet. 2017;389:941.

11. Halkitis PN, Wolitski RJ, Millett GA. A holistic approach to addressing HIV infection disparities in gay, bisexual, and other men who have sex with men. Am Psychol. 2013;68(4):261.
12. Warf CW, Clark LF, Desai M, et al. Coming of age on the streets: survival sex among homeless young women in Hollywood. J Adolesc. 2013;36(6):1205–13.
13. Singer M, Bulled N, Ostrach B, Mendenhall E. Syndemics and the biosocial conception of health. Lancet. 2017;389:941.
14. Stall R, Mills TC, Williamson J, et al. Association of co-occurring psychosocial health problems and increased vulnerability to HIV/AIDS among urban men who have sex with men. Am J Public Health. 2003;93:939.
15. DiClemente RJ, Salazar LF, Crosby RA. A review of STD/HIV preventive interventions for adolescents: sustaining effects using an ecological approach. J Pediatr Psychol. 2007; 32(8):888.
16. Sieving RE, Bernat DH, Resnick MD, et al. A clinic-based youth development program to reduce sexual risk behaviors among adolescent girls: prime time pilot study. Health Promot Pract. 2012;13(4):462.
17. Upchurch DM, Mason WM, Kusunoki Y, et al. Social and behavioral determinants of self reported STD among adolescents. Perspect Sex Reprod Health. 2004;36(6):276.
18. Charest M, Kleinplatz PJ, Lund JI. Sexual health information disparities between heterosexual and LGBTQ+ young adults: implications for sexual health. Can J Hum Sex. 2016;25:74.
19. Garcia CK. Sexual health education in Quebec schools: a critique and call for change. Can J Hum Sex. 2015;24:197.
20. Dbouba G, Shannon A. In: Chown S, editor. Sex ed is our right. Vancouver: YouthCO HIV & Hep C Society; 2018.
21. Cohen JN, Byers ES, Sears HA. Factors affecting Canadian teachers' willingness to teach sexual health education. Sex Educ. 2011;12:1.
22. Manzer D, O'Sullivan LF, Doucet S. Myths, misunderstandings, and missing information: experiences of nurse practitioners providing primary care to lesbian, gay, bisexual, and transgender patients. Can J Hum Sex. 2018;27:157.
23. Smith A, Stewart D, Poon C, Peled M, Saewyc EM. Our communities, our youth. Vancouver: McCreary Centre Society; 2015.
24. Saewyc EM, Drozda C, Rivers R, MacKay L, Peled M. Which comes first: sexual exploitation or other risk exposures among street-involved youth? In: Youth homelessness in Canada: implications for policy and practice. Toronto: Canadian Homelessness Research Network; 2013.
25. Abramovich AI. No fixed address: young, queer, and restless. In: Gaetz S, et al., editors. Youth homelessness in Canada: implications for policy and practice. Toronto: Canadian Observatory on Homelessness; 2013.
26. Remafedi G, Resnick M, Blum R, Harris L. Demography of sexual orientation in adolescents. Pediatrics. 1992;89:714.
27. Forhan SE, Gottlieb SL, Sternberg MR, et al. Prevalence of sexually transmitted infections among female adolescents aged 14 to 19 in the United States. Pediatrics. 2009;124:1505.
28. CDC. Sexually transmitted disease surveillance 2013. Atlanta: US Department of Health and Human Services; 2014.
29. Tu W, Batteiger BE, Wiehe S, et al. Time from first intercourse to first sexually transmitted infection diagnosis among adolescent women. Arch Pediatr Adolesc Med. 2009;163(12):1106.
30. Kahn JA, Rosenthal SL, Succop PA, Ho GY, Burk RD. Mediators of the association between age of first sexual intercourse and subsequent human papillomavirus infection. Pediatrics. 2002;109(1):E5.
31. Shew ML, Fortenberry JD, Miles P, Amortegui AJ. Interval between menarche and first sexual intercourse, related to risk of human papillomavirus infection. J Pediatr. 1994;125(4):661.
32. Burstein GR, Gaydos CA, Diener-West M, Howell MR, Zenilman JM, Quinn TC. Incident Chlamydia trachomatis infections among inner-city adolescent females. JAMA. 1998; 280(6):521.

33. Niccolai LM, Ethier KA, Kershaw TS, Lewis JB, Meade CS, Ickovics JR. New sex partner acquisition and sexually transmitted disease risk among adolescent females. J Adolesc Health. 2004;34(3):216.
34. Fortenberry JD. Adolescent substance use and sexually transmitted diseases risk: a review. J Adolesc Health. 1995;16(4):304.
35. Leigh BC. Alcohol and condom use: a meta-analysis of event-level studies. J Adolesc Health. 1995;16(4):304
36. Kleppa E, Holmen SD, Lillebø K, et al. Cervical ectopy. associations with sexually transmitted infections and HIV. A cross-sectional study of high school students in rural South Africa. Sex Transm Infect. 2015;91(2):124.
37. Hwang LY, Ma Y, Moscicki AB. Biological and behavioral risks for incident Chlamydia trachomatis infection in a prospective cohort. Obstet Gynecol. 2014;124(5):954.
38. McGrath JW, Strasburger VC, Cushing AH. Secretory IgA in cervical mucus. J Adolesc Health. 1994;15(5):423.
39. Hickey RJ, Zhou X, Settles ML, Erb J, Malone K, Hansmann MA, Shew ML, Van Der Pol B, Fortenberry JD, Forney LJ. Vaginal microbiota of adolescent girls prior to the onset of menarche resemble those of reproductive-age women. MBio. 2015;6(2):pii: e00097-15.
40. Seth P, Patel SN, Sales JM, DiClemente RJ, Wingood GM, Rose ES. The impact of depressive symptomatology on risky sexual behavior and sexual communication among African American female adolescents. Psychol Health Med. 2011;16(3):346.
41. Duron S, Panjo H, Bohet A, et al. Prevalence and risk factors of sexually transmitted infections among French service members. PLoS One. 2018;13(4):e0195158.
42. Trecker MA, Dillon JR, Lloyd K, Hennink M, Jolly A, Waldner C. Can social network analysis help address the high rates of bacterial sexually transmitted infections in Saskatchewan? Sex Transm Dis. 2017;44(6):338.
43. Cheng T, Johnston C, Kerr T, Nguyen P, Wood E, Debeck K. Substance use patterns and unprotected sex among street-involved youth in a Canadian setting: a prospective cohort study. BMC Public Health. 2016;16(10):4.
44. Gamarel KE, Brown L, Kahler CW, Fernandez MI, Bruce D, Nichols S. Prevalence and correlates of substance use among youth living with HIV in clinical settings. Drug Alcohol Depend. 2016;169:11.
45. Public Health Agency of Canada. Report on sexually transmitted infections in Canada: 2013–2014. Retrieved from: https://www.canada.ca/en/public-health/services/publications/diseases-conditions/report-sexually-transmitted-infections-canada-2013-14.html. Accessed 10 Aug 2018.
46. Centers for Disease Control and Prevention. STDs in adolescents and young adults. Available: https://www.cdc.gov/std/stats16/adolescents.htm. Accessed 10 Aug 2018.
47. Stamm WE. Chlamydia trachomatis infections of the adult. In: Holmes KK, Sparling PF, Mardh PA, et al., editors. Sexually transmitted diseases. 4th ed. New York: McGraw-Hill; 2008.
48. Cecil JA, Howell MR, Tawes JJ, et al. Features of Chlamydia trachomatis and Neisseria gonorrhoeae infection in male Army recruits. J Infect Dis. 2001;184(9):1216.
49. McCormack WM, Stumacher RJ, Johnson K, Donner A. Clinical spectrum of gonococcal infection in women. Lancet. 1977;1(8023):1182.
50. Sherrard J, Barlow D. Gonorrhoea in men: clinical and diagnostic aspects. Genitourin Med. 1996;72(6):422.
51. Handsfield HH, Lipman TO, Harnisch JP, Tronca E, Holmes KK. Asymptomatic gonorrhea in men. Diagnosis, natural course, prevalence and significance. N Engl J Med. 1974;290(3):117.
52. Klouman E, Masenga EJ, Sam NE, Klepp KI. Asymptomatic gonorrhoea and chlamydial infection in a population-based and work-site based sample of men in Kilimanjaro, Tanzania. Int J STD AIDS. 2000;11:666.

53. Geisler WM, Wang C, Morrison SG, Black CM, Bandea CI, Hook EW. The natural history of untreated Chlamydia trachomatis infection in the interval between screening and returning for treatment. Sex Transm Dis. 2008;35(2):119.
54. Fode M, Fusco F, Lipschultz L, Weidner W. Sexually transmitted disease and male infertility: a systematic review. Reprod Health. 2017;14(1):5.
55. Lieberman A, Badolato GM, Tran J, et al. Frequency of prescription filling among adolescents prescribed treatment for sexually transmitted infections in the emergency department. JAMA Pediatr. 2019; published online May 28, 2019. https://doi.org/10.1001/jamapediatrics.2019.1263.
56. Burchell AN, Allen VG, Gardner SL, et al. High incidence of diagnosis with syphilis co-infection among men who have sex with men in an HIV cohort in Ontario, Canada. BMC Infect Dis. 2015;15(1):356.
57. United States Centers for Disease Control and Prevention. Sexually transmitted disease surveillance. 2016. Available at: https://www.cdc.gov/std/stats16/Syphilis.htm. Accessed 10 Aug 2018.
58. Tramont EC. Treponema pallidum (Syphilis). In: Mandell GL, Bennett JE, Dolin R, editors. Principles and practice of infectious diseases. Philadelphia: Churchill-Livingstone; 2010. p. 3035–53.
59. Chapel TA. The signs and symptoms of secondary syphilis. Sex Transm Dis. 1980; 7(4):161.
60. Young MF, Sanowski RA, Manne RA. Syphilitic hepatitis. J Clin Gastroenterol. 1992;15(2):174.
61. Risser WL, Hwang LY. Problems in the current case definitions of congenital syphilis. J Pediatr. 1996;129(4):499.
62. Dobson SR, Sanchez PJ. Syphilis. In: Cherry JD, Harrison GJ, Kaplan SL, et al., editors. Feigin and Cherry's textbook of pediatric infectious diseases. 7th ed. Philadelphia: Elsevier Saunders; 2014. p. 1761.
63. The Lancet. Congenital syphilis in the USA. Lancet. 2018;392(10154):1168. https://doi.org/10.1016/S0140-6736(18)32360-2.
64. Reyes MP, Hunt N, Ostrea EM Jr, George D. Maternal/congenital syphilis in a large tertiary-care urban hospital. Clin Infect Dis. 1993;17(6):1041.
65. Caddy SC, Lee BE, Sutherland K, et al. Pregnancy and neonatal outcomes of women with reactive syphilis serology in Alberta, 2002 to 2006. J Obstet Gynaecol Can. 2011; 33(5):453.
66. Koutsky L. Epidemiology of genital human papillomavirus infection. Am J Med. 1997;102(5A):3.
67. Bonnez W, Reichman RC. Papillomaviruses. In: Mandell GL, Bennett JE, Dolin R, editors. Principles and practice of infectious diseases. Philadelphia: Churchill-Livingstone; 2010. p. 2035–49.
68. De Villers EM. Cross-roads in the classification of papillomaviruses. Virology. 2013;445:2.
69. Bouvard V, Baan R, Straif K, et al. A review of human carcinogens – part B: biological agents. Lancet Oncol. 2009;10:321.
70. Franco EL, Duarte-Franco E, Ferenczy A. Cervical cancer: epidemiology, prevention and the role of human papillomavirus infection. CMAJ. 2001;164(7):1017.
71. Forman D, de Martel C, Lacey CJ, et al. Global burden of human papillomavirus and related diseases. Vaccine. 2012;30(Suppl 5):F12.
72. Backes DM, Kurman RJ, Pimenta JM, Smith JS. Systematic review of human papillomavirus prevalence in invasive penile cancer. Cancer Causes Control. 2009;20(4):449.
73. Hoots BE, Palefsky JM, Pimenta JM, Smith JS. Human papillomavirus type distribution in anal cancer and anal intraepithelial lesions. Int J Cancer. 2009;124(10):2375.
74. Mork J, Lie AK, Glattre E, et al. Human papillomavirus infection as a risk factor for squamous-cell carcinoma of the head and neck. N Engl J Med. 2001;344(15):1125.
75. Brotherton JM, Fridman M, May CL, Chappell G, Saville AM, Gertig DM. Early effect of the HPV vaccination programme on cervical abnormalities in Victoria, Australia: an ecological study. Lancet. 2011;377(9783):2085.

76. Markowitz LE, Hariri S, Lin C, et al. Reduction in human papillomavirus (HPV) prevalence among young women following HPV vaccine introduction in the United States, National Health and Nutrition Examination Surveys, 2003–2010. J Infect Dis. 2013;208(3):385.
77. Smith LM, Strumpf EC, Kaufman JS, Lofters A, Schwandt M, Lévesque LE. The early benefits of human papillomavirus vaccination on cervical dysplasia and anogenital warts. Pediatrics. 2015;135(5):e1131.
78. Giuliano AR, Palefsky JM, Goldstone S, et al. Efficacy of quadrivalent HPV vaccine against HPV infection and disease in males. N Engl J Med. 2011;364(5):401.
79. An advisory Committee Statement (ACS) National Advisory Committee on Immunization. Available: https://www.canada.ca/en/public-health/services/publications/healthy-living/9-valent-hpv-vaccine-clarification-minimum-intervals-between-doses-in-hpv-immunization-schedule.html. Accessed 10 Aug 2018.
80. Petrosky E, Bocchini JA, Hariri S, et al. Use of 9-valent human papillomavirus (HPV) vaccine: updated HPV vaccination recommendations of the advisory committee on immunization practices. Available: https://www.cdc.gov/mmwr/preview/mmwrhtml/mm6411a3.htm. Accessed 10 Aug 2018.
81. Canada's provincial and territorial routine (and catch-up) vaccination program for infants and children. Available: https://www.canada.ca/content/dam/phac-aspc/documents/services/provincial-territorial-immunization-information/childhood_schedule-05-2017.pdf. Accessed 10 Aug 2018.
82. Paul P, Fabio A. Literature review of HPV vaccine delivery strategies: considerations for school- and non-school based immunization program. Vaccine. 2014;32:320.
83. Oliver SE, Unger ER, Lewis R, et al. Prevalence of human papillomavirus among females after vaccine introduction-National Health and Nutrition Examination Survey, United States, 2003–2014. J Infect Dis. 2017;216(5):594.
84. Ogilvie GS, Remple VP, Marra F, et al. Parental intention to have daughters receive the human papillomavirus vaccine. Can Med Assoc J. 2007;177:1506.
85. Hendry M, Lewis R, Clements A, et al. "HPV? Never heard of it!": a systematic review of girls' and parents' information needs, views and preferences about human papillomavirus vaccination. Vaccine. 2013;31:5152.
86. Ogilvie GS, Phan F, Pedesen HN, Dobson SR, Naus M, Saewyc EM. Population-level sexual behaviours in adolescent girls before and after introduction of the human papillomavirus vaccine (2003–2013). Can Med Assoc J. 2018;190(41):E1221.
87. Kissinger P. Epidemiology and treatment of trichomoniasis. Curr Infect Dis Rep. 2015;17(6):484.
88. Landers DV, Wiesenfeld HC, Heine RP, Krohn MA, Hillier SL. Predictive value of the clinical diagnosis of lower genital tract infection in women. Am J Obstet Gyncol. 2004; 190(4):1004.
89. United States Centers for Disease Control and Prevention. 2015 Sexually transmitted diseases treatment guidelines. 2015. Available at: https://www.cdc.gov/std/tg2015/trichomoniasis.htm. Accessed 28 Mar 2019.
90. Krieger JN, Tam MR, Stevens CE, et al. Diagnosis of trichomoniasis. Comparison of conventional wet-mount examination with cytologic studies, cultures, and monoclonal antibody staining of direct specimens. JAMA. 1988;259(8):1223.
91. Miller JM, Binnicker MJ, Campbell S, et al. A guide to utilization of the microbiology laboratory for diagnosis of infectious diseases: 2018 update by the Infectious Diseases Society of America and the American Society for Microbiology. Clin Infect Dis. 2018;67(6):e1.
92. Ko CJ, Elston DM. Pediculosis. J Am Acad Dermatol. 2004;50:1.
93. Heukelbach J, Feldmeier H. Scabies. Lancet. 2006;367(9524):1767.
94. World Health Organization. HIV and youth. Available: www.who.int/maternal_child_adolescent/topics/adolescence/hiv/en/. Accessed 10 Aug 2018.
95. Bourgeois AC, Edmunds M, Awan A, et al. HIV in Canada – surveillance report, 2016. Can Commun Dis Rep. 2017;43:248.

96. Centers for Disease Control and Prevention (CDC). Vital signs: HIV infection, testing, and risk behaviors among youths – United States. MMWR Morb Mortal Wkly Rep. 2012;61(47):971.
97. Society for Adolescent Health and Medicine. HIV pre-exposure prophylaxis medication for adolescents and young adults: a position paper of the Society for Adolescent Health and Medicine. J Adolesc Health. 2018;63:513.
98. Matthews DD, Herrick AL, Coulter RW, et al. Running backwards: consequences of current HIV incidence rates for the next generation of Black MSM in the United States. AIDS Behav. 2016;20:7.
99. Grant RM, Lama JR, Anderson PL, et al. iPrEx Study Team. Preexposure chemoprophylaxis for HIV prevention in men who have sex with men. N Engl J Med. 2010;363(27):2587.
100. Baeten JM, Donnell D, Ndase P, et al. Partners PrEP Study Team. Antiretroviral prophylaxis for HIV prevention in heterosexual men and women. N Engl J Med. 2012;367(5):399.
101. Thigpen MC, Kebaabetswe PM, Paxton LA, et al. TDF2 Study Group. Antiretroviral pre-exposure prophylaxis for heterosexual HIV transmission in Botswana. N Engl J Med. 2012;367(5):423.
102. Grant RM, Anderson PL, McMahan V, et al. iPrEx study team. Uptake of pre-exposure prophylaxis, sexual practices, and HIV incidence in men and transgender women who have sex with men: a cohort study. Lancet Infect Dis. 2014;14(9):820.
103. McCormack S, Dunn DT, Desai M, et al. Pre-exposure prophylaxis to prevent the acquisition of HIV-1 infection (PROUD): effectiveness results from the pilot phase of a pragmatic open-label randomised trial. Lancet. 2016;387(10013):53.
104. Liu AY, Cohen SE, Vittinghoff E, et al. Preexposure prophylaxis for HIV infection integrated with municipal- and community-based sexual health services. JAMA Intern Med. 2016;176(1):75.
105. Molina JM, Capiatant C, Spire B, et al. On-demand preexposure prophylaxis in men at high risk for HIV-1 infection. N Engl J Med. 2015;373:2273.
106. Hosek SG, Landovitz RJ, Kapogiannis B, et al. Safety and feasibility of antiretroviral pre-exposure prophylaxis for adolescent men who have sex with men aged 15 to 17 years in the United States. JAMA Pediatr. 2017;171:1063.
107. LeFevre ML, US Preventive Services Task Force. Screening for chlamydia and gonorrhea: US Preventive Services Task Force recommendation statement. Ann Intern Med. 2014;161(12):902–10.
108. Michielsen K, De Meyer S, Ivanova O, et al. Reorienting adolescent sexual and reproductive health research: reflections from an international conference. Reprod Health. 2016;13:3.
109. Halpern CT. Same-sex attraction and health disparities: do sexual minority youth really need something different for healthy development? J Adolesc Health. 2011;48:5.

Chapter 13
Human Immunodeficiency Virus and Acquired Immunodeficiency Syndrome

Jonathan D. Warus and Marvin E. Belzer

Etiology and Pathogenesis

Acquired immunodeficiency syndrome (AIDS) is the term initially used by the Centers for Disease Control and Prevention (CDC) in 1981 to describe the phenomenon of young homosexual men in New York and San Francisco dying from infections that individuals with healthy immune systems could fight off easily. Although many suspected a viral cause, this was not confirmed until 1983. The viral cause of AIDS was given the name "human immunodeficiency virus" (HIV), and researchers later identified that AIDS is a late manifestation of this infection [1].

HIV is an RNA retrovirus that is able to attach to and enter CD4+ immune cells in humans (including T cells, T helper cells, dendritic cells, and macrophages) and integrate itself into the host genome. The virus has a complex life cycle that then leads to viral propagation and constant generalized immune system activation. Over time, these immune cells decrease in number and in function, leaving individuals vulnerable to opportunistic infections and tumor growth due to impaired immune system protection, still referred to as AIDS [1, 2].

J. D. Warus (✉) · M. E. Belzer
Department of Pediatrics, University of Southern California, Division of Adolescent and Young Adult Medicine, Children's Hospital Los Angeles, Los Angeles, CA, USA
e-mail: jwarus@chla.usc.edu; mbelzer@chla.usc.edu

C. Warf, G. Charles (eds.), *Clinical Care for Homeless, Runaway and Refugee Youth*, https://doi.org/10.1007/978-3-030-40675-2_13

Clinical Presentation and Natural History of HIV

The presentation and course of HIV infection may vary widely between individuals. The CDC divides HIV infection into three different stages of disease.

Stage 1: Acute HIV Infection

In early HIV infection, the virus is actively replicating within immune cells in the bloodstream and lymph nodes [3]. Some people may be asymptomatic during this time, while others show signs and symptoms of mild illness, often mimicking the common cold or other minor infections. Common signs and symptoms during this stage of infection are shown in Table 13.1 and are sometimes collectively referred to as acute retroviral syndrome. As these findings can be very nonspecific, practitioners must maintain a high level of suspicion for acute HIV infection [4]. Individuals can be highly infectious during this stage of illness as the viral load can be very high, making transmission to others more efficient.

Stage 2: Clinical Latency

During the second stage of HIV infection, individuals are largely asymptomatic and may not have any clinical signs or symptoms of HIV. During this time, the viral load initially drops as the immune system works to suppress the infection. Over time, HIV weakens the immune system by infecting and killing CD4+ immune cells, which progressively decrease in number. The viral load starts to increase again as the immune system is unable to suppress the infection. When the CD4+ T cell count

Table 13.1 Clinical signs and symptoms of acute HIV infection

Sign/symptom	Frequency in presentation of acute HIV (%)
Fever	75
Fatigue	68
Myalgia	49
Skin rash	48
Headache	45
Pharyngitis	40
Cervical adenopathy	39
Arthralgia	30
Night sweats	28
Diarrhea	27

Adapted from Daar et al. [4]

drops below 500 cells/μL, some individuals may start to develop symptoms such as fatigue, fever, weight loss, and chronic diarrhea. They may also start to develop some mild opportunistic infections such as oral thrush and may manifest oral hairy leukoplakia associated with Epstein-Barr virus infection [5].

Stage 3: AIDS

Once the CD4+ T cell count drops below 200 cells/μL or a person is diagnosed with a characteristic opportunistic infection (see Table 13.2), they are classified as stage 3 disease, or AIDS. In untreated HIV, the incubation period before the onset of AIDS ranges from 1 to 14 years with an average of 6 years. Of those infected, 50–70% are referred to as *typical progressors* and may progress to AIDS over 8–10 years. Five to ten percent are referred to as *rapid progressors* and can develop AIDS within 2–3 years. *Long-term nonprogressors* are individuals who have not yet developed any symptoms of AIDS after 10 or more years since the initial infection (about 5% of those infected) [5].

Epidemiology

Prevalence

According to the CDC, an estimated 1.12 million persons aged 13 years or older were living with HIV in the United States at the end of 2015. Of these individuals, 162,500 (14.5%) were undiagnosed and unaware of their infection [6].

Table 13.2 Examples of opportunistic illnesses and infections in stage-3 HIV

Opportunistic illnesses and infections in stage-3 HIV	
Bacterial sinusitis/pneumonia	Herpes zoster
Candidiasis	Histoplasmosis (disseminated)
Cerebral toxoplasmosis	Kaposi sarcoma
Cervical carcinoma, invasive	*Mycobacterium avium* complex
Coccidioidomycosis	*Mycobacterium tuberculosis*
Cryptococcosis	Non-Hodgkin lymphoma
Cryptosporidiosis	*Pneumocystis jiroveci* pneumonia
Cytomegalovirus disease	Progressive multifocal leukoencephalopathy
Central nervous system lymphoma	*Salmonella* septicemia, recurrent
Herpes simplex virus	Wasting syndrome attributed to HIV

Adapted from Selik et al. [61]

Incidence

Overall incidence of new HIV infection in the United States has been relatively stable from 2011 to 2016 with around 40,000 new infections per year. However, the incidence for those aged 25–34 years has been slowly *increasing* over this same time period, accounting for 34.3% of all new HIV infections in 2016 [7].

Age

As of 2015, there were an estimated 60,300 persons between the ages of 13 and 24 years of age living with HIV in the United States (making up 5.4% of the total prevalence of HIV). Of these youth, 51.4% were undiagnosed and unaware of their infection, making this the largest percentage of undiagnosed HIV infection compared to any other age group [6]. Given the higher incidence of new HIV infection in adolescents and young adults (AYAs), many strategies to address HIV in the United States have focused on this age group.

Gender

According to CDC data from 2016, males account for the majority of HIV diagnoses in all age groups, making up 84% of those 13–19 years old and 89% of those 20–24 years old who are diagnosed with HIV [8]. In the National Transgender Discrimination Survey in 2011, 2.64% of transgender adults reported a diagnosis of HIV, over four times the rate of HIV in the general US population [9].

Race/Ethnicity

New HIV infections continue to disproportionately affect individuals within communities of color. Of the estimated 8536 youth aged 13–24 years who were diagnosed with new HIV infections in 2016, 4629 (54.2%) identified as Black/African American and 2040 (23.9%) identified as Hispanic/Latinx [7].

Transmission Category

As seen in Table 13.3, the most common route of transmission in AYA males is male-to-male sexual contact, while the most common route in AYA females is heterosexual contact [8].

Table 13.3 Diagnoses of HIV infection among male and female adolescents and young adults, by age group and transmission category, 2016 – United States and six dependent areas

	Males				Females			
	13–19 years		20–24 years		13–19 years		20–24 years	
Transmission category	No.	%	No.	%	No.	%	No.	%
Male-to-male sexual contact	1321	92.7	5595	91.6	–	–	–	–
Injection drug use (IDU)	15	1.0	88	1.4	17	6.5	76	10.4
Male-to-male sexual contact and IDU	40	2.8	188	3.1	–	–	–	–
Heterosexual contact[a]	42	3.0	234	3.8	222	84.2	650	88.2
Other[b]	6	0.4	6	0.1	25	9.4	10	1.4
Total[c]	**1424**	**100**	**6111**	**100**	**264**	**100**	**737**	**100**

Adapted from the Centers for Disease Control and Prevention [8]

[a]Heterosexual contact with a person known to have, or to be at high risk for, HIV infection

[b]Includes hemophilia, blood transfusion, perinatal exposure, and risk factor not reported or not identified

[c]Because column totals for numbers were calculated independently of the values for the subpopulations, the values in each column may not sum to the column total

Homelessness

AYAs experiencing homelessness are at increased risk for HIV as well as other sexually transmitted infections (STIs). Some studies estimate that 2–11% of youth experiencing homelessness in the United States are living with HIV. This means that they are at 2–10 times the risk of acquiring an HIV infection when compared to the general youth population [10]. Much of this increased risk has been attributed to increased risk behaviors such as risky sexual practices, exchanging sexual acts for survival, injection drug use, and needle sharing. Those experiencing homelessness also often have other psychosocial stressors such as poverty, mental illness, and alcohol and drug use [11]. One study looking into social networks has shown that youth who are centrally associated with other youth experiencing homelessness have more sexual risk-taking behaviors than youth who have more peripheral social positions. This may indicate that exposure to and normalization of risk-taking behaviors of other youth experiencing homelessness may increase participation in these behaviors, placing individuals at higher risk for HIV [12].

Transmission

Modes of Transmission

The transmission of HIV infection occurs by the transfer of the virus in body fluids from an infected individual to an uninfected individual, specifically through blood, semen, pre-seminal fluid, vaginal secretions, rectal secretions, and breast milk. The virus in these fluids must come into contact with the uninfected person through a mucous membrane (found in the mouth, penis, vagina, and rectum), damaged tissue (i.e., cuts), or directly into the bloodstream (needle stick or placental transmission from mother to child) [13].

Rates of Transmission

Different modes of transmission have different rates of transferring the infection from the infected person to the uninfected person (see Table 13.4). These differences in transmission rates are often accounted for by the type of epithelium or protective lining of different anatomic sites and the potential for breakdown of this protection [14]. It is worth noting that although HIV has been found in saliva, tears, urine, and sweat, there have been no cases of HIV transmission occurring via these fluids.

HIV Testing

Consent and Confidentiality

HIV screening or testing should always be voluntary and only performed with the individual's knowledge and consent. Many settings have incorporated consent for HIV screening into the general informed consent for medical care, and a separate

Table 13.4 Estimated per-exposure risk for acquiring HIV from an infected source

Type of exposure	Rate of HIV acquisition per 10,000 exposures[a]
Blood transfusion	9250
Receptive anal intercourse	138
Needle sharing during injection drug use	63
Percutaneous needle stick	23
Insertive anal intercourse	11
Receptive penile-vaginal intercourse	8
Insertive penile-vaginal intercourse	4
Receptive oral intercourse	Low risk
Insertive oral intercourse	Low risk
Biting	Negligible risk
Spitting	Negligible risk
Throwing body fluids (including semen or saliva)	Negligible risk
Sharing sex toys	Negligible risk

Adapted from Centers for Disease Control and Prevention [14]

[a]Factors that may increase the risk of HIV transmission include sexually transmitted infections, acute- and late-stage HIV infection, and high viral load. Factors that may decrease the risk of HIV transmission include condom use, male circumcision, antiretroviral treatment with viral suppression, and preexposure prophylaxis. None of these factors are accounted for in the transmission rates shown

consent specific to HIV testing is not recommended. Patients should not only be advised of the confidential nature of testing results but also be informed of the requirement of HIV case reporting to the state or local health department. In many states, adolescents under the age of 18 can consent to HIV testing, but this may vary based upon the state in which the test is performed. Professionals should become familiar with the public health statutes in their specific state and strive to protect the privacy and confidentiality of the patient [15].

Pretest Counseling

Prior to HIV testing, patients should be given written or oral information including an explanation of HIV infection, the routine screening recommendations for all individuals, and the meanings of positive and negative results. The individual should also be given the opportunity to ask questions and the ability to decline testing. Any declined test should be documented in the medical record [15].

HIV Testing Recommendations

The CDC recommends that HIV screening be performed routinely in all healthcare settings for patients aged 13–64 years on an opt-out basis. This means that all patients are offered HIV screening as part of their regular medical care but have the option to decline the test [15]. The US Preventive Services Task Force (USPSTF) recommendations for screening are very similar to the CDC but recommend routine screening for those aged 15–65 years. Screening in youth less than 13–15 years of age should occur for those determined to be at increased risk [16].

All pregnant individuals should be screened for HIV early in each pregnancy, and any declined test should be documented in the medical record. All patients starting treatment for tuberculosis should also be screening for HIV. In addition, patients seeking testing or treatment for sexually transmitted infections (STIs) should be screened routinely for HIV during each visit [15].

Repeat screening (at least annually) is recommended for those who are likely to be at high risk for HIV. This includes those whose sexual partners are living with HIV and are not virally suppressed, those who use injection drugs and their partners, those who exchange sex for survival (money, food, shelter, drugs, etc.), men who have sex with men, and persons who themselves or whose sex partners have had more than one sexual partner since their most recent HIV test [15]. Youth who are on preexposure prophylaxis (PrEP) for HIV prevention must have an HIV screen every 3 months to safely administer the medication. A recent systemic review looking into the benefits and harms of more frequent than annual HIV screening in men who have sex with men revealed that there is insufficient evidence to change the recommendation to more frequent screening. However, several modeling studies in the review did predict that more frequent screening in this population (every 3–6 months) may be cost-effective compared with annual screening [17]. Repeat screening in those who are not likely to be at high risk for HIV should be performed based on the clinical judgment of the provider [15].

Diagnostic HIV testing should be conducted in all individuals with signs or symptoms of HIV infection or with an AIDS-defining opportunistic infection. If acute retroviral syndrome is possible, it is recommended to use a plasma RNA test in addition to an HIV antibody test [15].

HIV Testing Methods

Many tests have been developed for the detection of HIV infection. Over time, the tests have become easier to administer with quicker results and earlier detection from the time of infection. The currently available testing methods are shown in Table 13.5. Enzyme-linked immunoassay (EIA) methods are often available as rapid tests, giving results within 1–20 minutes of performing the test. These rapid tests (oral swabs or blood samples) are often used for HIV screening due to lower cost, easy administration in any setting, and the ability to provide the result during the same encounter. Western blot and viral load testing require analysis in a laboratory and are more expensive; thus, they are not recommended for HIV screening. Western blot may be used for confirmatory testing after a positive EIA test, but this has largely been replaced by HIV RNA PCR (viral load). Viral load testing can be used for initial HIV testing if there is a clinical suspicion for acute HIV infection that may be missed by other testing methods. Viral load testing is also used to monitor the course of treatment of HIV with the goal of suppressing the viral load to undetectable [18–20].

Table 13.5 HIV diagnostic testing windows

Testing method	Target of detection	Estimated window from infection to positive result, days
First-generation EIA	IgG antibody	35–45
Second-generation EIA	IgG antibody	25–35
Third-generation EIA	IgG and IgM antibody	20–30
Fourth-generation EIA	IgG and IgM antibody + p24 antigen	15–20
Western blot	IgG and IgM antibody	Indeterminate: 35–50
		Positive: 45–60
Viral load (cutoff 50 copies/mL)	HIV RNA	10–15
Viral load, ultrasensitive (cutoff 1–5 copies/mL)	HIV RNA	5

Adapted from: Branson and Stekler [18], Cohen et al. [19], Owen [20]

EIA enzyme-linked immunoassay, *IgG* immunoglobulin G, *IgM* immunoglobulin M, *RNA* ribonucleic acid

Posttest Counseling

HIV test results should be communicated to patients as soon as possible in order to maximize the number of individuals who are aware of their HIV status.

Negative Result

Testing results that are negative for HIV can be communicated to patients without direct personal contact between the patient and provider. Patients who are at increased risk for HIV should be given recommendations for repeat screening. Those who want assistance with modifying risk behaviors should also be provided with referrals to risk-reduction services. These may include prevention services (such as PrEP or PEP) or risk-reduction counseling (discussed in the section on prevention), treatment for STIs, substance use treatment, mental health treatment, or other supportive services [15].

Positive Result

Testing results that are positive for HIV should be communicated through personal contact by the provider with an emphasis on preserving confidentiality. Any positive rapid HIV test result is preliminary and must be confirmed by further testing before the diagnosis of HIV is established. Any individuals who have a confirmed diagnosis of HIV infection should be linked to clinical care as soon as possible and referred to supportive services. Rapid initiation of treatment improves retention in care and can reduce transmission of HIV. Practitioners should strongly encourage patients with HIV infection to disclose their diagnosis to their spouses as well as any current or previous sex partners and recommend that they also be tested for HIV. Health departments are able to assist patients in this process while preserving confidentiality. In addition, any positive HIV testing results must be reported to the state or local health department, and patients should be made aware that this report will be made [15].

HIV Testing Rates

Rates of testing for HIV among youth experiencing homelessness tend to be higher than the rates among youth in the general population. Many studies indicate that more than half of homeless youth have ever been tested for either HIV or STIs compared to 22.6% of sexually active youth in the general population. Some factors associated with increased rates of testing in youth experiencing homelessness include youth who self-identified as gay, identified as Hispanic, used injection drugs, and used drop-in centers. Many studies in this area use convenience samples of homeless youth and are not able to be generalized to youth outside of these samples. It is also difficult to determine the structural factors such as service utilization that likely impacts the rates of HIV testing [21].

HIV Prevention

Since the beginning of the HIV epidemic, many medical, scientific, and public health advances have decreased the number of new infections from an estimated 130,000 in 1985 down to an estimated 37,600 in 2014 [22].

Treatment as Prevention (TasP)

One major advance in preventing new HIV infections has been termed treatment as prevention (TasP). In 2016, in the landmark HIV Prevention Trials Network 052 study, it was shown that early initiation of antiretroviral therapy (ART) was associated with a 93% relative reduction in the risk of transmission when compared to delayed ART. This study also established that in participants who were stably virally suppressed throughout the study, there were zero linked infections observed [23]. In the same year, the PARTNERS study showed that in heterosexual couples who did not use condoms, there were no transmissions of HIV from partners living with HIV who were virally suppressed [24]. After the release of this information in 2016, the Prevention Access Campaign launched the slogan *Undetectable = Untransmittable* (*U = U*) [25]. In 2017, the CDC officially recognized that individuals who take ART and achieve an undetectable viral load do not sexually transmit the infection to their partners [26].

Preexposure Prophylaxis (PrEP)

Preexposure prophylaxis (PrEP) is a relatively new HIV prevention method. In order to work, an individual who is HIV-negative takes one daily pill in order to prevent HIV infection. The medication approved by the US Food and Drug Administration (FDA) in 2012 for use in adults for this purpose is called Truvada (a combination of two antiretroviral medications, tenofovir disoproxil fumarate and emtricitabine). This medication has been shown to be safe and is effective at reducing the risk of HIV from sexual transmission by more than 90% when taken daily [27]. Recently, in 2018, based on studies of medication safety and efficacy in AYAs, the FDA expanded the indication for Truvada for PrEP in any individuals, including minors, who weigh at least 35 kg [28]. In 2019, a second medication (Descovy) was approved by the FDA for use as PrEP in any individuals weighing at least 35 kg, excluding vaginal HIV exposures [29].

Table 13.6 Preexposure prophylaxis (PrEP) visit recommendations

Laboratory test or counseling	Initial visit	1 mo	3 mo	6 mo	9 mo	12 mo, etc.
HIV antibody, blood (every 3 mo)[a]	+	+/–[f]	+	+	+	+
Creatinine (every 6 mo)[b]	+		+/–[f]	+	+/–[f]	+
Weight (every 6 mo)[b]	+		+/–[f]	+	+/–[f]	+
Hepatitis B surface antibody[c]	+					
Hepatitis B surface antigen[c]	+					
Hepatitis C virus antibody[c]	+					
Urine pregnancy (if applicable)	+/–[f]	+/–[f]	+/–[f]	+/–[f]	+/–[f]	+/–[f]
RPR (every 3–6 mo)[d]	+	+/–[f]	+/–[f]	+	+/–[f]	+
GC/CT (every 3–6 mo)[d]	+	+/–[f]	+/–[f]	+	+/–[f]	+
Medication counseling[e]	+	+	+	+	+	+
Adherence counseling	+	+	+	+	+	+
Risk reduction counseling	+	+	+	+	+	+

RPR rapid plasma reagin test for syphilis, *GC* gonorrhea, *CT* chlamydia

[a]Rapid blood HIV testing is valid, but oral swabs are not adequate. A viral load may be sent if there have been possible symptoms of acute HIV in the prior 1–2 months

[b]Creatinine and weight are used to calculate creatinine clearance (CrCl must be ≥60 to be on Truvada without renal dosing)

[c]Hepatitis is not a contraindication to Truvada, but individuals must be counseled that their hepatitis may reactivate when discontinuing Truvada; consider referral to a specialist. Those who are nonimmune to hepatitis B should be vaccinated

[d]Frequency of STI screening should be based upon risk factors and patient preference. GC/CT screening should be performed at any sites of sexual contact (urine, vaginal, rectal, pharyngeal)

[e]Medication counseling should include discussions about time to efficacy (reaches maximum levels in rectal tissue in 7 days, maximum levels in other sites in 20 days), efficacy (reduces the risk of HIV from sex by >90% and from injection drugs by >70%), and side effects (i.e., headache, abdominal pain, and decreased appetite that usually resolve over time)

[f]More frequent screening should take place based upon clinical suspicion for the disease or condition

PrEP can be initiated by any prescribing practitioner and should be discussed with any patients who are at risk for HIV or who are requesting PrEP. The CDC has created guidelines and supplemental reports to assist providers in delivering this important service to prevent HIV infection [27, 30]. Please see Table 13.6 for an example of recommended tasks during PrEP visits.

Recent data from the IPERGAY study in 2017 showed that "on-demand" PrEP may be highly efficacious at preventing HIV among men who have sex with men at risk for the infection with a relative reduction of 97% in new HIV infections compared to placebo. This regimen consists of taking two tablets of Truvada 2–24 hours before sex and one tablet at both 24 and 48 hours after sex [31]. Since many individuals in the study were using on-demand PrEP frequently, many were taking an average of 15 doses per month. Thus, this efficacy may be confounded by the finding in previous PrEP studies that those who took 4 doses of PrEP per week were able to achieve 96% relative risk reduction [32]. However, the efficacy of on-demand PrEP is further supported by the pharmacology of Truvada dosing for men who have sex with men and transgender women in the Cell PrEP study. This study found that after 4 initial doses of Truvada, medication levels corresponded to a 98% relative risk reduction in 84% of participants [33]. The convenience of on-demand PrEP for those with infrequent sexual exposures must be balanced with the fact that the regimen must be started prior to sexual activity and would require future-oriented thinking. This may be difficult for younger patients or those who have psychosocial stressors that may impact adherence. Current evidence supports on-demand PrEP as an alternative dosing strategy in those with infrequent sexual exposures and offers much more protection than no PrEP at all.

With the emergence of new prevention methods and efforts to increase patient access and retention, many sites have incorporated PrEP and PEP "navigators" to assist with patient care for these prevention methods. These peer navigators can assist with engaging patients in care, providing information and counseling regarding HIV and PrEP/PEP, as well as helping patients to navigate the healthcare system (insurance, payment assistance, pharmacies, etc.). These services are essential, especially for youth seeking HIV prevention services.

Postexposure Prophylaxis (PEP)

While PrEP is a preventive medication that is taken all of the time to preemptively cover possible exposures to HIV, postexposure prophylaxis (PEP) is an emergency medical regimen given after a substantial possible exposure to HIV to decrease the risk of contracting HIV. In order to differentiate the two, some describe PrEP as the "birth control" for HIV and PEP as the "emergency contraception" for HIV infection. PEP must be started within 72 hours of the possible HIV exposure and consists of three antiretroviral medications (as opposed to two medications in PrEP). In occupational HIV exposure data, PEP demonstrated an 81% reduction in the odds of contracting HIV with 28 days of treatment [14].

PEP can also be initiated by any prescribing practitioner. The preferred medication regimen for adults and adolescents aged ≥13 years with normal kidney function is Truvada (tenofovir disoproxil fumarate and emtricitabine) once daily *with either* dolutegravir 50 mg once daily *or* raltegravir 400 mg twice daily. This combination is taken for 28 days to complete the course of PEP. At that time, those who are at continued risk for HIV should be transitioned to PrEP for continued protection against future possible exposures. The CDC has also created guidelines to assist providers in delivering PEP [14].

Risk-Reduction Counseling

In order to achieve primary prevention of HIV infection, providers must also effectively promote behavioral change through risk-reduction counseling. This method creates a dialogue between the patient and the provider to increase knowledge, skills, and self-efficacy while acknowledging the individual's feelings, beliefs, attitudes, and values [34].

In this patient-centered counseling session, the discussion is built around previously obtained information including sexual history (number of partners, gender of partners, sexual practices, patterns of condom use, and pregnancy prevention), drug and/or alcohol use prior to or during sexual activity, use of injection drugs, and history of STI/HIV testing and infection. The practitioner can ask them to identify any of these behaviors they would like to change. After assessing their willingness to change, the practitioner can assist the patient in identifying a safer goal behavior that can reduce or prevent the risk of HIV. This is followed by praising planned or accomplished efforts and helps them to identify any barriers to change. The final step for the session is for the patient to identify a specific step they can take to help create this change [34]. Many of the fundamentals of this counseling strategy are based in motivational interviewing (MI), and training in MI is advisable for those administering risk-reduction counseling. Risk-reduction counseling can take place in a 15- to 20-minute session and can be carried out by a variety of providers [35].

Other Barriers to Prevention

Despite having effective ways to prevent HIV, the literature shows that there are barriers to accessing these services and ideal outcomes. For example, TasP could have the potential to stop any new HIV infections if it were able to be fully implemented. One study, however, notes that this strategy alone has limitations in real-world populations where even slight delays in testing, treatment, and adherence would keep the transmission rate from reaching zero. This method must likely be combined with other existing HIV prevention methods in order to have the maximal effect on transmission. This required multifaceted approach may make financial allocation difficult in where to place priority [36].

There are also many barriers that exist for youth to access HIV prevention services. Compounded onto other baseline social determinants of health are the issues of consent and confidentiality, financial barriers, and even the stigma associated with sexual activity and HIV, even in seeking prevention services. One study examining barriers to HIV prevention for the young black MSM population identified that these youth have inadequate access to culturally competent prevention services including limited services in areas where they live and a deficiency of these services within correctional institutions. The authors recommend structural interventions to eliminate barriers to HIV testing and prevention and to provide these youth with skills to navigate the complex healthcare system [37].

Once programs are in place that youth can access, services must also be tailored to ensure completion of the interventions. One study examined if motivational barriers would predict youth retention in an HIV prevention counseling program. Those younger participants who felt pressured to attend the program as well as those who perceived the program as ineffective had lower rates of retention. The authors recommend that programs should ensure that younger clients do not feel coerced into participation and that practitioners make every effort to communicate the efficacy of the intervention. Programs should also help participants foster a sense of self-relevance with the intervention in order to improve retention [38].

HIV Prevention Research in Homeless Youth

A systematic review in 2011 looked at different interventions to modify HIV sexual risk behaviors in youth experiencing homelessness. The review only found three eligible studies and was unable to estimate the effectiveness of the interventions due to high variability in the studies and lack of rigorous methodology. This lack of evidence for prevention work is a large area for improvement within research on homeless youth [39].

Few studies have looked into identifying specific correlates or predictors of HIV risk behaviors in youth experiencing homelessness. One such study found that female sex, belonging to a sexual minority group, depression, alcohol use to intoxication, and frequent traveling between cities were associated with unprotected sex [40]. For homeless youth, Internet use and social networking that maintains connections to family or home-based peers has been associated with decreased unprotected sex and lower sexual risk behavior [41, 42]. In looking at factors associated with homeless youths' motivation to change HIV risk behaviors, shorter period of current homelessness was the only factor that predicted higher levels of motivation to change HIV risk behaviors [43]. Future studies should focus on ways to improve HIV prevention strategies for youth experiencing homelessness.

HIV Management

Since the first antiretroviral medication (zidovudine, "AZT") was developed and approved by the FDA in 1987, there have been many breakthroughs in the area of HIV management. One such advancement was the development of protease inhibitor medications that allowed for the first highly active antiretroviral treatment (HAART) in 1995 and led to the first decline in new HIV cases since the epidemic began. In 1990, the Ryan White Act was passed by the Congress allowing for the creation of a federal funding program to support community-based care and treatment services for HIV, which still allows for increased access to care for patients to this day [44].

Medication regimens continue to improve with fewer pills required per day, less side effects, and better suppression of the virus in individuals living with HIV. While the science of HIV treatment has advanced rapidly, many barriers remain in all areas of management that require continued investigation and development of improved treatment models.

HIV Care Continuum

Dr. Edward Gardner and his team first described the different levels of engagement in HIV care in 2011. They recognized that in order to fully benefit from antiretroviral medications, patients must not only be tested and treated but must also be regularly engaged in their medical care, receive medications, and adhere to the recommended treatment [45]. This "care continuum" (see Fig. 13.1) became more widely disseminated through the formation of the HIV Care Continuum Initiative, created via Execute Order by President Barack Obama in 2013. This framework has been adopted internationally and has been used to establish measurable indicators for HIV care. Using this continuum, the current National HIV/AIDS Strategy (NHAS) for the United States outlines measurable outcome indicators in order to assess the progress of improving HIV care [46].

Diagnosis and Testing

In order to first identify those who should receive HIV treatment, individuals must be tested for HIV and diagnosed with the infection. The recognition of this important step in treatment has prompted the previously discussed HIV screening recommendations from the CDC and USPSTF. However, despite these recommendations, many individuals living with HIV remain unaware of their infection with youth and young adults aged 13–34 years having the highest proportion of undiagnosed

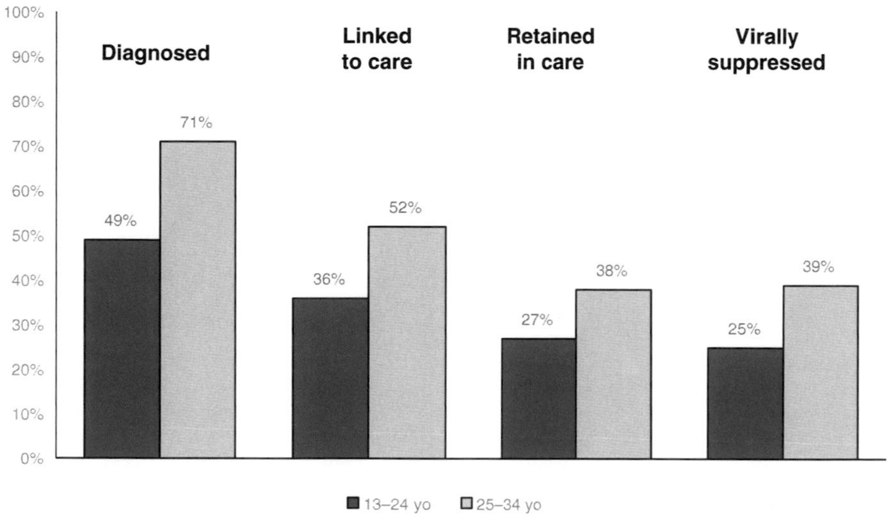

Fig. 13.1 HIV care continuum data in adolescents and young adults, 2015. (Adapted from Centers for Disease Control and Prevention [48])

HIV. These individuals are unable to proceed with any treatment until they are aware of the infection [47, 48]. To address this barrier, the NHAS has set the goal of increasing awareness of HIV status to 90% among those living with HIV by 2020 [46].

In order to continue to improve in this area, providers, clinics, and agencies serving youth experiencing homelessness should strive to offer HIV screening to all youth as recommended by the CDC. By using tests that allow for rapid results with a shorter time-to-positivity window, more youth will be able to find out their HIV status during the same visit, earlier in the course of infection. This is particularly important for youth who may be transiently housed or who move frequently between service providers.

Linkage to Care

This step of the continuum refers to connecting individuals who are diagnosed with HIV to a care provider. The NHAS goal for 2020 is to link 85% of people living with HIV to a care provider within 1 month of diagnosis. Care models that have had higher success with linkage to care in vulnerable populations involve the collaboration of interdisciplinary providers with multiple sites of service access [47].

Retention in Care

According to the CDC, individuals are considered "retained in care" if they have had at least two visits for HIV medical care, at least 3 months apart, within the past year [47]. It is often difficult to estimate the rates of retention in care in any population that may have more transient housing and changes sites of service utilization. Some areas of the country have established inter-agency partnerships (such as the Hollywood Homeless Youth Partnership) in order to help find and track youth who may move frequently between local service sites [49].

Viral Suppression

The primary goal of public health interventions in HIV management is achieving viral suppression (most recent viral load of <200 copies/mL, performed within the last year) using antiretroviral therapy [49]. The NHAS goal for 2020 is to achieve viral suppression in 80% of those diagnosed with HIV infection [46]. This final step of the continuum has the potential to improve the health of individuals living with HIV and prevent transmissions of the infection to others. Although this is the ultimate goal of management, individuals should be encouraged at every level of the continuum. Providers need to be aware of and to address the societal determinants of health for individuals living with HIV as these can have complex impacts on engagement in the HIV care continuum.

Components of HIV Treatment

As there is no current cure for HIV infection, the primary goal of treatment is to reduce associated morbidities and to improve the quality and length of life through suppression of the viral load and improvement in immune function. This section briefly reviews some principles of HIV treatment. Please note that patient care should involve the assistance of an HIV specialist when possible given the complexity of testing and medication selection.

Initial Testing

After the confirmed diagnosis of HIV infection, individuals should receive a CD4 cell count and percentage, HIV RNA level, HIV genotype (test for resistance), complete blood count with differential, complete metabolic panel including hepatic and renal function, fasting blood glucose and lipid panel, vitamin D level, urinalysis, tuberculosis screening, STI screening (syphilis, gonorrhea, chlamydia), viral hepatitis screening, and cervical and/or anal Pap testing if indicated. Additional laboratory tests may be sent for specific patients or if certain medications may be used for HIV treatment [50].

Principles of ART

The basic principle of ART is to use multiple mediations that are directed against different stages of the HIV life cycle in order to make treatment more effective and avoid the development of resistance to medications. There are currently six drug classes used to treat HIV. Usual medication regimens consist of using three different medications from at least two different drug classes. Medications are selected based upon the patient's HIV genotype, coexisting conditions, and potential medication interactions. Practitioners also try to choose a regimen that has the lowest number of pills per day and are more tolerable with less side effects [50].

Until relatively recently, providers often delayed treatment with ART until a patient's immune system began to weaken and approach the diagnosis of AIDS (CD4+ count of ≤350 cells/mL). The landmark START (Strategic Timing of Antiretroviral Treatment) study in 2015 showed that early initiation of ART provided net benefit over delayed treatment by decreasing rates of opportunistic infections, AIDS-related cancers, liver and renal disease, cardiovascular disease, and death [51]. Patients are now started on ART as early as possible after diagnosis with HIV in order to improve their health and prevent new HIV infections through TasP. Effective viral suppression and continued engagement in HIV care have the ability to extend the mortality of those living with HIV to that of the general population.

Although everyone with HIV should be on ART as much as possible, there are times when individuals are unable to adhere to their medical regimen. This may be due to difficulties with housing, money, insurance, healthcare access, stigma, mental health, substance use, or a multitude of other psychosocial stressors. At times, it may be advisable to take a break from ART and concentrate on addressing these other stressors. Individuals who are less adherent to their medications may be at higher risk of inducing resistance to the medications and may make continued HIV treatment much more difficult in the future.

Monitoring

Those who are asymptomatic and on ART should be monitored with bloodwork every 3–6 months with CD4+ cell count and percentage, HIV viral load, urinalysis, hepatic and renal function, as well as fasting lipids and glucose level [50]. Patients should also be monitored for side effects, adherence, opportunistic infections, and psychosocial stressors.

Risk Reduction

All individuals living with HIV should be counseled on the modes of transmission of HIV and ways to reduce the risk of transmitting the infection to others. It is safe for those living with HIV to be in close contact with others (HIV is only spread through sexual contact, exposure to infected blood or breast milk, and perinatal transmission). While bathroom facilities can be shared, it is important to note that those living with HIV should not share hygiene items such as toothbrushes or razors.

To decrease transmission, individuals should notify sexual partners and health providers of their HIV status, use condoms with sexual activity, encourage HIV-negative partners to use PrEP (or PEP if needed), avoid sharing any syringes or needles, perform screening for STIs regularly, and adhere to their ART medications. Those who are living with HIV are also not able to donate blood, semen, or body organs. Those who are or may become pregnant should be counseled on ways to decrease transmission to their partners during conception and methods for decreasing transmission to their future children. They should also be offered options for family planning and pregnancy prevention as indicated [50, 52].

Opportunistic Infections (OIs)

OIs (Table 13.2) are those infections that healthy individuals are usually able to fight off or prevent with an intact immune system but can cause severe or prolonged disease in those living with HIV and a compromised immune system.

Prophylaxis

Prophylaxis and treatment for opportunistic infections are guided by the CD4+ cell count and percentage as well as any signs or symptoms of infection. Patients often become vulnerable to some of these infections (such as *Pneumocystis* pneumonia) when their CD4+ cell count approaches or drops beneath 200 cells/mL. The risk of infections associated with end-stage AIDS (such as *Mycobacterium avium* complex) increases when the CD4+ cell count goes below 75 cells/mL. Prophylaxis for these conditions may be discontinued once the CD4+ cell count has been above 200 cells/mL for at least 3 months [50].

Evaluation

Professionals who do not routinely work with patients living with HIV may become overly concerned by any sign of potential infection. It is important to remember that all people occasionally experience fever, sore throat, cough, diarrhea, or other common indications of mild infection. Patients living with HIV who have signs or symptoms of acute infection should first have a standard evaluation by a medical provider as is recommended for any individual living with or without HIV infection. If there is suspicion for a possible OI, the patient's CD4+ cell count should be measured. Those with a normal cell count and mild symptoms should be treated as any other individual. If symptoms are severe and prolonged or if the CD4+ cell count is less than 200 cells/mL, the patient should be further evaluated for an OI and may require consultation with an HIV or infectious disease specialist.

Vaccination

In an effort to decrease opportunistic and other infections in those living with HIV, certain immunizations are recommended. Some must be given when the CD4+ cell count is above 200 cells/mL, particularly live viral vaccines. These vaccines include *Streptococcus pneumoniae*, influenza (inactivated), hepatitis A and B series, human papillomavirus (HPV) series, varicella series, tetanus/diphtheria/pertussis (TdaP), and meningococcus [50].

Addressing Barriers to Care

As previously described, engagement in all levels of the HIV care continuum is required for successful viral suppression in HIV treatment. There are many barriers to optimal HIV care for youth and young adults that are further amplified in those experiencing homelessness. As with many areas of medicine, the societal determinants of health must be addressed in order to increase access to and engagement in care [53].

Adherence

Many barriers to care can have a direct or indirect effect on the ability of a patient to adhere to their medical treatment plan. Table 13.7 outlines examples of barriers that can affect adherence to HIV treatment in adolescents and young adults. AYAs experiencing homelessness often have many of the barriers listed that overlap based on their psychosocial development, support system, and comorbid conditions.

In order to address these barriers to adherence, many intervention models have been trialed for efficacy in improving patient adherence. A recent systematic review and meta-analysis on adherence found that interventions focusing on behavioral strategies, particularly habit-based interventions, were more effective than cognitive strategies to change participants' knowledge and/or beliefs [54]. A pilot study examined the use of a cell phone support intervention to improve adherence and psychosocial outcomes for youth living with HIV. This study found preliminary data that supports this intervention for decreasing perceived stress, substance use, depression, and increasing self-efficacy in comparison to those who received standard care [55].

A recent randomized control trial looked into using mindfulness-based stress reduction (MBSR) in youth living with HIV. Results suggest that those who participated in the intervention reported improved problem-solving coping and life satisfaction with lower levels of aggression. Individuals in the MBSR group also had significantly lower viral load measurements which may indicate improved medication adherence as well [56]. As of particular concern for youth experiencing homelessness, a recent meta-analysis looked into the effect of housing stability on medication adherence in HIV treatment. The study found that patients with more

Table 13.7 Barriers to adherence in AYAs living with HIV

Medical barriers	*Developmental barriers*
Lack of understanding about condition or medications	Underdeveloped problem-solving skills
Complexity of the medical regimen (i.e., number of pills, frequency)	Preoccupation with self-image
Adverse effects of treatment	Need for peer acceptance
If asymptomatic, difficulty accepting implications of the disease	Difficulty with future-directed thinking (present oriented)
Psychosocial barriers	Desire to establish independence and self-sufficiency
Lack of adult and peer social support	*HIV stigma barriers*
Busy or unstructured life or schedule	Fear of disclosure of HIV status to others
Lack of stable housing	Difficulty coming to terms with a life-threatening illness
Co-occurring mental health or substance use condition	Distrust of healthcare providers and systems

Adapted from Simons and Belzer [62]

stable housing had better adherence to their medications, but this difference was small. Some treatment guidelines and practitioners advocate for deferring HIV treatment until after housing and other psychosocial needs are met, which may need to be reconsidered based upon these new findings [57].

Psychosocial Support and Trauma-Informed Care

Youth experiencing homelessness who have acquired HIV through risk behaviors often experience rejection, stigma, violence, and discrimination after disclosure of their HIV status. Many are at increased risk for substance use, mental health conditions, and sexual victimization. Specific actions can be taken in order to provide high-quality care for these youth and young adults and to establish comprehensive multifaceted services [58].

Services should be structured to be youth-friendly and focus on confidentiality, stigma, and HIV disclosure. Improved outcomes are reported when confidentiality and privacy policies are discussed during each visit and implemented for all youth. Services should address ways that youth can cope with their diagnosis of HIV in a developmentally appropriate fashion that works to destigmatize their illness. Case management and interdisciplinary care teams (physicians, nurses, mental health providers, dieticians, social workers, etc.) should be available to provide a medical home to address all societal determinants of health and strive to provide continuity of care. Secure messaging that is Health Information Portability and Accountability Act (HIPAA)-compliant through mobile phones, the Internet, and social media can also be used to improve engagement in care and adherence to medications [58].

The Ryan White HIV/AIDS Program (RWHAP) currently provides support for direct healthcare services and support for more than 50% of all people living with diagnosed HIV in the United States. These services are patient-centered and coordinated with city, state, and local community-based organizations to provide efficient linkage to care, healthcare services, and supportive services for low-income individuals living with HIV. This program is essential to ensuring that people living with HIV are able to fully participate in the HIV care continuum by striving to address the psychosocial determinants of health [59].

Current Status of HIV Care and Homelessness

Data on the current status of HIV care in the United States is constantly updating and changing. Specific HIV data on youth experiencing homelessness can be difficult to assess, but the RWHAP's most recent report included data on housing status for all individuals living with HIV served by the program. In 2016, among those who reported stable housing, 86.1% were virally suppressed, compared to 78.9% of those reporting temporary housing, and 72.0% of those reporting unstable housing. This percentage of viral suppression in those reporting unstable housing has, however, increased since 2010 from 54.8%. Viral suppression among youth aged 13–24 years has also improved from 46.6% in 2010 to 71.1% in 2016 [59].

The impact of housing status on engagement in the HIV care continuum has been demonstrated in several studies, and those who are experiencing homelessness have also been shown to be less likely to adhere to HIV treatment. Participants in studies of supportive housing programs have reported the greatest benefit from positive relationships with case managers and assistance with changing health behaviors, improving adherence, maintaining stable housing, and improving overall well-being. Through continuous improvement in patient-centered supportive housing program development and interventional research, more adolescents and young adults will have the resources and support for engagement in the full HIV care continuum [60].

Take-Home Points

1. Despite improvements in HIV care and prevention, new infections continue to disproportionately affect marginalized populations at the highest rates, including adolescents and young adults, those experiencing homelessness, LGBTQ populations, and people of color.
2. Over time, HIV infection can cause a decrease in immune system function and resultant vulnerability to opportunistic infections.
3. All youth experiencing homelessness should be offered screening for HIV and other sexually transmitted infections at least annually.
4. All youth should receive information about recent advances in HIV prevention strategies such as TasP, PrEP, and PEP and linked to appropriate services.
5. Risk reduction strategies including condom use should be encouraged in order to minimize the risk for HIV and other STIs.
6. Providers should be aware of the signs and symptoms of HIV infection and have a high index of suspicion for acute HIV in at-risk populations.
7. Those with a new diagnosis of HIV should be linked to care as soon as possible to optimize continued engagement in care, adherence to ART, and viral suppression.
8. Programs should strive to provide comprehensive case management and interdisciplinary care to support youth living with or at risk for HIV.
9. HIV care and prevention has advanced rapidly in the past 35 years and HIV surveillance data has reflected improvements in the epidemic.
10. Continued improvement in housing resources is essential for ending homelessness and HIV in the United States.

References

1. Rowland-Jones SL. AIDS pathogenesis: what have two decades of HIV research taught us? Nat Rev Immunol. 2003;3:343–8.
2. Simon V, Ho DD, Karim QA. HIV/AIDS epidemiology, pathogenesis, prevention, and treatment. Lancet. 2006;368(9534):489–504.
3. Naif HM. Pathogenesis of HIV infection. Curr Infect Dis Rep. 2013;5(s1e6):26–30.
4. Daar ES, Pilcher CD, Hecht FM. Clinical presentation and diagnosis of primary HIV-1 infection. Curr Opin HIV AIDS. 2008;3:10–5.
5. Natural history of HIV Infection. In: Kartikeyan S, Bharmal RN, Tiwari RP, Bisen PS, editors. HIV and AIDS: basic elements and priorities. Dordrecht: Springer; 2007.
6. Centers for Disease Control and Prevention. Estimated HIV incidence and prevalence in the United States, 2010–2015. HIV surveillance supplemental report 2018;23(No. 1). http://www.cdc.gov/hiv/library/reports/hiv-surveillance.html. Published March 2018. Accessed 20 Aug 2018.
7. Centers for Disease Control and Prevention. HIV surveillance report 2016;28. http://www.cdc.gov/hiv/library/reports/hiv-surveillance.html. Published November 2017. Accessed 22 Aug 2018.
8. Centers for Disease Control and Prevention. National Center for HIV/AIDS, Viral Hepatitis, STD, and TB Prevention. Division of HIV/AIDS Prevention. HIV surveillance – adolescents and young adults. Slide set available online at http://www.cdc.gov/hiv/pdf/library/slidesets/cdc-hiv-surveillance-adolescents-young-adults-2016.pdf. Accessed 20 Aug 2018.
9. Grant JM, Mottet LA, Tanis J, et al. Injustice at every turn: a report of the National Transgender Discrimination Survey. Washington, DC: National Center for Transgender Equality and National Gay and Lesbian Task Force; 2011.
10. Young SD, Rice E. Online social networking technologies, HIV knowledge, and sexual risk and testing behaviors among homeless youth. AIDS Behav. 2011;15:253–60.
11. Kidder DP, Wolitski RJ, Campsmith ML, et al. Health status, health care use, medication use, and medication adherence among homeless and housed people living with HIV/AIDS. Am J Public Health. 2007;97(12):2238–45.
12. Rice E, Barman-Adhikari A, Milburn NG, et al. Position-specific HIV risk in a large network of homeless youths. Am J Public Health. 2012;102(1):141–7.
13. Shaw GM, Hunter E. HIV transmission. Cold Spring Harb Perspect Med. 2012;2:a006965.
14. Centers for Disease Control and Prevention. Updated guidelines for antiretroviral postexposure prophylaxis after sexual, injection drug use, or other nonoccupational exposure to HIV – United States, 2016. Table 1 (Page 25).
15. Centers for Disease Control and Prevention. Revised Recommendations for HIV Testing of Adults. Adolescents, and pregnant women in health-care settings. MMWR. 2006;55(No. RR-14):1–13.
16. Moyer VA, on behalf of the U.S. Preventive Services Task Force. Screening for HIV: U.S. preventive services task force recommendation statement. Ann Intern Med. 2013;159:51–60.
17. DiNenno EA, Prejean J, Delaney KP, et al. Evaluating the evidence for more frequent than annual HIV screening of gay, bisexual, and other men who have sex with men in the United States: results from a systematic review and CDC expert consultation. Public Health Rep. 2018;133(1):3–21.
18. Branson BM, Stekler JD. Detection of acute HIV infection: we can't close the window. J Infect Dis. 2012;205:521–4.
19. Cohen MS, Gay CL, Busch MP, Hecht FM. The detection of acute HIV infection. J Infect Dis. 2010;202(S2):S270–7.

20. Owen SM. Testing for acute HIV infection: implications for treatment as prevention. Curr Opin HIV AIDS. 2012;7:125–30.
21. Ober AJ, Martino SC, Ewing B, Tucker JS. If you provide the test, they will take it: factors associated with HIV/STI testing in a representative sample of homeless youth in Los Angeles. AIDS Educ Prev. 2012;24(4):350–62.
22. Trent-Adams S. Charting the course to end HIV transmission in the United States. Public Health Rep. 2017;132(6):603–5.
23. Cohen MS, Chen YQ, McCauley M, et al. Antiretroviral therapy for the prevention of HIV-1 transmission. N Engl J Med. 2016;375(9):830–9.
24. Rodger AJ, Cambiano V, Bruun T, et al. Sexual activity without condoms and risk of HIV transmission in serodifferent couples when the HIV-positive partner is using suppressive antiretroviral therapy. JAMA. 2016;316(2):171–81.
25. U = U taking off in 2017. Lancet. 2017;4:e475.
26. Centers for Disease Control and Prevention. Dear Colleague. September 27, 2017. Available at https://www.cdc.gov/hiv/library/dcl/dcl/092717.html. Published 2017. Accessed 26 Aug 2018.
27. Centers for Disease Control and Prevention, Department of Health & Human Services. Preexposure prophylaxis for the prevention of HIV infection in the United States – 2017 update. A clinical practice guideline. Available online at https://www.cdc.gov/hiv/pdf/risk/prep/cdc-hiv-prep-guidelines-2017.pdf. Published 2017. Accessed 26 Aug 2018.
28. United States Food and Drug Administration. Highlights of prescribing information: Truvada. Available online at https://www.accessdata.fda.gov/drugsatfda_docs/label/2018/021752s055lbl.pdf. Published 2018. Accessed 26 Aug 2018.
29. United States Food and Drug Administration. Highlights of prescribing information: Descovy. Available online at https://www.accessdata.fda.gov/drugsatfda_docs/label/2019/208215s012lbl.pdf. Published 2019. Accessed 1 Feb 2019.
30. Centers for Disease Control and Prevention, Department of Health & Human Services. Preexposure prophylaxis for the prevention of HIV infection in the united states – 2017 update. Clinical providers' supplement. Available online at https://www.cdc.gov/hiv/pdf/risk/prep/cdc-hiv-prep-provider-supplement-2017.pdf. Published 2017. Accessed 26 Aug 2018.
31. Molina JM, Charreau I, Spire B, et al. Efficacy, safety, and effect on sexual behaviour of on-demand pre-exposure prophylaxis for HIV in men who have sex with men: an observational cohort study. Lancet HIV. 2017;4:e402–10.
32. Glidden DV, Anderson PL, Grant RM. Pharmacology supports "on-demand" PrEP. Lancet HIV. 2016;3(9):e405–6.
33. Seifert GM, Glidden DV, Meditz AL, et al. Dose response for starting and stopping HIV pre-exposure prophylaxis for men who have sex with men. Clin Infect Dis. 2015;60:804–10.
34. National Network of STD/HIV Prevention Training Centers Curriculum Committee. Behavioral counseling for STD/HIV risk-reduction. Available online at http://nnptc.org/wp-content/uploads/Behavioral-Counseling-Risk-Reduction-Curriculum-Module-2011.pdf. Published 2011. Accessed 31 Jan 2017.
35. Project Inform and Please PrEP Me. Helping people access pre-exposure prophylaxis. A front-line provider manual on PrEP research, care and navigation. Available online at https://www.projectinform.org/wp-content/uploads/2018/06/PPM-PrEP-Manual-Eng.pdf. Published 2018. Accessed 26 Aug 2018.
36. Wilson DP. HIV treatment as prevention: natural experiments highlight limits of antiretroviral treatment as HIV prevention. PLoS Med. 2012;9(7):e1001231.
37. Levy ME, Wilton L, Phillips G. Understanding structural barriers to accessing HIV testing and prevention services among black men who have sex with men (BMSM) in the United States. AIDS Behav. 2014;18:972–96.
38. Liu J, Jones C, Wilson K. Motivational barriers to retention of at-risk young adults in HIV-prevention interventions: perceived pressure and efficacy. AIDS Care. 2014;26(10):1242–8.

39. Naranbhai V, Abdool KQ, Meyer-Weitz A. Interventions to modify sexual risk behaviours for preventing HIV in homeless youth. Cochrane Database Syst Rev. 2011;1:CD007501. https://doi.org/10.1002/14651858.CD007501.pub2.
40. Logan JL, Frye A, Pursell HO, et al. Correlates of HIV risk behaviors among homeless and unstably housed young adults. Public Health Rep. 2013;128:153–60.
41. Rice E, Monro W, Barman-Adhikari A, et al. Internet use, social networking, and HIV/AIDS risk for homeless adolescents. J Adolesc Health. 2010;47:610–3.
42. Rice E. The positive role of social networks and social networking technology in the condom-using behaviors of homeless young people. Public Health Rep. 2010;125:588–95.
43. Collins J, Slesnick N. Factors associated with motivation to change HIV risk and substance use behaviors among homeless youth. J Soc Work Pract Addict. 2011;11(2):163–80.
44. AIDS.gov. A timeline of HIV/AIDS. Available online at https://www.hiv.gov/sites/default/files/aidsgov-timeline.pdf. Published 2016. Accessed 29 Aug 2018.
45. Gardner EM, McLees MP, Steiner JF, et al. The spectrum of engagement in HIV care and its relevance to test-and-treat strategies for prevention of HIV infection. Clin Infect Dis. 2011;52(6):793–800.
46. The Office of National AIDS Policy. The national HIV/AIDS strategy: updated to 2020. Available online at https://files.hiv.gov/s3fs-public/nhas-update.pdf. Published 2015. Accessed 26 Aug 2018.
47. Kay ES, Batey DS, Mugavero MJ. The HIV treatment cascade and care continuum: updates, goals, and recommendations for the future. AIDS Res Ther. 2016;13:35.
48. Centers for Disease Control and Prevention. National Center for HIV/AIDS, Viral Hepatitis, STD, and TB Prevention. Selected national HIV prevention and care outcomes. Available online at https://www.cdc.gov/hiv/pdf/library/slidesets/cdc-hiv-prevention-and-care-outcomes.pdf. Published 2017. Accessed 27 Aug 2018.
49. Hollywood Homless Youth Partnership. Available online at http://hhyp.org/. Updated 2018. Accessed 29 Aug 2018.
50. Feinberg J, Keeshin S. Management of newly diagnosed HIV infection. Ann Intern Med. 2017;167(1):ITC1–ITC16.
51. Lundgren JD, Babiker AG, Gordin F, et al. Initiation of antiretroviral therapy in early asymptomatic HIV infection. N Engl J Med. 2015;373(9):795–807.
52. Matthews LT, Smit JA, Cu-Uvin S, Cohan D. Antiretrovirals and safe contraception for HIV-serodiscordant couples. Curr Opin HIV AIDS. 2012;7(6):569–78.
53. Secretary's Advisory Committee on Health Promotion and Disease Prevention Objectives for 2020. Healthy people 2020: an opportunity to address the societal determinants of health in the United States. Available online at http://www.healthypeople.gov/2010/hp2020/advisory/SocietalDeterminantsHealth.htm. Published 2010. Accessed 30 Aug 2018.
54. Conn VS, Ruppar TM. Medication adherence outcomes of 771 intervention trials: systematic review and meta-analysis. Prev Med. 2017;99:269–76.
55. Sayegh CS, MacDonell KK, Clark LF, et al. The impact of cell phone support on psychosocial outcomes for youth living with HIV nonadherent to antiretroviral therapy. AIDS Behav. 2018; https://doi.org/10.1007/s10461-018-2192-4.
56. Webb L, Perry-Parrish C, Ellen J, Sibinga E. Mindfulness instruction for HIV-infected youth: a randomized controlled trial. AIDS Care. 2018;30(6):688–95.
57. Harris RA, Xue X, Selwyn PA. Housing stability and medication adherence among HIV-positive individuals in antiretroviral therapy: a meta-analysis of observational studies in the United States. J Acquir Immune Defic Syndr. 2017;74(3):309–17.
58. Martinez J, Chakraborty R, and the Committee on Pediatric AIDS. Psychosocial support for youth living with HIV. Pediatrics. 2014;133:558–62.

59. Health Resources and Services Administration. Ryan White HIV/AIDS program annual client-level data report 2016. Available online at http://hab.hrsa.gov/data/data-reports. Published November 2017. Accessed 28 Aug 2018.
60. Hilvers J, George CC, Bendixen AV. HIV housing helps end homelessness and HIV/AIDS in the United States. In: Write E, Carnes N, editors. Understanding the HIV/AIDS epidemic in the United States. The role of syndemics in the production of health disparities. Cham: Springer; 2016.
61. Selik RM, Mokotoff ED, Branson B, et al. Revised surveillance case definition for HIV infection – United States, 2014. MMWR. 2014;63(No. RR-3):10.
62. Simons LK, Belzer ME. Human immunodeficiency virus infections and acquired immunodeficiency syndrome. In: Neinstein LS, editor. Adolescent and young adult health care a practical guide. Philadelphia: Wolters Kluwer; 2016. p. 292.

Chapter 14
Medical Care of Youth After Acute Sexual Assault

Margaret Colbourne and Tracy Ann Pickett

Introduction

The American Academy of Pediatrics defines sexual assault as "any nonconsensual sexual act", which may include both non-voluntary sexual contact and sexual interactions that occur when a victim is unable to consent due to age, cognitive challenges or substance use [1]. Sexual assault need not involve physical injury, but due to the use of intimidation, fear and violation of trust, it almost always involves significant psychological trauma.

Sexual assault and intimate partner violence are relatively common in the adolescent population, whether disclosed or not. The US national data indicate that adolescents ages 12–17 years have the highest rates of being sexually assaulted of any age group [2]. This is particularly true for youth who have left traditional family situations and are living on the street or "couch-surfing" with friends or acquaintances. Homeless, runaway and transgender youth are at particular risk for commercial sexual exploitation [3]. Numerous factors may contribute to youth not initially disclosing sexual assault, including the fact that the assailant may be well known to the youth, even a related family member; the youth may be struggling with issues of gender identity and may feel that this somehow contributed to the events; and knowledge that they may face threat of future harm or repercussions if a forensic assessment is completed.

M. Colbourne (✉)
Department of Paediatrics, University of British Columbia, Vancouver, BC, Canada
e-mail: mcolbourne@cw.bc.ca

T. A. Pickett
Department of Emergency Medicine, University of British Columbia, Vancouver, BC, Canada
e-mail: Tracy.Pickett@cw.bc.ca

C. Warf, G. Charles (eds.), *Clinical Care for Homeless, Runaway and Refugee Youth*, https://doi.org/10.1007/978-3-030-40675-2_14

Consent and the Introduction to the Assessment

Healthcare providers (HCP) should remember that the medical care of youth following acute sexual assault must take priority over the forensic assessment. Patients must be fully informed of all aspects of the medical assessment, as well as details and the purpose of any forensic evidence collection. Although medical assessment and forensic evaluation may occur concurrently, it is important to emphasize that both examinations serve different roles. Obtaining separate consent for examination, treatment and forensic evidence collection can be the first step in healing as the HCP is returning some of the power/choice back to a person who has had this taken from them. Youth should be permitted the presence of a support person for part, or all, of the exam if desired; however, for homeless or runaway youth that may be victims of commercial sexual exploitation, beware of "handlers" who may present as friends or partners, whose purpose is to intimidate and limit any patient disclosure of the assault. If at all possible, the offer of whether to have a friend or support person present for the assessment should occur during a private conversation between the examiner and the youth.

Management begins with introductions and a brief explanation of the purposes of the emergency assessment; that is to address any physical or psychological trauma the youth may have sustained, management of any potential medical concerns such as pregnancy and infections, as well as to ensure wellness following discharge with respect to medical complications and mental health issues.

The HCP should also be aware of the current reporting requirements related to sexual assault within their jurisdiction and should inform the youth of this duty at the outset. The concept of the forensic assessment as a vehicle to document and provide evidence for criminal prosecution should be offered; however, this should be considered a secondary goal, and the youth may require some time to consider the ramifications of consent for this process. It is very important that the youth understands they will get appropriate medical care, even if they should choose not to undergo a forensic evaluation. Some jurisdictions will have Forensic Nurse Examiners (FNEs), Sexual Assault Nurse Examiners (SANEs), Sexual Assault Response Teams (SARTs) or forensically trained physicians to provide forensic assessments. Early involvement of these teams may facilitate appropriate documentation and collection of specimens as well as communication with the necessary forensic investigators such as child welfare social workers and police.

It is important early in the assessment to understand what specifically the youth may be most concerned about, as this may not be initially obvious. This may range from concerns for pregnancy, future sexual activities, infection, concurrent substance use, threat of future violence by the perpetrator, family response/dysfunction following disclosure, knowledge of the event by the youth's parent/family/friends and potential social media repercussions. While the youth may not fully share all their concerns when initially asked, it is important to return to these issues at various points throughout the assessment and explore the patient's thoughts on how they see things unfolding.

For refugee youth, acknowledging and sharing the details of sexual assault may be particularly difficult due to cultural differences and taboos often associated with sexual activity. If an interpreter is required, it is important to ensure that they are professionally trained and not known to the patient in any other capacity. The gender of the interpreter may be a factor in ensuring the youth's comfort or confidence with the assessment process. Refugee youth may be reluctant to report sexual assault due to prior negative experiences with the criminal justice system, fear of deportation or separation and/or concerns regarding repercussions from family.

History

Acknowledge that both the history and the examination processes take time and that the patient may wish to stop or rest when desired. Questioning patients about an assault history can be challenging. Maintain a calm, non-judgemental and reassuring manner throughout. Patients often feel shame or guilt about the circumstances of the assault and have typically never before recounted such details. Ask simple, open-ended questions, inviting the patient to begin the story of what happened where they feel it is appropriate. Information should be gathered about who the assailant was, where and when the assault occurred, what happened during the course of the assault and what events have occurred since the assault. The HCP may need to clarify specific details about concurrent physical assault to other non-genital body parts and the nature of the sexual abuse (actual or attempted oral, vaginal or anal penetration, use of foreign objects, ejaculation or use of condom). The history is meant to guide the subsequent examination and treatment.

Inquire as to past medical and social history with use of the H.E.A.D.S.S. assessment (home, education/employment, activities, drugs, sexuality, suicide/depression) to guide content. Consider that youth may be victims of human trafficking, which may require more direct questioning of their concerns for safety and support [4]. Some questions which may be helpful when there are suspicions of commercial sexual exploitation are listed in Table 14.1.

Table 14.1 Questions to consider when suspecting commercial sexual exploitation

Home/work:
Are you able to come and go freely from home/work? Have you ever run away from home/work? Has anyone at home/work ever physically hurt or threatened to hurt you or your family?
Family/friends:
Has anyone ever forced you to do things you do not want to do? Has anyone ever taken your identification or cell phone? Have you or the family/friends you live with ever been involved with law enforcement?

Physical Examination

Ideally the physical examination is performed concurrently with the forensic evaluation, provided the patient has consented to both. Examination should involve a complete head-to-toe assessment even if the patient has not indicated concern for non-genital physical injury. Attend to any areas of active bleeding as needed. Be alert to signs of occult intracranial or intra-abdominal injury. Use appropriate draping throughout to minimize exposure at any one time. Reassure the patient that a speculum examination may not be necessary. Documentation should include the following:

- Vital signs, general appearance and level of alertness
- Skin:
  - Examine all areas carefully for bruising, abrasion, lacerations, bite marks, burns or scars
  - Record all areas of tenderness even if no obvious sign of bruising
  - Document any tattoos or other skin markings, as these may indicate involvement in trafficking or commercial sexual exploitation
- Head and neck:
  - Evidence of hair loss to the scalp
  - Oral injury
  - Strangulation marks/petechiae to face/neck/behind ears
- Trunk:
  - Injury to the breasts
  - Abdominal tenderness or distension
- Extremities:
  - Particular attention to the upper arms and thighs
  - Hands and fingernails
- Genitalia and anus:
  - Injury to the labia, posterior fourchette or hymen
  - Injury to the penis, foreskin or scrotum
  - Injury to the anus/rectum

Standardized body diagrams are helpful for documentation purposes, but all injuries should be described clearly in the medical record as well. In some areas, photo-documentation of injuries is performed routinely; however, patients must clearly consent to this prior to examination as photographs may be used later in court proceedings. If obtained, all photographs should include documentation with a standardized forensic measurement tool and colour-bar code.

Forensic Evaluation

In general, forensic evidence collection is recommended if the assault has occurred in the past 72 hours; however, many jurisdictions extend the potential window 7–10 days after the event. The forensic aspects of an evaluation are those elements that pertain to the criminal investigation and, as sexual assault laws may vary between jurisdictions, forensic evaluations and the kits provided for evidence collection may also vary to some degree. Any evidence collected must follow clearly documented chain of custody and storage requirements. Once specimens are released to the police, neither the HCP nor the patients have any control over their processing. The HCP should be aware of, and familiar with, the kit available in their area.

Not all parts of the sexual assault kit may need to be collected in all cases, and in some areas, prepackaged kits may not be available. Forensic specimens may still be collected with attention to a few specific areas outlined in Table 14.2. If collected, all specimens should be labelled with the correct patient information, speci-

Table 14.2 Forensic evidence collection

Clothing:
1. Pants and underwear – remove in unison, package together so as not to dislodge evidence 2. If other clothing articles are collected, bag separately (non-waxed paper bag)
Swabs for perpetrator evidence:
1. Areas of possible sperm/semen contamination generally include the perineum, posterior vaginal pool, rectum or oropharynx. History should guide swab collection, as other areas (face, abdomen, umbilicus or back) may contain forensic evidence 2. Swabs for salivary secretions from "hickey" or bite marks should be processed with the "double swab" technique: swab suspicious area with sterile water-moistened swab and then again with dry swab; label and package separately (use dry, sterile swab, preferably with breathable membrane sleeve to permit air-drying) 3. Tampon or sanitary pad: place in sterile urine container with air-permeable lid, or in breathable envelope or paper bag, and stored in freezer
Swab for patient's DNA profile:
Single buccal swab
Pubic hair combings:
Collect on sterile gauze and place, along with comb, in labelled envelope
Fingernail clippings/scrapings/swabs:
Generally only helpful in stranger assaults. If clippings/scrapings are not possible, obtain wet swabs from finger tips (1 swab per hand)
Toxicology/drug screen
1. Urine (if DFSA suspected): first available void post SA, if possible. Urine should be frozen if not immediately processed 2. Blood if quantitative sample required – grey-top Vacutainer, label with date and time collected. Blood should be frozen if not immediately processed

If immediately handed to police, notify them of biologic contents requiring expedient processing

men site, date/time of collection and initials of who collected the sample, and packaged in a separate envelope within a clearly labelled kit (box or envelope). All forensic swabs should have a mechanism to be air-dried (i.e. using breathable membranous swab) prior to packaging in separate envelopes. An ultraviolet light source (wavelength 430–500 nm) may assist site selection for swab collection but has variable success [5]. The traditional Wood's lamp (360 nm), present in many emergency departments, is inadequate for forensic evaluation of sexual assault. Clothing, particularly underclothes, may also need to be collected in non-waxed paper bags.

Once collected, all forensic evidence should be placed in a large brown forensic envelope or collection kit, sealed, labelled and either given to police investigators or immediately securely stored, depending upon patient request and services available in your region. Biologic samples (urine and/or blood for toxicology), if collected, will need expedient processing or freezing to limit sample degradation. If police are not immediately available, the evidence kit must be stored in a secure cupboard until they are able to accept custody. Proper chain of custody procedures must be followed to ensure documentation of an unbroken chain of evidence.

Laboratory Investigations

Laboratory investigations are rarely needed for the acute medical management of a sexual assault patient, with the rationale being to try and limit further trauma to the patient. A urine pregnancy test is important prior to giving emergency contraception.

Routine baseline HIV testing has limited value; however, it should be offered if desired. Blood work for HIV status, hepatitis B, syphilis, complete blood count (CBC), electrolytes, BUN and creatinine are recommended if initiating HIV post-exposure prophylaxis (PEP).

Some laboratory investigations are typically performed within hospitals, rather than the forensic labs. If drug-facilitated sexual assault (DFSA) is suspected, the first urine produced post assault it most ideal for qualitative toxicological analysis. Blood is generally most useful for quantitative analysis (grey-top Vacutainer). Many of the drugs used in DFSA are not included in the routine drug-screening panels and must be specifically requested.

Management

While adolescents who have been sexually assaulted may have evidence of minor physical injuries elsewhere, most will have an unremarkable anogenital examination. Following the examination, the HCP should review any abnormal findings, discuss any injuries that may require further treatment and provide the youth with some reassurance that physically they are likely to do well. Most centres are able to provide appropriate fresh clothing, as much of the youth's clothing may have been sequestered as part of the forensic evidence kit.

(A) Emergency contraception:

Emergency contraception should be offered to all female youth if there is risk of pregnancy and the assault has occurred within the previous week. If pharmacologic prophylaxis is provided, consider antiemetics to mitigate associated nausea and vomiting.

(B) Sexually transmitted infection (STI) prophylaxis:

Routine testing for chlamydia, gonorrhoea and trichomonas is not required as STI treatment is recommended as part of the emergency assessment [6].

Tetanus and hepatitis B vaccination should be provided if needed. HPV vaccination is also now recommended in both male and female patients if not previously received [6].

HIV post-exposure prophylaxis (PEP):

Some issues faced by vulnerable or homeless youth may put them at higher risk of HIV exposure. HIV transmission following a single sexual assault, while very unlikely, is possible; thus, PEP should be considered and recommended as per the Center for Disease Control (CDC) guidelines [6]. If considering PEP, it should be initiated within 72 hours of sexual assault and continued for 28 days.

Mental Health

Throughout the assessment, the HCP will be evaluating for concerns of emotional trauma. Once the physical examination is complete, it is very important that the HCP once again explore any potential negative emotional feelings that the youth may be experiencing. Thoughts of self-blame, anxiety, depression, suicidal ideation and self-harm should be addressed. A more formal psychiatric assessment may be indicated. Some centres may have access to trained social workers or sexual assault counsellors who can initiate crisis counselling at first presentation within the emergency department or clinic.

The HCP should explore what the youth will face following discharge from the hospital environment and whom they specifically identify as members of their support network. Inquire as to with whom, and how, the youth intends to share knowledge of the assault. If any supporters are present in the emergency department and the youth wishes to share information with them, offer to assist them with this process. Some youth may identify a community social worker or other resource that has been helpful to them in the past and may prove useful for ongoing support.

A note for respite from school or work ("for medical reasons" and not detailing the assault) is often appreciated and may provide the patient the opportunity to process the emotional sequelae of the assault.

Follow-Up Care and Support

All victims of sexual assault should be provided options for follow-up care; however, it is well known that adolescents are among the least reliable at attending follow-up clinic appointments. Review the reasons for reassessment, and explore the barriers that might be present to attendance at future appointments. Unfortunately many youth do not have a regular HCP, and if they do, they may be reluctant to follow-up there due to concerns for confidentiality from other family members. Many centres have community clinics, youth health clinics or specialty medical teams that provide follow-up medical care and counselling services for youth who have been victims of sexual assault. Proximity of the follow-up clinic to the youth's community may facilitate successful follow-up attendance.

Follow-up typically occurs 1–2 weeks following the initial presentation but should be sooner in the rare instance where HIV-PEP is provided. The goals of this assessment include the following:

1. Document healing of any physical injuries.
2. Assessment of adequacy of pregnancy and STI prophylaxis.
3. Arrange remainder of HIV-PEP, if initiated.
4. Review the recommended STI blood tests according to CDC guidelines:
   (a) Syphilis and HIV tests at 4–6 weeks and 3 months.
5. Schedule for completion of hepatitis B and HPV immunizations, if needed.
6. Mental health assessment and counselling services should be strongly encouraged as victims of sexual assault are at high risk of subsequent emotional distress and post-traumatic stress disorder.

References

1. Crawford-Jakubiak JE, et al. Committee on Child Abuse and Neglect, Committee on Adolescence, American Academy of Pediatrics. Care of the adolescent after an acute sexual assault. Pediatrics. 2017;139(3):e20164243. Available at: http://pediatrics.aappublications.org/content/139/3/e20164243. Accessed 28 Aug 2018.
2. Planty M, Langton L, Krebs C, et al. Female victims of sexual violence, 1994-2010. Washington, DC: US Department of Justice, Office of Justice Programs, Bureau of Justice Statistics; 2013. Available at: www.bjs.gov/content/pub/pdf/fvsv9410.pdf. Accessed 28 Aug 2018.
3. Hampton MD, Lieggi M. Commercial sexual exploitation of youth in the US: a qualitative systematic review. Trauma Violence Abuse. 2020;21:57–70. https://doi.org/10.1177/1524838017742168.
4. Becker HJ, Bechtel K. Recognizing victims of human trafficking in the pediatric emergency department. Pediatr Emerg Care. 2015;31(2):144–50.
5. Mackenzie B, Jenny C. The use of alternative light sources in the clinical evaluation of child abuse and sexual assault. Pediatr Emerg Care. 2014;30:207–10.
6. Centers for Disease Control and Prevention. Sexually transmitted diseases treatment guidelines: sexual assault and abuse and STDs. 2015. Available at: www.cdc.gov/std/tg2015/sexual-assault.htm. Accessed 28 Aug 2018.

Chapter 15
Suicide Risk and Intervention Among Homeless and Precariously Housed Youth

Sara Sherer, Bridgid Mariko Conn, and Mari Radzik

A young person who dies by suicide leaves a wake of pain with family members, friends, and others dealing with the loss and often questioning what they might have been able to do or if their loved one's death could have been prevented. For youth who are homeless or have a fractured relationship with their family, there are even more limited means for support and addressing suicide risk such that providers often take on a larger role in suicide prevention for these vulnerable, marginalized, and isolated youth.

According to the World Health Organization [1], suicide is the second leading cause of death globally among 15- to 29-year-olds. In the United States (USA), suicide is one of the most concerning and preventable areas of public health concern, leading to the development of a multitude of interventions targeting the individual, family, and community level [2]. Adolescent and young adult suicide prevalence rates show that suicide is the second leading cause of death among individuals between the ages of 10 and 34. Between 2007 and 2016, suicide rates for youth between ages 10 and 19 years old rose to fifty-nine percent with greater increases for females compared to males [3]. The impact of depression and suicidal ideation becomes more deleterious when youth are homeless or precariously housed due to complex psychosocial stressors and limited supports and resources [4]. With the total homeless population in the USA being comprised of many of

S. Sherer (✉) · M. Radzik
Department of Pediatrics, Keck School of Medicine, University of Southern California, Los Angeles, CA, USA

Division of Adolescent and Young Adult Medicine, Children's Hospital Los Angeles, Los Angeles, CA, USA
e-mail: SSherer@chla.usc.edu; MRadzik@chla.usc.edu

B. M. Conn
Division of Adolescent and Young Adult Medicine, Children's Hospital Los Angeles, Los Angeles, CA, USA
e-mail: bconn@chla.usc.edu

C. Warf, G. Charles (eds.), *Clinical Care for Homeless, Runaway and Refugee Youth*, https://doi.org/10.1007/978-3-030-40675-2_15

children or families with children, recent estimates have indicated that there may be over 2.5 million homeless youth in the USA. Additionally, there are more than 3 million young adults (ages 18–25 years old) in the USA who experience homelessness each year [5]. Thus, homeless adolescents and young adults are considered a crucial, underserved group for suicide prevention and intervention initiatives.

Individuals experiencing homeless or unstable housing are more likely to have a history of adversity and mental health problems and are more likely to be exposed to adversity, stress, and high-risk situations. Significant literature has documented the link between adverse childhood experiences (ACEs); maladaptive coping, including suicidal behavior; and long-term social and medical difficulties [6, 7]. Prior research has also well-documented numerous risk factors that are associated with suicide, including a history of psychiatric disorders, particularly schizophrenia and bipolar disorder; self-harm and prior suicide attempts; personality disorders; history of family violence/abuse and/or intimate partner violence; family history of suicide; and medical conditions including chronic pain [8, 9, 10, 6, 11]. Further, comorbid substance use or abuse often further intensifies risk and decreases inhibition necessitating early and proactive intervention.

Sources of resilience and coping are developed throughout childhood and adolescence as youth learn to adjust and adapt to a range of adverse experiences. How an individual response to early childhood trauma is influenced by their own internal resiliency, as well as protective factors including supportive relationships with others. “Social capital,” or the gains felt by youth from supportive homeless or non-homeless individuals, builds resiliency across multiple domains such as increased future orientation and housing stability and decreased likelihood of victimization [12, 13]. For youth who have intact family structures, family cohesion and school and community connectedness or belongingness support the development of internal sources of resiliency, including their sense of worth and confidence. Further, academic achievement, social engagement in meaningful life activities, and cultural and spiritual/religious beliefs also function as adaptive coping strategies which increase reasons for living and support healthy management of emotional distress. In their review article, Cronley and colleagues [14] identified that homeless youth often receive support from fictive or non-related kin and may engage in activities and behaviors viewed as negative or maladaptive in order to cope with particularly adverse conditions. Another model, the Multimodal Social Ecological Model [15], encourages the use of a trauma-informed approach to understand the effects of the environment, family, and social interactions on an individual. Using multiple layers of intervention, it creates an understanding of the impact of trauma, and where to intervene, from an individual, social, environmental, and community perspective. Previous literature highlights how understanding adaptive coping and sources of resiliency remains crucial in developing appropriate resources and interventions to serve the unique needs of diverse homeless and precariously housed youth.

Suicide Among Homeless LGBTQ Youth

Sexual minority youth, or youth who identify as lesbian, gay, bisexual, transgender, or queer (LGBTQ), are disproportionately at risk for homeless compared to their heterosexual peers, largely due to familial rejection, being "kicked out" of the home, or running away from home [16]. Recent estimates indicate that past-year rates of homelessness among LGBTQ youth may be as high as 30–45% [17]. One of the major factors identified as increasing suicide risk for LGBTQ youth is having an unsupportive social environment, including family, friends, and school [18]. Many LGBTQ youth report having experienced homelessness directly related to their sexual or gender identity. Further, these LGBTQ youth experiencing homelessness are also more likely to have a past history of trauma and to be at increased risk for trauma. For instance, research has found that homeless LGBTQ youth are more likely to stay with strangers for shelter which was associated with engaging in more high-risk sexual behavior [19]. Barr et al. [20] found that such trauma experiences were linked to increased suicidal ideation and symptoms of post-traumatic stress disorder were associated with suicide attempts among these youth.

Sexual minority youth demonstrate significantly higher rates of suicidal ideation and suicide attempts. Some estimates say that LGB adolescents and adults are twice as likely to have suicidal ideation compared to heterosexual peers. Recent data estimate that rates of suicide attempts among LGB youth in the past 12 months were approximately 29.4% compared to 6.4% of their heterosexual peers [21]. Though the research is still limited, rates are estimated to be even higher for gender minority youth [22].

In identifying sources for protective support and resiliency, social and parental support and acceptance, lower experienced transphobia or homophobia, possessing personal identification reflecting gender identity, and access to medical intervention, as well as legislative and societal policies which support LGBTQ individuals, have been found to mitigate risk [23–25]. Thus, interventions that address the vulnerabilities among this community of youth are much needed. To address suicide risk and promote resilience and hope for the future, several grassroots organizations have developed to meet this need, including The Trevor Project (www.thetrevorproject.org) and the It Gets Better Project (https://itgetsbetter.org) [26].

Assessment

When addressing suicide risk, a thorough assessment of past and present suicidal thoughts, planning, and action is essential. The term "suicidal ideation" (SI) refers to thoughts of wanting to die or ending one's life. Oftentimes, providers are wary or uncomfortable with assessing suicide risk due to the concern that talking to the youth may increase their level of risk or "give them ideas." This belief is a harmful fallacy which has contributed to stigma, shame, and continued silence around suicide. If youth share that they have been experiencing SI, chances are they have been struggling with disclosing about their emotional distress and are trying to reach out for help because they do not want to act on their thoughts. Care in assessment needs to be taken, because abrupt, intrusive questions could result in a reduction of rapport and a lower likelihood of the adolescent sharing mental health concerns. This is especially true during a brief encounter for an unrelated concern. Initial questions should be open-ended and relatively nonthreatening, such as "Aside from your housing issues, how have you been doing?" "I know that a lot of people your age have a lot going on. What kinds of things have been on your mind or stressing you lately?" and "How have things been going with [school, friends, work]?"

Suicidal thoughts or comments should never be dismissed as unimportant. Assessing SI will not increase the likelihood of suicide and can only help youth to access the support they need. Statements such as "You've come really close to killing yourself" may acknowledge the deep despair of the youth and communicate to the adolescent that the provider understands how serious he or she has felt about dying or even escaping their life situation. Such disclosures should be met with reassurance that the youth's pleas for assistance have been heard and that help will be sought.

Suicidal ideation is viewed to exist on a spectrum from more passive and low-risk thoughts to chronic, intrusive high-risk thoughts. There are several dimensions that are assessed when determining where SI might fall on this continuum, including frequency, intensity, content, and perseverance, or the ability of an individual to push the thought from their mind and not have it return readily. Research indicates that the presence or absence of ideation has little predictive value by itself; rather, SI in addition to planning and preparation is more predictive of suicide attempts [27]. A thorough suicide risk assessment should include three major areas of inquiry: how often is the youth experiencing SI (i.e., several times a minute? An hour? A week?); what is the thought content focused on; and is the youth able to make the thoughts go away with effort. Figure 15.1 shows key questions that assess these three major areas of inquiry.

In the course of a suicide risk assessment, if the youth discloses having thought of a plan, it is imperative to follow-up with questions to further understand the functionality of the suicidal urge. Specifically, the provider should inquire about their

Fig. 15.1 Key questions to ask to assess frequency, content, and perseverance

How many times have you had these thoughts?

When you have these thoughts how long do they last?

Can you stop thinking about killing yourself if you want to?

Are there things you can do to stop the thoughts or wanting to die?

What sort of reasons do you have for wanting to die?

intentionality; their hoped-for aim or goal for attempting suicide, such as escape or relieving a burden for themselves or others; as well as their desire – what is the subjective expectation and is their desire for the outcome to be death. Asking whether a youth has come up with a plan for suicide is unlikely to prompt them to consider a plan and will not "give them ideas" for a suicide plan. It is important to ask about their plans as this information contributes greatly to understanding the youth's level of suicide risk.

While it may be disconcerting, providers must follow-up and inquire about the method they are planning to use to be able to determine the level of lethality and rescuability, which will indicate the likelihood that a fatal outcome could have occurred. A youth who planned to use over-the-counter pain killers at their shelter or group home during a time when someone might witness or intervene presents with a different level of risk than a youth who planned to use a noose after waiting for everyone to leave or at night when everyone is asleep. It is important to remember that past behavior is a strong predictor of future behavior. While not all youth who may have attempted once will go on to attempt again, there is evidence to suggest that having attempted suicide does significantly increase risk for future attempts [28]. Thus, asking about past history of suicidal ideation, planning, and attempts remains crucial. Figure 15.2 illustrates examples of questions that assess for past and present suicidal behavior and suicide attempts.

Finally, a thorough suicide risk assessment also considers the influence of additional risk factors and will inquire about current emotional difficulties, use of drugs and alcohol, impairment of functioning, and significant psychosocial stressors, such as academic or vocational challenges, housing disruption, and trauma.

Does the patient have a plan?

How detailed is the plan?

Do they have the means to carry it out?

Have they used this method before?

*Capability? Past history of self-harm? **not all self-harm is a suicidal gesture*

Have they acquired the means to carry out the plan?

Have they started preparations?

What did person expect would be consquence of behaviour?

Have you ever made preparations to kill yourself?

Have you made a suicide attempt? what did you do?

Did you want to die (even slightly) when you did it?

Have you ever tried to kill yourself but been interrupted?

Have you ever started to kill yourself but stopped or been stopped?

Fig. 15.2 Questions to assess present and past suicidal behaviour and suicide attempts

Measurement Tools

Self-administered scales can be useful for screening because adolescents may disclose information about suicidality on self-report that they deny in person. Scales, however, tend to be oversensitive and under-specific and lack predictive value. Adolescents who endorse suicidality on a scale should always be assessed clinically. Screening tools useable in primary care settings have not been shown to have more than limited ability to detect suicide risk in adolescents.

Depression screening instruments shown to be valid in adolescents include the Patient Health Questionnaire (PHQ-9 and PHQ-2) ([29]; https://www.ncbi.nlm.nih.gov/pmc/articles/PMC1495268/). Other recommended assessment screeners include the Suicidal Ideation Questionnaire ([30]; https://www.parinc.com/Products/Pkey/413), Suicide Behaviors Questionnaire – Revised (http://www.integration.samhsa.gov/images/res/SBQ.pdf), University of Texas Health Care Center's Evaluation of Suicide Risk for Clinicians (http://www.cqaimh.org/pdf/tool_suicide_risklevl.pdf), and Columbia Suicide Severity Rating Scale (http://www.integration.samhsa.gov/clinical-practice/Columbia_Suicide_Severity_Rating_Scale.pdf).

Management/Interventions

Working with a suicidal adolescent can be very difficult for those who are providing treatment. Suicide risk can only be reduced, not eliminated, and risk factors provide no more than guidance. Cumulative risk is not a sufficient determinant of severity or intent for suicide; rather, it is important to consider the balance of factors that might increase suicide risk and those that may protect against it. In addition, adolescents may have their own "agendas" or goals in the discussion which may influence the content and level of self-disclosure regarding suicide. Thus, all providers need to be attuned to their own personal reactions to these disclosures to prevent any interference or bias in evaluation and intervention, including overreaction or underreaction. While there is no prescriptive approach to suicide management, strategies will be provided to guide the development of comprehensive, tailored safety plans and interventions.

Levels of Suicide Intervention

Immediate

Based on the risk assessment, a provider may conclude that hospitalization is necessary to maintain a client's safety as they are unable or unwilling to develop a safety plan, adhere to their safety plan, or feel incapable of keeping themselves safe. There are a number of considerations when recommending hospitalization as the next step in care. The first consideration will be whether the client agrees to be hospitalized voluntarily. In cases whether clients refuse hospitalization and safety is assessed to be in imminent risk, the provider will need to follow-up with connecting psychiatric emergency teams or local law enforcement for assistance in transporting and admitting clients for evaluation and observation according to state laws.

Other considerations for hospitalization include the following: specific plan with high lethality and intent, presence of psychosis or a major psychiatric disorder, past attempts (especially if they were medically serious), medical condition, limited family and/or social support including lack of stable living situation, limited and/or inadequate clinician-patient relationship, and limited access to timely outpatient follow-up.

Planning for discharge from hospitalization is crucial, particularly in terms of communication between the hospital team and any providers or family members who will support the client post-discharge. Discharge planning works best when it is collaborative, takes into account the strengths and limitations of the client and their support network, and accurately reflects the client's clinical needs. Fostering a supportive, sustained environment following discharge can help a client to transition more successfully back into their day-to-day life.

Short Term

The goals of safety planning ideally focus on addressing risk factors, decreasing vulnerabilities, and increasing protective factors. Safety plans are developed collaboratively and revisited often to ensure that they remain reflective of clients' current needs and resources. Frequently safety plans will include warning signs or "red flags" which could indicate greater risk for suicide, such as noticing more suicidal thoughts, isolating or withdrawing from others, or losing motivation. They will also include a list of crisis survival skills (e.g., distracting, writing, drawing) or preferred coping skills to use when in feeling more suicidal. Several evidence-based interventions focus on the utilization of safety planning to reduce risk of suicide and address key capacities of emotion regulation and distress tolerance. For example, in Seeking Safety, Lisa Najavits [31] focuses on the use of grounding and self-soothing techniques to address symptoms of trauma and reduce maladaptive coping (i.e., substance use). Marsha Linehan's cognitive behavioral intervention, originally developed for individuals with borderline personality disorder, also incorporates these types of coping strategies focused on reducing self-injurious or suicidal behavior and increasing internal coping resources [32].

Safety plans may also include additional strategies to reinforce behavioral activation, such as activity scheduling and making appointments to see therapists, friends, or other supports in the future. Increasing levels of activity has been shown to significantly impact feelings of depression and provide much needed structure for a young person's life during an emotional crisis [33]. Previous literature has identified the beneficial approach to address both feelings of perceived burdensomeness and impeded sense of belongingness, as well as increasing sources of support (e.g., [2]). Such interpersonal interventions aim to help individuals increase their sense of purpose and reasons for living. Identifying sources of support is always essential for any thorough safety plan, which should incorporate a survey of potential resources, from family and friends to religious institutions and national organizations. Further, including reasons to live can also serve as a visual reminder of their goals and values, as well as the potential impact that their loss will bring. Finally, each plan must also consider reasonable steps for follow-up in order to provide continuity of care and ensure linkage to appropriate services. Clinicians should check-in with the client and any significant others involved to determine their capacity for and commitment to following the safety plan. Psychoeducation regarding managing risk and supporting a young person through their emotional distress can also help to build a more sustainable support system.

Continued Intervention

Following a hospitalization or crisis, clinicians can help clients to follow up with appointments and follow-through on discharge recommendations. It is imperative that following a period of suicidal ideation or urges clinicians continue to monitor and assess for risk as well as continue to adjust safety plans based on clients' needs, presentations, and available resources. Therapeutic work can also focus on eliciting hope and supporting clients in future-oriented planning.

Research indicates that past or current suicidal ideation or suicide attempts are a significant predictor of future ideation or attempts [28]; thus, clinicians should continue to check-in with clients and help clients develop the critical skills necessary to cope with such thoughts and feelings in the future. Finally, it is important to consider program or agency-wide trainings on suicide assessment and intervention in order to prepare all staff for potential contact with youth experiencing suicidal ideation. Concepts and tools grounded in the postvention literature may be particularly helpful. Postvention refers to intervention conducted with survivors, schools, or communities once a suicide has occurred, which includes staff and providers. Postvention includes providing structure for understanding the death and alleviating some of the guilt and isolation experienced by survivors, minimizing the scapegoating that can affect survivors, and reducing the likelihood of imitation or "contagion" within a community such as schools, clinics, or shelters. Postvention also serves as a preventative intervention to mitigate risk of suicide for those impacted.

Appendix

https://www.cdc.gov/mmwr/preview/mmwrhtml/00031525.htm

http://www.suicidology.org/ncpys youth site

https://afsp.org/about-suicide/suicide-statistics/

http://www.suicidology.org/Portals/14/docs/NSPW/WS%20Press%20Release%20Final.pdf

https://www.eachmindmatters.org/SPW2018/

http://homelesshub.ca/blog/infographic-adverse-childhood-experiences-and-adult-homelessness

https://www.ncbi.nlm.nih.gov/pubmed/15261471

http://hhyp.org/wp-content/uploads/2012/02/A-guide-to-suicide-assessment-and-prevention.pdf

https://www.nn4youth.org/

References

1. World Health Organization (2016) Suicide. http://www.who.int/mediacentre/factsheets/fs398/en/
2. Buchman-Schmitt JM, Chiurliza B, Chu C, Michaels MS, Joiner TE. Suicidality in adolescent populations: a review of the extant literature through the lens of the interpersonal theory of suicide. Int J Behav Consult Therapy. 2014;9(3):26–34.
3. Shain B, Committee on Adolescence. Suicide and suicide attempts in adolescents. Pediatrics. 2016;138(1, PII: e20161420.) https://doi.org/10.1542/peds.2016-142.
4. Barnes AJ, Gilbertson J, Chatterjee D. Emotional health among youth experiencing family homelessness. Pediatrics. 2018;141(4):e20171767. https://doi.org/10.1542/peds.2017-1767.
5. Morton MH, Dworsky A, Samuels GM. Missed opportunities: youth homelessness in America. National estimates. Chicago, IL: Chapin Hall at the University of Chicago; 2017.. Accessed on 1 Nov 2018 at: http://voicesofyouthcount.org/wp-content/uploads/2017/11/VoYC-National-Estimates-Brief-Chapin-Hall-2017.pdf.
6. Hadland SE, Wood E, Dong H, Marshall BD, Kerr T, Montaner JS, DeBeck K. Suicide attempts and childhood maltreatment among street youth: a prospective cohort study. Pediatrics. 2015;136(3):440–9. https://doi.org/10.1542/peds.2015-1108.
7. Rebbe R, Nurius PS, Ahrens KR, Courtney ME. Adverse childhood experiences among youth aging out of foster care: a latent class analysis. Child Youth Serv Rev. 2017;74:108–16. https://doi.org/10.1016/j.childyouth.2017.02.004.
8. Brent DA. Risk factors for adolescent suicide and suicidal behavior: mental and substance abuse disorders, family environmental factors, and life stress. Suicide Life Threat Behav. 1995;25(Supplement):52–63.
9. Davies BR, Allen NB. Trauma and homelessness in youth: psychopathology and intervention. Clin Psychol Rev. 2017;54:17–28. https://doi.org/10.1016/j.cpr.2017.03.005.
10. Dong M, Anda RF, Felitti VJ, Dube SR, Williamson DF, Thompson TJ, et al. The interrelatedness of multiple forms of childhood abuse, neglect, and household dysfunction. Child Abuse Negl. 2004;28(7):771–84.
11. Kidd SA. Factors precipitating suicidality among homeless youth: a qualitative follow-up. Youth Soc. 2006;37(4):393–422. https://doi.org/10.1177/0044118X05282763.
12. Barman-Adhikari A, Bowen E, Bender K, Brown S, Rice E. A social capital approach to identifying correlates of perceived social support among homeless youth. Child Youth Care Forum. 2016;45(5):691–708. https://doi.org/10.1007/s10566-016-9352-3.
13. Wright ER, Attell BK, Ruel E. Social support networks and the mental health of runaway and homeless youth. Soc Sci. 2017;6(4):117. https://doi.org/10.3390/socsci6040117.
14. Cronley C, Evans R. Studies of resilience among youth experiencing homelessness: a systematic review. J Human Behav Soc Environ. 2017;27(4):291–310. https://doi.org/10.1080/10911359.2017.1282912.

15. Hopper EK. The Multimodal Social Ecological (MSE) Approach: a trauma-informed framework for supporting trafficking survivors' psychosocial health. In: Chisolm-Straker M, Stoklosa H, editors. Human trafficking is a public health issue: a paradigm expansion in the United States. Cham: Springer; 2017. p. 153–83.
16. Rhoades H, Rusow JA, Bond D, Lantelgne A, Fulginiti A, Goldbach JT. Homelessness, mental health and suicidality among LGBTQ youth accessing crisis services. Child Psychiatry Hum Dev. 2018;49(4):643–51. https://doi.org/10.1007/s10578-018-0780-1.
17. Rice E, Fulginiti A, Winetrobe H, Montoya J, Plant A, Kordic T. Sexuality and homelessness in Los Angeles public schools. Am J Public Health. 2012;102(2):200a–3201. https://doi.org/10.2105/AJPH.2011.300411.
18. Haas AP, Eliason M, Mays VM, Mathy RM, Cochran SD, D'Augelli AR, et al. Suicide and suicide risk in lesbian, gay, bisexual, and transgender populations: review and recommendations. J Homosex. 2011;58(1):10–51. https://doi.org/10.1080/00918369.2011.534038.
19. Rice E, Barman-Adhikari A, Rhoades H, Winetrobe H, Fulginiti A, Astor R, et al. Homelessness experiences, sexual orientation, and sexual risk taking among high school students in Los Angeles. J Adolesc Health. 2013;52(6):773–8. https://doi.org/10.1016/j.jadohealth.2012.11.011.
20. Barr N, Fulginiti A, Rhoades H, Rice E. Can better emotion regulation protect against suicidality in traumatized homeless youth? Arch Suicide Res. 2017;21(3):490–501. https://doi.org/10.1080/13811118.2016.1224989.
21. Hill RM, Rooney EE, Mooney MA, Kaplow JB. Links between social support, thwarted belongingness, and suicide ideation among lesbian, gay, and bisexual college students. J Fam Strengths. 2017;17(2):1–23.. Accessed on 25 Sept 2018 at: http://digitalcommons.library.tmc.edu/jfs/vol17/iss2/6.
22. Goldblum P, Testa RJ, Pflum S, Hendricks ML, Bradford J, Bongar B. The relationship between gender-based victimization and suicide attempts in transgender people. Prof Psychol Res Pract. 2012;43(5):468–75. https://doi.org/10.1037/a0029605.
23. O'Brien KHM, Putney JM, Hebert NW, Falk AM, Aguinaldo LD. Sexual and gender minority youth suicide: understanding subgroup differences to inform interventions. LBGT Health. 2016;3(4):248–51. https://doi.org/10.1089/lgbt.2016.0031.
24. Raifman J, Moscoe E, Austin SB, McConnell M. Difference-in-differences analysis of the association between state same-sex marriage policies and adolescent suicide attempts. JAMA Pediatr. 2017;171(4):350–6. https://doi.org/10.1001/jamapediatrics.2016.4529.
25. Russell ST, Pollitt AM, Li G, Grossman AH. Chosen name use is linked to reduced depressive symptoms, suicidal ideation, and suicidal behavior among transgender youth. J Adolesc Health. 2018;63:503–5. https://doi.org/10.1016/j.jadohealth.2018.02.003.. Available online 30 Mar 2018.
26. Anand P. Mental health as an advocacy priority in the lesbian, gay, bisexual, and transgender communities. J Psychiatr Pract. 2014;20(3):225–7. https://doi.org/10.1097/01.pra.0000450322.06612.a1.
27. Klonsky ED, May AM. The three-step theory (3ST): a new theory of suicide rooted in the 'Ideation-to-Action' framework. Int J Cogn Ther. 2015;8(2):114–29. https://doi.org/10.1521/ijct.2015.8.2.114.
28. Horwitz AG, Czyz EK, King CA. Predicting future suicide attempts among adolescent and emerging adult psychiatric emergency patients. J Clin Child Adolesc Psychol. 2015;44(5):751–61. https://doi.org/10.1080/15374416.2014.910789.
29. Kroenke K, Spitzer RL, Williams JB. The PHQ-9: validity of a brief depression severity measure. J Gen Intern Med. 2001;16(9):606–13. https://doi.org/10.1046/j.1525-1497.2001.016009606.x.
30. Reynolds WM. Suicidal Ideation Questionnaire (SIQ). Odessa, FL: Psychological Assessment Resources. 1987.
31. Najavits LM, Gallop RJ, Weiss RD. Seeking safety therapy for adolescent girls with PTSD and substance use disorder: a randomized controlled trial. J Behav Health Sci Res. 2006;33(4):453–63. https://doi.org/10.1007/s11414-006-9034-2.

32. Linehan MM, Comtois KA, Murray AM, Brown MZ, Gallop RJ, Heard HL, Lindenboim N. Two-year randomized controlled trial and follow-up of dialectical behavior therapy vs therapy by experts for suicidal behaviors and Borderline Personality Disorder. Arch Gen Psychiatry. 2006;63(7):757–66. https://doi.org/10.1001/archpsyc.63.7.757.
33. Ritschel LA, Ramirez CL, Jones M, Craighead WE. Behavioral activation for depressed teens: results of a pilot study. Cogn Behav Pract. 2011;18(2):281–99. https://doi.org/10.1016/j.cbpra.2010.07.002.

Chapter 16
Common Dermatology Problems Among Youth Experiencing Homelessness

Saud A. Alobaida and Wingfield E. Rehmus

Common Skin Conditions

Common skin conditions are seen in homeless just as they are in the community at large, but presentations may be more severe and treatment may be more difficult than in other cohorts due to challenges with routine skin care as well as decreased access to medical care [1]. The five most common skin conditions are acne, eczema, seborrheic dermatitis, skin cancer, and psoriasis. Fortunately, skin cancer is rare in teens, but the other conditions are very common in this age group.

Atopic Dermatitis (Eczema)

Background Atopic dermatitis (AD) is a common, chronic skin problem caused by deficits in the skin barrier and an inflammatory response to irritants, allergens, and infections on the skin. AD runs in families and in individuals alongside other "atopic" diseases such as environmental allergies, food allergies, and asthma.

Presentation Atopic dermatitis in adolescence is usually characterized by poorly defined erythematous and scaly plaques (Fig. 16.1). These may develop lichenification (Fig. 16.2) or erosions. The most common locations are the folds of the elbows, behind the knees, the hands, and the neck. Some teens have widespread involvement with very dry skin. AD is very itchy and can cause sleep disturbance as well as increase the risk of skin infections (Fig. 16.3).

S. A. Alobaida · W. E. Rehmus (✉)
Departments of Pediatrics and Dermatology, University of British Columbia, Vancouver, BC, Canada
e-mail: WRehmus@cw.bc.ca

C. Warf, G. Charles (eds.), *Clinical Care for Homeless, Runaway and Refugee Youth*, https://doi.org/10.1007/978-3-030-40675-2_16

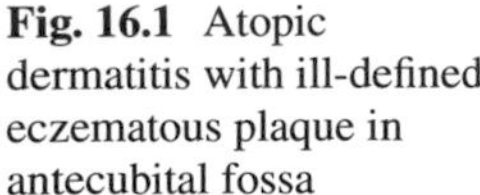

Fig. 16.1 Atopic dermatitis with ill-defined eczematous plaque in antecubital fossa

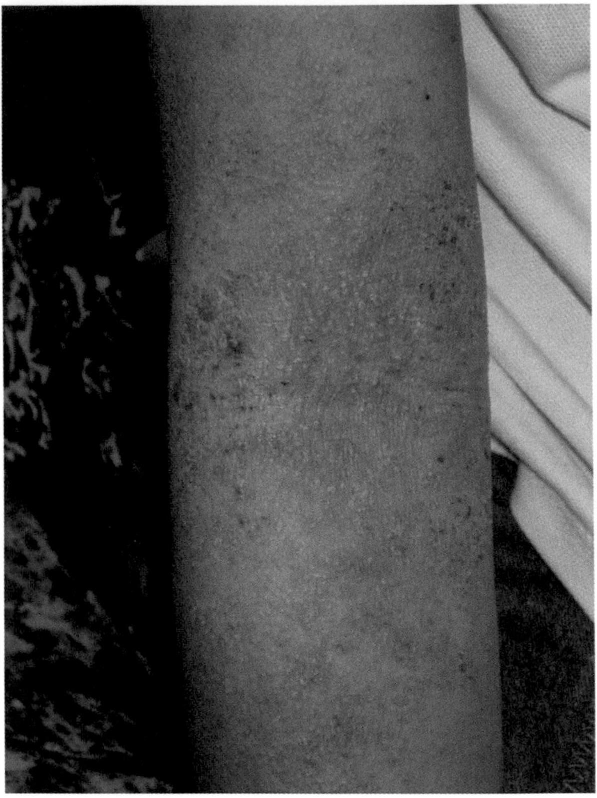

Treatment Treatment of AD requires a lot of work, which might be particularly difficult for vulnerable teens to manage. People affected by AD should avoid contact with irritants such as fragrance and harsh soaps. They need to apply moisturizer several times per day if possible.

Low-potency corticosteroids such as hydrocortisone can be used on the face and diffusely on the body. Medium-potency corticosteroids such as triamcinolone, betamethasone valerate, and mometasone should be used on more severe areas of involvement, but should not be routinely used on the face. Potent corticosteroids such as clobetasol and halobetasol should be reserved for the very thickest areas on hands and feet. Medications should generally be applied twice a day [2, 3].

Practical tips:

- Very low-potency cortisone such as hydrocortisone 1% can be used in place of moisturizer and might be more accessible for homeless teens and refugees than plain moisturizer is if it is covered as a medical expense.
- Ointment-based products do not sting as much as creams when applied and tend to be more effective than creams.

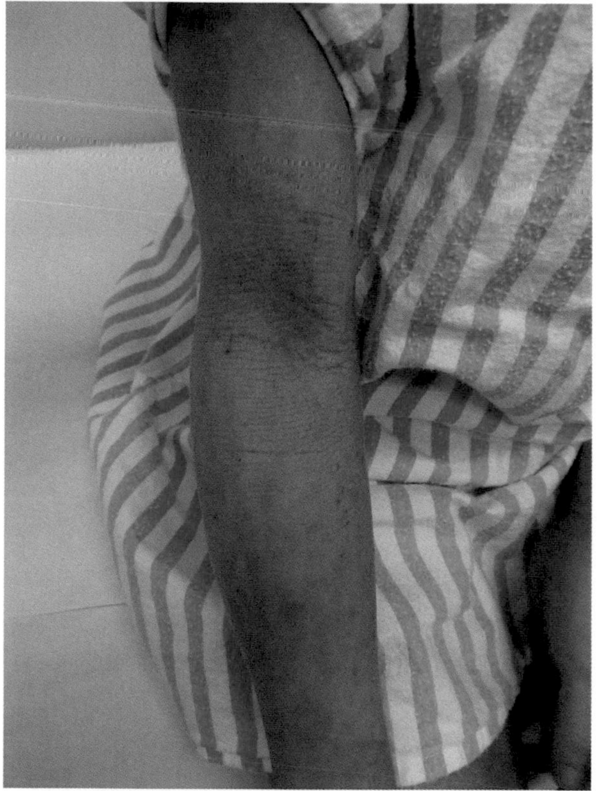

Fig. 16.2 Atopic dermatitis with lichenification

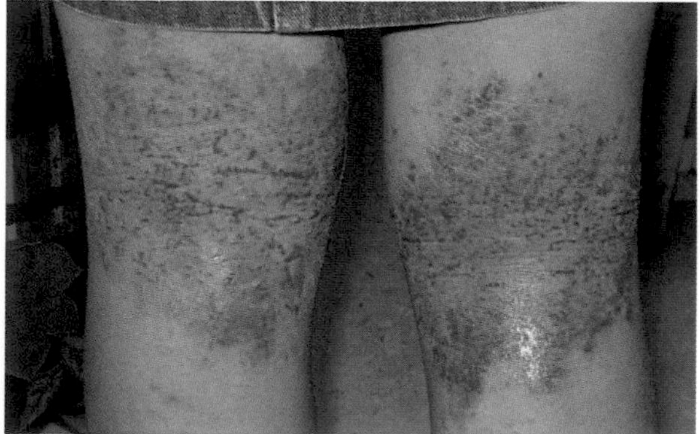

Fig. 16.3 Atopic dermatitis with superficial infection

- Moisturizers do not need to be expensive. Petroleum jelly, mineral oil, cooking oil, hair grease, and even vegetable shortening can all be used as moisturizer when necessary.
- Some teens do not tolerate the feel of creams and ointments. Oils are a reasonable substitute and are faster and easier to apply.

- Wrapping topical cortisones with plastic wrap will significantly increase the potency. This may be helpful for very severe plaques but also increases the risk of skin thinning and stretch mark formation and so should be carefully monitored.
- If a bathtub is available, the addition of ¼-½ cup of household bleach to a bathtub full of water and soaking for 10 minutes twice a week may lower the chance of secondary infection.

Psoriasis

Background Psoriasis is an inflammatory skin condition that is mediated by T cells. It often runs in families and is associated with arthritis. People with psoriasis are now known to also be at higher risk for obesity and hypertension.

Presentation Psoriasis causes well-demarcated erythematous plaques with thick scale that often has a silvery hue (Fig. 16.4). It is seen most commonly on the

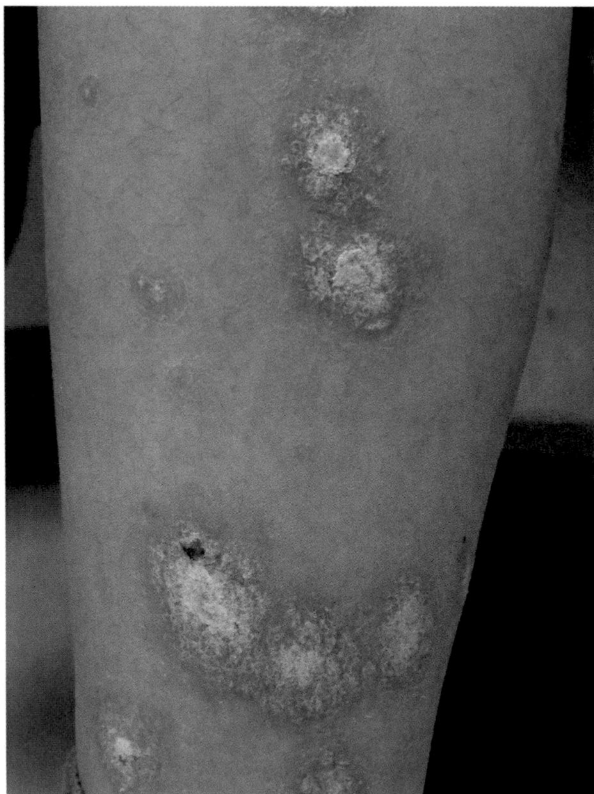

Fig. 16.4 Typical example of plaque psoriasis with well-demarcated plaques with scale

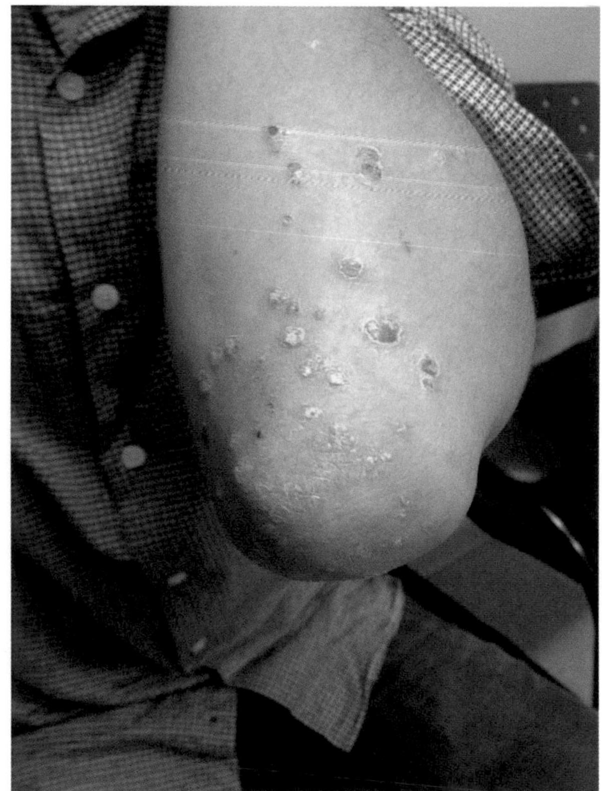

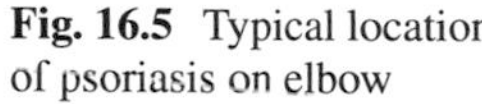
Fig. 16.5 Typical location of psoriasis on elbow

elbows, knees, and scalp (Fig. 16.5). It can flare with many small (guttate) plaques in a widespread distribution after infections with *group A streptococcus* and has both pustular and inverse variants.

Treatment Localized psoriasis is treated with mid-high potency topical corticosteroids such as triamcinolone, betamethasone valerate, mometasone, or fluocinonide applied twice a day to the affected areas. Other topical products that may be helpful in treating psoriasis include calcipotriene, tazarotene (pregnancy category X), and salicylic acid. More widespread and severe psoriasis often requires systemic therapy for management. Potential treatment options include narrow-band UVB light therapy, methotrexate, cyclosporine, and biologics such as TNFα, IL 12/23, and IL17 inhibitors.

Practical tips: Oil treatments on the head (massage oil into scalp several hours before showering) can help to remove scale from the scalp.

- If systemic treatment is required and cost-coverage is available, ustekinumab may be a good alternative for adolescents with severe psoriasis because it is dosed only once per quarter.

- As with atopic dermatitis, covering topical corticosteroids with plastic wrap will increase their potency and might be helpful for very thick plaques but should be done with caution.
- In the setting of acute and widespread flare of psoriasis, a throat swab may be able to identify *streptococcal* infection.

Seborrheic Dermatitis

Background Seborrheic dermatitis is the cause of common dandruff.

Presentation Seborrheic dermatitis causes widespread erythema with fine or greasy scale on the scalp. The areas of involvement are usually not as red, localized, or scaly as is seen in psoriasis. Seborrheic dermatitis also can affect the eyebrows, nasal ala, axilla, central chest, and groin.

Treatment Anti-dandruff shampoos often contain an anti-yeast preparation such as selenium sulfide, ketoconazole, or ciclopirox. Other dandruff shampoos contain keratolytics such as salicylic acid. Low-potency corticosteroids in liquid form such as hydrocortisone scalp lotion and fluocinolone oil can be applied daily as needed.

Practical tips:
- Dandruff shampoos can be used on affected areas of the body as a face or body-wash when needed.
- Shampoos should be left on for a few minutes before rinsing.
- Oil treatments for the scalp can be useful.

Contact Dermatitis

Background Contact dermatitis can be either allergic or irritant in nature. Allergic contact dermatitis is a type IV-mediated allergic response to contact with an allergen to which a person is sensitized. The most common causes of contact dermatitis are contact with nickel, plants such as poison ivy/oak, fragrances, and preservatives such as formaldehyde and quaternium 15. Irritant contact dermatitis is caused by contact with chemicals (including soaps) that dry the skin and elicit nonspecific inflammation in the skin or cause direct skin injury.

Presentation Allergic contact dermatitis presents with geographic shapes that are well demarcated. After acute contact with the allergen, the skin is often red, blisters, and is very itchy. Chronic contact with an allergen may resemble irritant dermatitis and present with dry, red, cracking inflamed skin in the areas of exposure (Figs. 16.6 and 16.7).

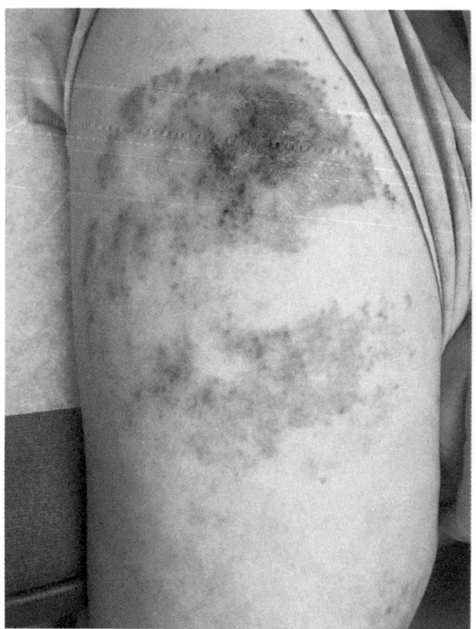

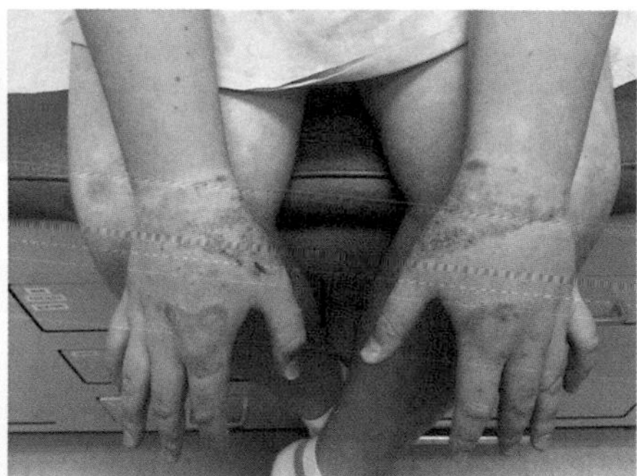

Figs. 16.6 and 16.7 Contact dermatitis with clear margins showing area of exposure

Treatment The mainstay of contact dermatitis treatment is avoiding contact with the allergen or irritant. Sleuthing and patch testing aid in the determination of the cause of contact dermatitis. Dermatitis can be treated with mid-potency cortisones, and some find the drying effect of calamine lotion helpful for acute allergic contact dermatitis. Severe episodes of allergic contact dermatitis may require a 2-week taper of oral corticosteroids [4].

Practical tips:

- Nickel is a common allergen and is found in watches and belt buckles. Contact with the nickel can be prevented by painting clear nail polish over the exposed metal.

Acne

Background Acne is common among teenagers as hormonal changes lead to increased oil production and blockage of pores especially over the face, chest, and back. This allows for increased growth of *P. acnes* bacteria and leads to inflammation at the affected areas. Acne has been proven to have a significant impact not only on self-esteem but also on the way teens are perceived by others, even leading to lower employment rates among those most significantly affected.

Presentation Acne varies widely in severity. Inflammatory papules, pustules, cysts, and nodules can be seen in the affected areas depending on severity

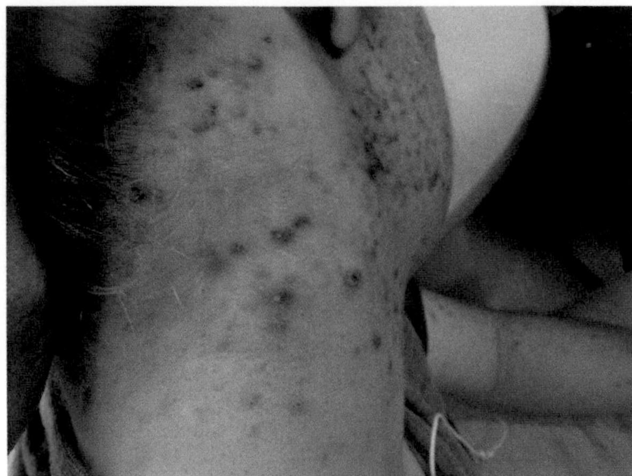

Fig. 16.8 Inflammatory papules and pustules typical for acne vulgaris

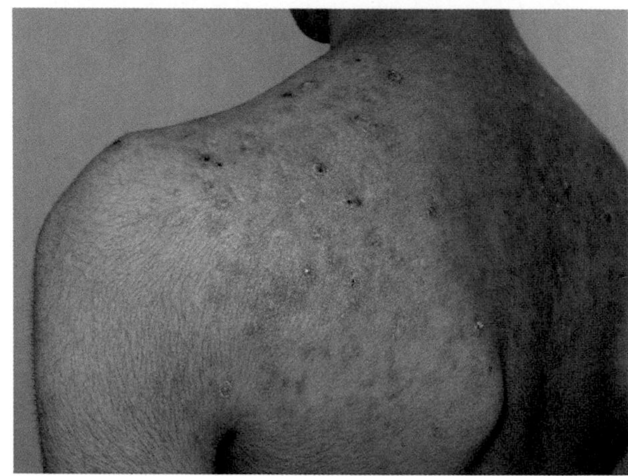

Fig. 16.9 Scaring and post-inflammatory pigment change due to acne vulgaris

(Fig. 16.8). The primary lesion is the comedone which can be open (blackhead) or closed (white head). The mildest acne is comedonal in nature and presents with scattered skin colored papules on the forehead particularly in preteens. Severe acne caused deep nodules and cysts to develop and can lead to scarring (Fig. 16.9).

Treatment Comedonal acne is best treated with a retinoid such as adapalene or tretinoin. Mild inflammatory acne responds well to topical antibiotics such as benzoyl peroxide or clindamycin. Moderate-severe acne is generally treated with systemic therapy: antibiotics such as doxycycline 100 mg daily, oral contraceptive pills for females, or isotretinoin at 0.5–1 mg/kg/day are examples of frequently used systemic therapy. Patients taking isotretinoin must be carefully monitored because of the side-effect profile that includes teratogenicity, effects on the liver, dry skin and lips, nose bleeds, and mood changes [5].

Practical tips:

- Therapies are best applied to affected zones and not as spot therapy.
- Combination products containing a retinoid and an antibiotic are often more expensive than single-ingredient products but may be easier for teens for adherence.
- Topical clindamycin should be used along with benzoyl peroxide or a retinoid to prevent antibiotic resistance in the *P. acnes* bacteria.
- Stress, contact with greasy substances, and occlusion by hats/headbands may increase outbreaks of acne.

Infections and Infestations

Infections and infestations are common among the homeless, runaways, and refugees due to lack of access to bathing facilities, potential for living in crowded facilities, and often particular challenges with foot care. When present, HIV infection, drug use, or having multiple sexual partners also increase the risk of infections and infestations. Refugees may arrive with chronic infections that are uncommon in their new homes.

Bacterial Infections

Impetigo

Background Impetigo is a superficial bacterial infection of the skin. It is most often caused by *Staphylococcus aureus* but may also be caused by streptococcal species. The risk of impetigo is increased when there is a break in the skin barrier due to a dermatologic disease such as atopic dermatitis, an infestation such as scabies, or physical breaks in the skin such as scratches or drug injection sites.

Presentation Impetigo presents with weepy crusted plaques with honey-colored crust. It may present with blisters, can lead to deeper ulcerations (ecthyma), and sometimes spreads to other areas of the body (Figs. 16.10 and 16.11).

Treatment Localized impetigo: Topical therapy applied twice to three times daily may suffice. Options include bacitracin, polymyxin, neomycin, fusidic acid, and mupirocin.

Widespread lesions, large plaques, or recurrent infections: Systemic therapy for 7–10 days is recommended. Options include cephalosporins, clindamycin, and trimethoprim/sulfamethoxazole depending on the organism causing the infection.

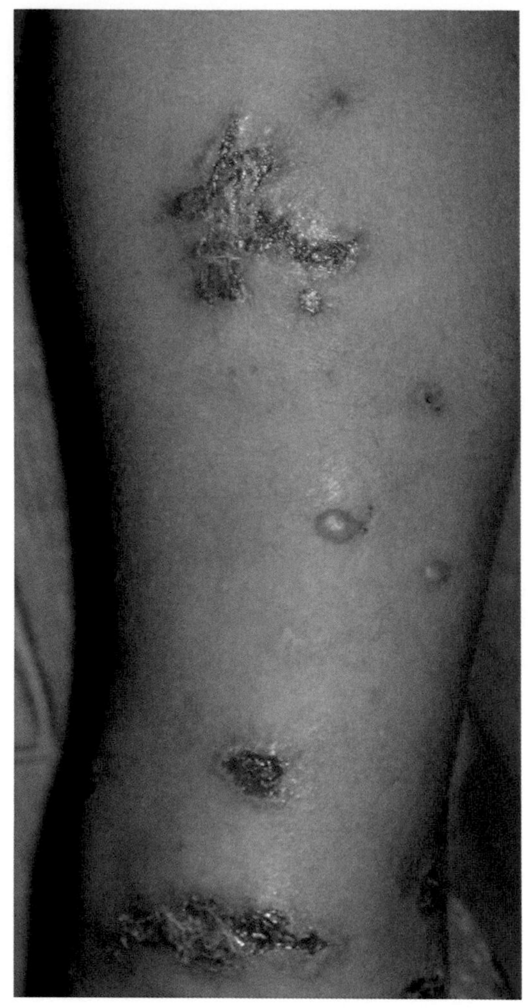

Fig. 16.10 Crusted lesions with some bullae due to impetigo

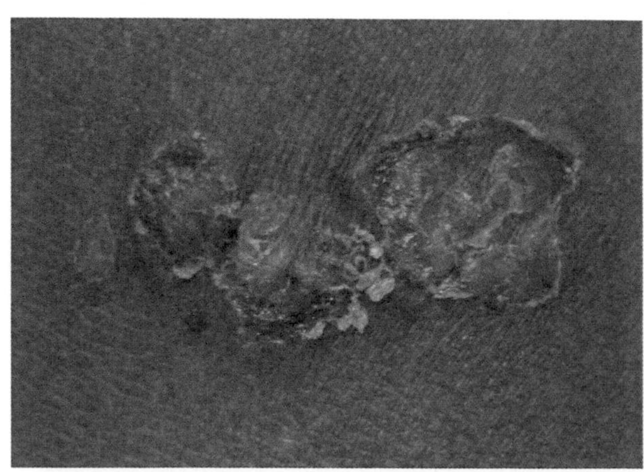

Fig. 16.11 Close-up of honey-colored crust in impetigo

Practical tips:

- Taking a swab from the affected area before initiation of antibiotics will help guide changes in antibiotic coverage if necessary. Damping the swab with sterile water or saline before rubbing on the skin may increase the yield, especially if the skin is dry.
- Dilute bleach solution (1tsp bleach per 2 L of water) or saline (1 tsp salt per 2 cups of water) applied with a washcloth for several minutes just before the application of topical antibiotics may help remove the crust.

Folliculitis and Abscess

Background Folliculitis is an inflammation of the hair follicle which can be associated with a number of different skin conditions and infections. One of the most common forms of folliculitis is bacterial. If the infection is more severe and the deeper portions of the hair follicle are affected, a painful boil or furuncle may form. A furuncle is the most common form of abscess, but abscesses can develop after trauma and do not always center around a hair follicle. *S. aureus* is the most common bacteria to cause folliculitis and abscesses. Community-acquired methicillin-resistant *Staphylococcus Aureus* (MRSA) is commonly identified in recurrent furunculosis.

Presentation Folliculitis presents with multiple erythematous papules and tiny pustules, each of which is centered around a hair follicle. They appear commonly on the back, thighs, and buttocks but can be seen in any hair-bearing areas. Abscesses are larger erythematous nodules that may be fluctuant or drain.

Treatment Folliculitis and abscesses are best treated with systemic antibiotics geared toward the organism causing the infection. Wound swabs can identify the causative organism and guide management. Negative swabs from folliculitis suggest a noninfectious cause of the folliculitis as can be seen in folliculitis barbae. Abscesses often require drainage in addition to antibiotic therapy.

Practical tips:

- Antibiotic washes or dilute bleach baths along with mupirocin application to the nares may help prevent outbreaks in patients who are experiencing frequent recurrences.
- Buttock folliculitis is very common and may be difficult to cure but is often less symptomatic than in other locations.
- Irritant folliculitis that develops due regrowing hair after shaving or waxing is not infectious in nature. The treatment is to stop hair removal for a few months and resume using gentle skin care.

Fungal Infections

Pityriasis Versicolor

Background Pityriasis versicolor is caused by an overgrowth of the *Malassezia furfur* yeast which is a commensal organism on human skin. It is not contagious and is seen in higher rates in teens, those who are frequently sweaty, the malnourished,

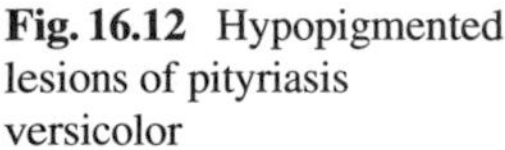

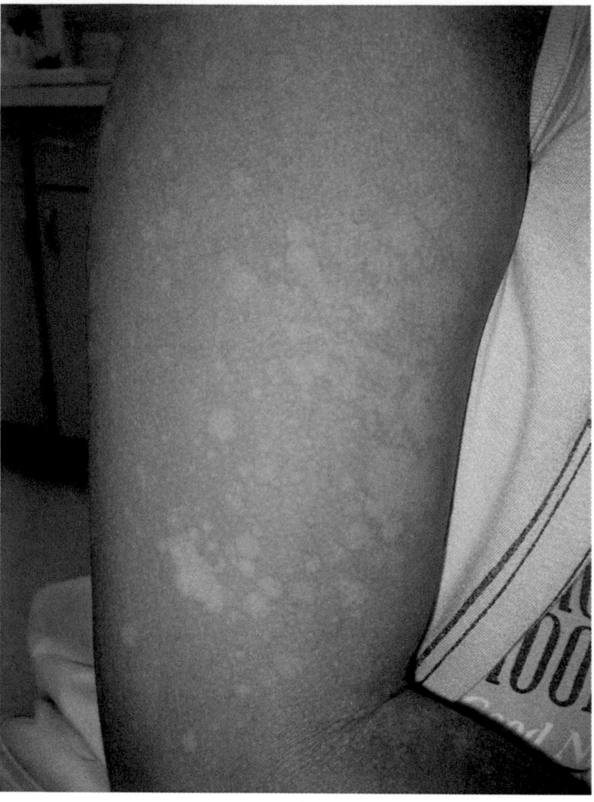

Fig. 16.12 Hypopigmented lesions of pityriasis versicolor

and those with weakened immune systems. It is often more noticeable and may be slightly itchy or stinging after sun exposure.

Presentation As the name versicolor implies, pityriasis versicolor can have a different appearance in different people. It causes small approximately dime-sized macules especially on the chest, upper back, and upper arms that can be hypopigmented, hyperpigmented, or slightly pink (Fig. 16.12). The involved areas often have very subtle scale that is more visible if the skin is scratched. Diagnosis can be confirmed on KOH preparation.

Treatment Anti-yeast preparations will decrease the amount of yeast on the skin, which controls the scaling and the symptoms. Topical therapies should be used for 2 weeks and include creams such as ketoconazole or clotrimazole applied twice daily, or anti-dandruff shampoos such as selenium sulfide and ketoconazole as a bodywash. Oral fluconazole has also been demonstrated to be effective therapy.

Practical tips:

- Because the yeast tend to flourish in certain conditions, people with pityriasis versicolor are prone to recurrences. Weekly maintenance with anti-dandruff shampoos as a bodywash may help prevent recurrence.

- Treatment will fairly quickly relieve the symptoms and scale associated with pityriasis versicolor, but the color may take months to return to normal.

Tinea Capitis/Corporis

Background Tinea is a skin condition caused by dermatophytes such as *Microsporum canis* and *Trichophyton* species. They are generally acquired through contact with other people or animals that have the condition, though they can be passed through fomites as well.

Presentation On the skin, tinea corporis presents with round plaques with an accentuation of scale, elevation, and redness at the border (Figs. 16.13 and 16.14). These plaques are often less inflamed than atopic dermatitis and less scaly than psoriasis. On the scalp (tinea capitis), individuals may have areas of hair loss, red papules, or swelling at the site (Fig. 16.15). In the nails (onychomycosis), dermatophyte infections lead to thickening, white discoloration, and crumbling of the nail plate.

Treatment Localized skin involvement: Topical antifungals such as terbinafine, ketoconazole, and clotrimazole applied twice daily for 2–4 weeks.

Widespread skin involvement, tinea capitis, and onychomycosis all require systemic therapy. Most commonly, terbinafine is utilized. For adults, a dose of 250 mg/day is standard with 2 weeks treatment for the body, 4–6 weeks for the scalp, and

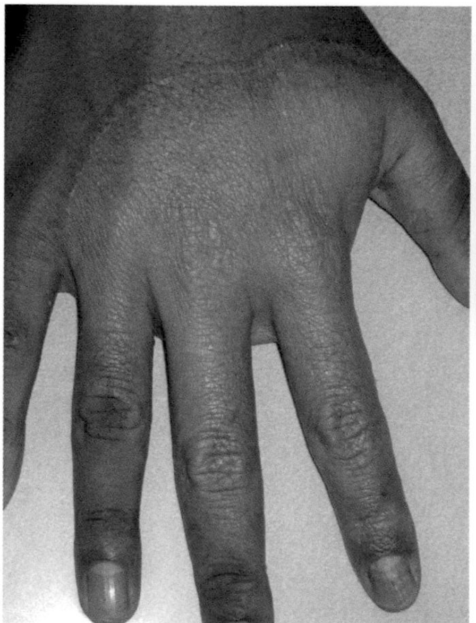

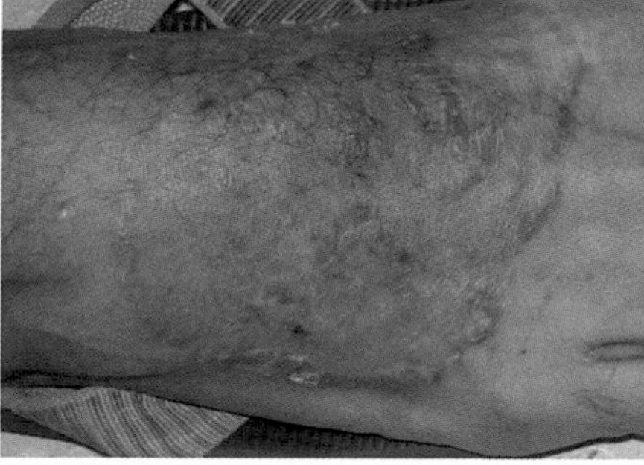

Figs. 16.13 and 16.14 Annular plaques with scale and redness at the active border

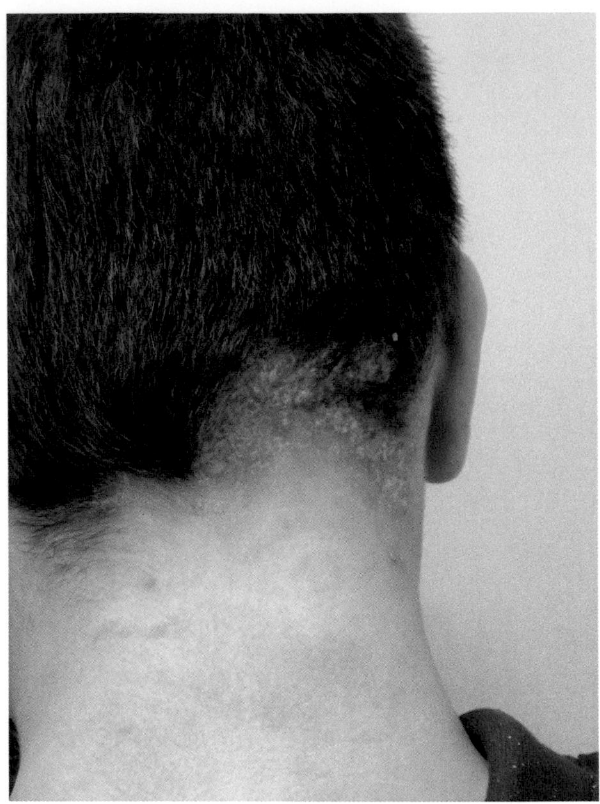

Fig. 16.15 Tinea capitis

3 months for the nails. Alternative treatments include itraconazole and fluconazole. Terbinafine is metabolized through the liver. Alcohol consumption should be minimized during the treatment course and liver function tests evaluated for courses of treatment longer than 6 weeks.

Practical tips:

- While concomitant use of topical steroids may help decrease symptoms quickly, their use also increases the risk of incomplete response of the therapy as well as development of tinea incognito, so they should be used judiciously or avoided.
- Nystatin is beneficial in the treatment of yeast infections but is ineffective in treating dermatophyte infections.

Sexually Transmitted Infections

(See chapter in this book on Sexually Transmitted Infections and Sexual Health Care of Homeless and Street-Involved Youth)

Sexually transmitted infections are covered in more detail elsewhere in the text. Many of these diseases present with dermatologic manifestations such as ulcerations. A few notable skin findings outside of genital ulcerations may be seen in patients with sexually transmitted infections and some common skin infections may be occurring as a sexually transmitted infection when seen in the genital area.

Syphilis Syphilis is a sexually transmitted disease that presents in phases with latent periods between phases of involvement.

- Primary syphilis: Painless genital sore that heals in 4–8 weeks without treatment or 1–2 weeks with appropriate treatment.
- Secondary syphilis: 3 weeks to 3 months after the genital sore heals, patients present with a widespread rash that includes the trunk, palms, and soles. The rash is characterized by red or red-brown macules then papules and is not pruritic. It might be associated with hair loss, raw mucosal surfaces, constitutional symptoms, and/or gray-white moist raised plaques in the groin, axilla, or umbilicus or under the breasts.
- Tertiary syphilis: 3–10 years after the initial infection, people affected by untreated syphilis can develop solitary granulomatous lesions, nodules, and ulcers that are usually painless when they appear in the skin. Bone changes, neurological alterations, and spinal cord disease all can occur in the tertiary phase.

Treatment is with penicillin by injection with close follow-up to monitor for treatment failure.

Gonorrhea Gonorrhea is caused by *Neisseria gonorrhoeae* and is transmitted through sexual contact. Localized symptoms include creamy or green discharge, painful urination, and itching/irritation of the penis or vulva. Initial symptoms may be quite minimal and not come to medical attention. Disseminated gonococcal infection leads to joint pain with decreased mobility and a widespread rash. The skin findings are diffuse, but spare the face and scalp, and include small papules that turn into pustules on an erythematous base and may develop necrotic centers. Gonorrhea is diagnosed by swabs taken for Gram staining and culture. Treatment is with antibiotics depending on sensitivities.

Human papillomavirus Human papillomavirus is common in adolescents. Nongenital HPV are frequently found on the hands and feet. HPV can be passed to the genital area from the hand by touching. Certain strains are found most commonly in the genital area and are spread through sexual contact. The HPV vaccine may decrease the frequency of genital warts over time; however, they remain prevalent. Treatment is often difficult. Topical imiquimod is approved for the treatment of genital warts and can be applied three times weekly. Destructive therapies such as liquid nitrogen are helpful but can be painful.

Molluscum contagiosum Molluscum contagiosum is caused by a pox virus and is spread by direct contact. It is characterized by individual pearly papules, many of which have central umbilication and may develop a white core. Molluscum is most commonly seen in preschool and early school-aged children but also appears in adolescents as a sexually transmitted disease. In this setting, lesions are most commonly seen in the suprapubic region. They will self-resolve over a matter of months but can be treated with curettage, a single application of a thin coating of cantharidin (which must be washed off in 2–4 hours), or with a short cycle of liquid nitrogen therapy.

Human immunodeficiency virus There are a myriad of skin conditions that are seen in association with HIV. Because of the immune effects of the virus, people who are infected with HIV may have increased number or more severe presentation of skin infections. For example, widespread warts and molluscum contagiosum may be the presenting illness in patients with HIV. Recurrent episodes of herpes simplex infections and varicella zoster are common. Common immune-driven dermatologic problems may be more prevalent or severe in those affected by HIV. Seborrheic dermatitis, psoriasis, and eczema are all seen in increased frequency in patients with HIV infection. Eosinophilic folliculitis causes development of very itchy papules and pustules especially over the neck, back, and scalp. In the era of antiretroviral therapy, drug effects such as lipodystrophy, drug rashes, and development of xanthoma occur commonly. Finally, there are malignant skin conditions such as Kaposi sarcoma and cutaneous lymphoma that are seen in increased frequency in HIV *(See chapter in this book on Human Immunodeficiency Virus and Acquired Immune Deficiency Syndrome).*

Infestations

Scabies

Background Scabies is caused by the mite *Sarcoptes scabiei* var. hominis. It can be seen in all socioeconomic groups and more commonly in overcrowded communities like refugee camps and shelters. The mite lives in the epidermis where it can complete the regular life cycle. Scabies infestation is limited to the skin and systemic involvement is not seen. Transmission occurs through direct human contact or contact with infected fomites. Higher incidence is seen in children and sexually active individuals. Patients with immune deficiency, e.g., HIV and organ transplant recipients, are at risk of developing crusted scabies with very high number of mites.

Presentation Symptoms of intractable pruritus are the main presentation of scabies. Secondary signs of pruritus including excoriations and erosions are the most visible signs of infestation. Burrows are classic findings of scabies; however, they can be difficult to detect, particularly in patients who are actively scratching. Burrows present as linear wavy tracks on the skin; they tend to occur more frequently in the webs of the fingers and toes (Figs. 16.16 and 16.17). Erythematous

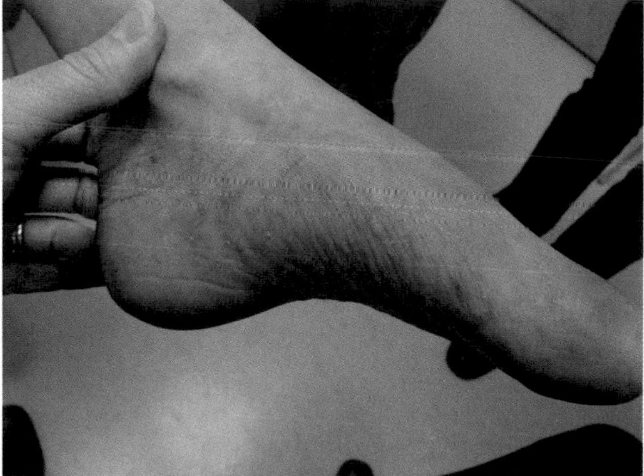

Fig. 16.16 Scabies on the side of the foot, a common location for burrows and inflammatory papules

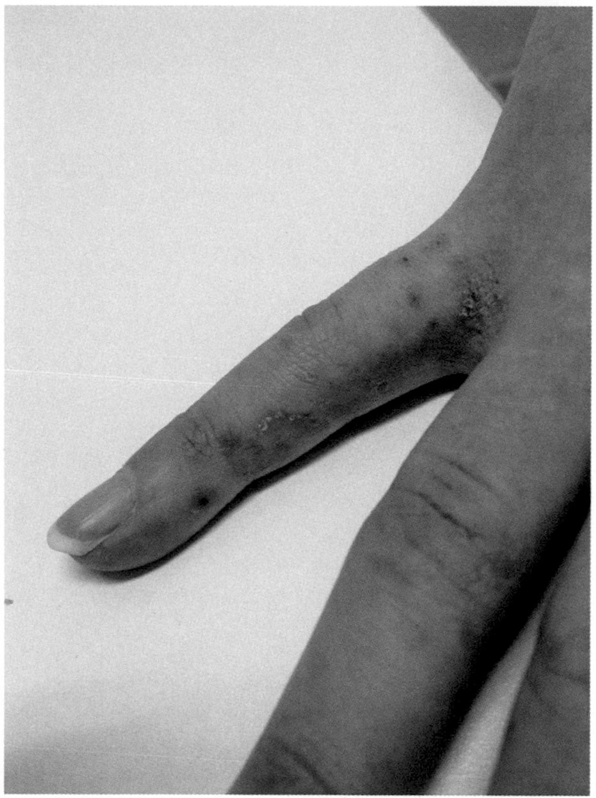

Fig. 16.17 Scabies burrow on the side of the finger

nodules may develop in the axilla and on the scrotum. Secondary infections with *Staphylococcus aureus* and *Streptococcus pyogenes* can be seen. Recurrence of scabies can be related to insufficient treatment, reinfestation from fomites, and failure of close contacts to be treated [6].

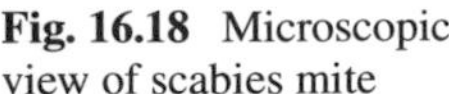

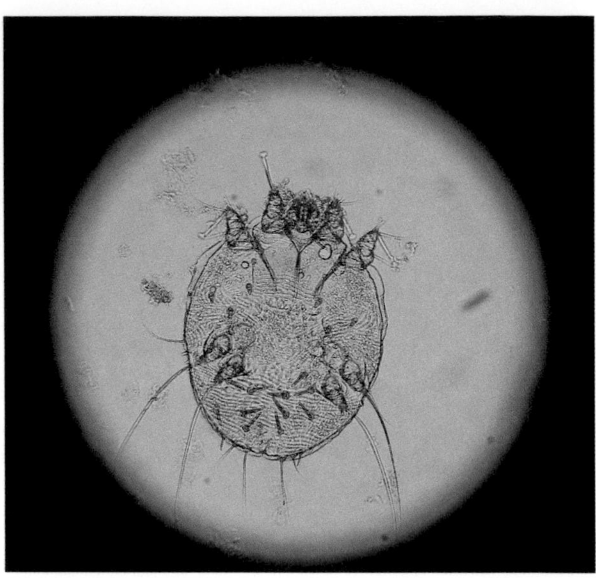

Fig. 16.18 Microscopic view of scabies mite

Diagnosis can be established clinically and if a microscope is available and confirmed microscopically by scraping the skin of the burrows using a 15-blade scalpel and placing the scrapings on a glass slide. The sample is fixed using different media including mineral oil, potassium hydroxide, and cryostat. Diagnosis is made by visually inspecting the eight-legged mite or its remnants under microscopy (Fig. 16.18) [7].

Treatment Treatment includes two applications of topical treatments 1 week apart and should be recommended for all close contacts of an affected person. Topical permethrin 5% is the most commonly used treatment for scabies. It is applied and left on overnight from the neck downward with concentration of the body folds, web spaces, and genitals. Other topical agents including crotamiton cream 10%, 5–10% precipitated sulfur in ointment base are used less frequently. Where available, oral ivermectin 200 μg/kg dose given in two doses 1 week apart can also be effective.

Towels, clothes, and bed linens should be washed in hot water and dried or stored in a bag for 5–7 days. The mite is unable to survive long outside the epidermis.

Pediculosis/lice infestation

Background Lice are ectoparasites that live on the human body. They feed on human blood by using sharp mouth pieces. During their meal, they inject saliva that causes an allergic reaction and pruritus. Lice are wingless insects that grasp strongly to the hair shaft where they can be seen crawling. Female lice place nits (eggs) daily; they are firmly adherent to the hair or fibers of clothes in cases of body lice. The nits hatch in 10–12 days and form nymphs that grow to adult lice. Nits can live and hatch outside the host for 10 days [6].

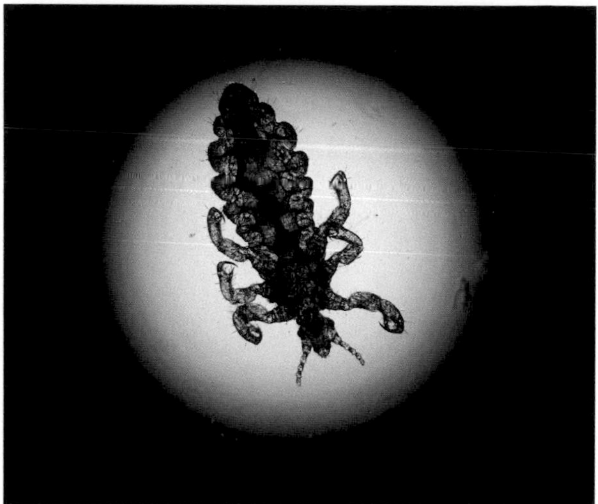

Fig. 16.19 Head louse

Head lice Head lice are the most common cause of human infestation. They are unable to survive outside the human host for more than 1–2 days, and transmission is by head-to-head contact, sharing grooming tools or headwear, and less commonly by couches and chairs that recently had been in contact with an infested person. Head lice involve the scalp and can extend to involve the neck and behind the ears. Pruritus develops after an immune response to louse saliva leading to evidence of excoriations, secondary bacterial infection, and lymph node enlargement. Lice and nits can be seen on examination (Fig. 16.19). Nits can be distinguished from scale by their firm adherence to the hairs. Nits more than 2 cm from the base of the hair are not likely to be viable and may be remnants of a past infestation.

Head lice are managed using different chemical and physical agents that help eradicate the lice. Resistance to treatment is a developing problem. Treatments should be repeated to assure all nits that hatch are treated. Treatment options include permethrin 1%, malathion, benzyl alcohol lotion, dimethicone, spinosad 0.9%, and ivermectin.

Treatments are repeated in 7–9 days. The use of nit comb and physically removing visible nits are helpful, and some find the use of petrolatum or heavy conditioner along with careful nit combing sufficient for curing lice [6].

Body lice Because body lice (or pediculosis corporis) cannot survive long without human contact and do not reside on the skin, they are primarily seen in areas of overcrowding where there is poor access showers and washing machines, most commonly among people who are homeless, refugees or incarcerated. Unlike other lice, the body louse is a vector for different infections including epidemic typhus, trench fever, and epidemic relapsing fever. On clinical exam, the lice are not seen on the skin but are usually seen along the clothing seams. Bites cause pruritus and present as small erythematous papules, excoriations, and crusts [6].

Crab lice Infestation with *Pthirus pubis*, the crab louse, involves mainly the hairs in the pubic region but may involve the scalp, eyelashes, eyebrows, and axillary hair. In most cases, it is considered a sexually transmitted infestation, particularly when lice are found in the eyebrows or eyelashes. Evaluating for other sexually transmitted infections in patients with crab lice is recommended. Shared fomites and towels can also be a route of infestation. Patients present with pruritus which can be disturbing, secondary bacterial infections, and lymph node enlargement. Crab louse is diagnosed clinically and can be confirmed with direct visualization under microscopy. Treatment of crab lice is similar to other forms of lice, which includes using topical permethrin 1 or 5% overnight to the affected area; the treatment is repeated in 7–10 days. Other options include topical ivermectin or, less commonly, lindane. For eyelashes, an ophthalmic-grade petrolatum ointment used twice to four times daily for 10 days is effective [6].

Clothing, towels, and bedding of all who have been in contact with the patient over the last 2–3 days must be machine washed and machine dried. Sexual partners should be treated or there continues to be a significant risk of reinfestation.

Bedbugs are small parasites that are commonly encountered in crowded places with transient populations such as shelters, single-resident occupancy hotels, and in some low-income housing. They are small in size, are less than 1 cm, and can leave behind red-brown excrement. A sweaty, musty odor can be associated with heavy infestations. Bedbugs are nocturnal; during the daytime they hide in crevices, mattress seams, under paint peels, and bed boards. Edematous papules with a hemorrhagic center following a linear pattern "breakfast-lunch-dinner" is typically seen on exposed skin. No known human infection is transmitted by bedbugs.

Management tips include vacuuming, heat treatments, laundering, mattress and box spring encasements, and destroying or removing infested objects such as bedding. Heated pitfall traps are available to collect the bugs and can help with diagnosis and evaluation but are not helpful for treatment. Washing and drying items in a dryer on a hot setting is sufficient to kill bedbugs in clothing or linen. With heavy infestation, in shelters or continued transient housing, an exterminator assessment and intervention is commonly necessary [8].

Dermatological Signs of Systemic Diseases

Lupus erythematosus Cutaneous lupus erythematosus can present with or without systemic findings associated with systemic lupus erythematosus (SLE). Cutaneous findings of SLE are divided into acute cutaneous lupus erythematosus (ACLE), subacute cutaneous lupus erythematosus (SCLE), and chronic lupus erythematosus (CCLE). ACLE presents as erythematous indurated papules and plaques with occasional erosions and telangiectasia, in the malar area (malar rash). Other forms include generalized maculopapular eruption, photosensitivity, and blisters. SCLE commonly presents in a photo-distributed pattern, either annular papules and plaques or papulosquamous eruption (eczema or psoriasis like); it tends to spare the central face. Lesions can resemble more common dermatoses like psoriasis, atopic dermatitis, and photoallergic contact dermatitis. A neonatal form of lupus erythematosus is considered a subtype of SCLE and presents with multiple annular papules and plaques mainly on the scalp and periorbital region. The disease is seen in infants up to 3 months of age; early recognition is important for early detection of cardiac involvement: heart block, and cardiomyopathy. Other systemic findings include thrombocytopenia and hepatic involvement. Mothers of infants with neonatal lupus erythematosus have circulating autoantibodies to Ro/SSA, La/ SSb and/or U1RNP.

Different forms are categorized as CCLE, discoid lupus erythematosus, being the prototype of this group. Skin lesions present in sun-exposed and sun-protected areas as multiple well-circumscribed plaques with adherent scales. The plaques develop a characteristic finding of central scarring, atrophy, and hypopigmentation and a peripheral rim of hyperpigmentation. Lesions most commonly involve the head and neck areas including the scalp and mucous membranes.

Practical tips:

- Sun protection, with broad-spectrum sunscreen, clothing, and seeking shade are crucial.
- Topical medium-potency corticosteroids can be applied on the active lesions.
- Intralesional triamcinolone (5–10 mg/ml) for DLE lesions helps reduce inflammation.

Diabetes Mellitus

Cutaneous findings associated with diabetes mellitus (DM) include common findings like acanthosis nigricans. Lesions present as velvety brown-black papules and plaques that mainly involve the lateral neck and axilla. They are often seen in obese patients with insulin resistance.

Necrobiosis Lipoidica

Yellow thin atrophied plaques that are seen on the shins. They can ulcerate and cause pain and are most commonly associated with DM.

Pyoderma Gangrenosum

A painful ulcer with a pustular base and violaceous-gray rim that often occurs on the lower legs. PG is commonly associated with systemic diseases. The most common associations are inflammatory bowel disease, hematological malignancies, and autoimmune conditions like connective tissue diseases. Lesions can be confused with skin infections, and skin biopsy might be necessary to rule out other diseases.

Aphthous Ulcers

Painful ulcers in the oral cavity with yellow pseudomembranous center. They can be seen in multiple systemic diseases including IBD, SLE, Behçet disease, and periodic fever syndromes. Herpes simplex virus infection should be ruled out by sending a swab sample for PCR.

Cutaneous Vasculitis

Cutaneous small-vessel vasculitis (CSVV, also known as leukocytoclastic vasculitis) presents as palpable and nonpalpable purpura, pustules, necrotic bullae, and urticarial plaques. It often involves the lower limbs, and widespread lesions can be seen. There are numerous causes of CSVV: infections, autoimmune diseases, medications (beta lactam, sulfonamide), and street drugs (adulterated cocaine with levamisole), more than 50% remain idiopathic. Systemic involvement including the kidneys can rarely be seen; urinalysis and 24-hour urine collection may be necessary to rule out kidney involvement. A full history and physical examination should be performed to rule out other systemic involvement.

Henoch-Schonlein purpura (HSP): IgA-induced small-vessel vasculitis. HSP classic tetrad consists of palpable purpura, arthritis, abdominal pain, and hematuria. The purpura usually starts on the feet and distal legs and ascends to involve the thighs and trunk. The eruption is usually preceded by an upper respiratory tract infection. Topical steroid therapy and supportive therapy are usually sufficient to control skin symptoms. Systemic therapies like dapsone, colchicine, and prednisone may be required for more advanced disease.

Nutritional Deficiency

Homeless youth and refugees are at increased risk of nutritional deficiencies. These can be related to poor food security, disordered eating, or alcohol and drug abuse. Crash diets are trends that can be seen in teens and may be associated with cutaneous changes including in hair and nails.

Anorexia and bulimia nervosa Skin findings include telogen effluvium (diffuse nonscarring hair loss), lanugo-like hair growth, and skin hyperpigmentation. Vasomotor instability can lead to acrocyanosis, perniosis, and livedo reticularis. Other findings include enlarged salivary glands, erosions of the tooth enamel from gastric reflux, and calluses or scars on the knuckles or dorsal hand from purging (Russell's sign).

Pellagra Niacin (vitamin B1) deficiency causes pellagra. The common mnemonic "4 Ds" includes the following: diarrhea, dermatitis, dementia, and death. It can be associated with chronic alcoholism, medications (isoniazid), and other conditions associated with low levels of niacin. The skin lesions are photodistributed plaques, with a shellac like surface. The characteristic Casals necklace can also be seen. Niacin replacement therapy and treatment of the underlying cause are the main aspects of management.

Acrodermatitis enteropathica Zinc deficiency may be either acquired or congenital. It presents with a persistent eczematous dermatitis involving skin around the peri-oral, perianal regions, and distal upper extremities and can be seen in patients with chronic malabsorption, HIV, alcoholism, or strict vegan diet. The congenital form presents few days to weeks after weaning off breast milk. Diagnosis can be made by low zinc levels; alkaline phosphatase, a zinc-dependent enzyme, is also decreased.

Scurvy Vitamin C deficiency can lead to spongy gingiva with easy bleeding and erosions, petechiae around hair follicles, and corkscrew hairs. Scurvy is a serious risk factor for hemorrhage; these changes are from poor collagen formation, which leads to fragile blood vessels.

Iron deficiency anemia Iron deficiency can lead to alopecia (telogen effluvium), brittle and fragile nails, koilonychia (spoon-shaped nails), and angular cheilitis. This can result from poor nutrition or internal bleeding.

Exposures and External Factors

Homeless, runaway, and refugee youth are at risk of environmental exposures that stable housing would otherwise help to prevent. Exposure to sun, cold, and localized sources of heat can all lead to skin changes. Other "exposures" that may lead to dermatologic findings include drug use, physical abuse, and self-injury.

Sun Exposure

Sunburn Acute excessive sun exposure can lead to first- or second-degree burns. Sun-exposed areas commonly affected include the face, ears, arms, and chest. While more common in fair-skinned individuals, all skin types can burn. Because midday sun is the strongest, those without access to adequate shelter are particularly at risk. Chronic excessive sun exposure increases the risk of skin cancer and photoaging. Hats, long sleeves and pants, and shade all aid in protection from sun exposure and may be more accessible for youth than sunscreens.

Polymorphous light eruption (PMLE) PMLE is not uncommon in teens and is more commonly seen in females. It is an inflammatory reaction that occurs on exposed skin usually the dorsal hands and arms. It appears after the first strong sun exposure on previously unexposed skin such as in the spring and early summer. PMLE presents with stinging and itching, but symptoms do not appear immediately on exposure to the sun. It tends to improve throughout the course of the summer and may recur the following spring. It is prevented by protection from exposure to UVA radiation through the use of sunscreens, long clothing, and shade seeking.

Phytophotodermatitis Certain plants such as lemon, lime, hogweed, and fig can make the skin more sensitive to the sun after contact. After exposure to the plant and then the sun, the skin may become red and painful and blister and then turns profoundly brown. Phytophotodermatitis usually presents with odd geographic patterns that correspond to the areas where contact occurred (Fig. 16.20).

Sunscreens are divided into organic (soluble) and inorganic (insoluble) and previously were named chemical and physical sunscreens, respectively. They provide protection against sun-induced skin change, most importantly skin cancer. There are lots of sunscreen choices in the market, with a wide range of price. The FDA recommends choosing sunscreens with broad-spectrum activity (UVB+UVA), SPF (sun protection factor) of 30 and above, and water resistance. The inorganic sunscreens (e.g., zinc oxide and titanium dioxide) provide a wide spectrum of UV protection but are less cosmetically favored, due to the white appearance of the skin.

Sunscreens should be applied 15–30 minutes before getting exposed to the sun. The total amount of sunscreen required to cover the whole body is around 1 ounce. Repeat application in 2–4 hours and more frequently with excessive sweating and immersion in water. Sunscreen can cause skin irritation; therefore, switching between brands may be necessary to find a more tolerable sunscreen.

Cold Exposure

Frostbite Exposure to subfreezing temperatures can lead to cell death and frostbite. Areas affected are usually appendages such as the fingers, toes, ears, and nasal tip. Drug and alcohol use may predispose to developing frostbite as they may decrease sensation of the affected areas and lower heat-seeking behavior.

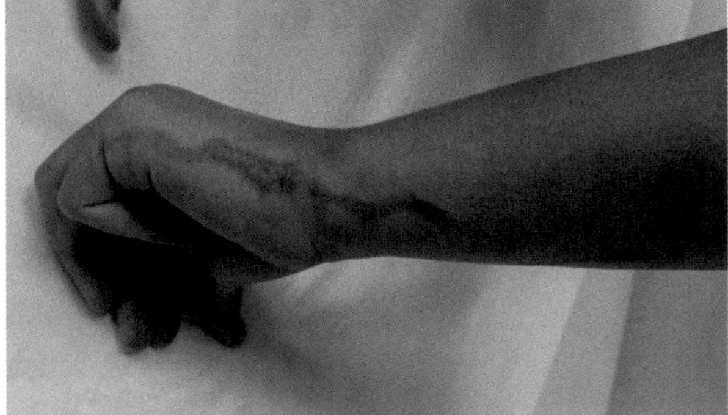

Fig. 16.20 Phytophotodermatitis with profound hyperpigmentation in area of contact with plant prior to sun exposure

The mechanism of injury involves vascular instability, inflammation, thrombosis, and tissue damage.

- The first phase involves freezing, which presents with woody induration and blanching.
- The second phase presents with pain, swelling with red-blue discoloration, and blister formation. It corresponds to vasodilation that occurs in the injured vessel.
- The third phase involves the extension of injury and is variable depending on the extent of the cold injury.
- The fourth phase is the healing or amputation stage, where the process terminates and is contained to the site of involvement.

Frostbites are classified similar to burns depending on the level of injury. First-degree frostbite is called frostnip and resolves completely with no scarring. Second-degree causes blistering and neurological sequelae may persist. Third-degree and fourth-degree carry a poor prognosis.

Gentle rewarming with warm water is the intervention of choice for frostbite. Wound care management and pain control are the other aspects of management for frostbite. Evaluation and treatment by a health professional is recommended for all frostbite more severe than frostnip.

Chilblains/pernio Chilblains is caused by an abnormal inflammatory response in acral skin (fingers and toes) in response to cold exposure. It occurs in areas in the world where the weather is cold and damp. Unlike frostbite which occurs after exposure to extreme cold, chilblains occurs in the setting of prolonged contact with damp chilly weather. It is seen most commonly on the fingers and toes and presents with multiple red-blue papules, nodules, and erosions (Fig. 16.21). It is often initially painful then becomes very pruritic. In severe cases, blistering and ulceration is seen. Cigarette smoking can worsen the symptoms [9].

Prevention of chilblains is through avoidance of exposure to cool damp weather and wearing proper clothing. Water-proof boots and wool socks are best for keeping the feet warm. Ensuring that the toe box of the shoe is wide enough helps to prevent restriction of blood flow to the toes. Treatment of active lesions is mid-high-potency topical corticosteroids. Those who suffer recurrent episodes may be treated with calcium channel blockers such as nifedipine.

Raynaud phenomenon Raynaud phenomenon is caused by vasospasm in response to cold exposure. Primary Raynaud's typically begins before the age of 25 and is more common than secondary Raynaud's, which is found in associated with connective tissue diseases. In Raynaud phenomenon, the affected areas, usually the fingers, turn white and numb when exposed to cold temperatures and cold water. They will become red-blue and tingle when rewarmed. Prevention is through avoidance of cold exposure and wearing appropriate clothing to keep fingers and toes warm. Smoking contributes to vasoconstriction and should be stopped. Swinging the affected hands can increase blood flow to the fingertips and may hasten rewarming. For very severe and recurrent cases, calcium channel blockers may be helpful.

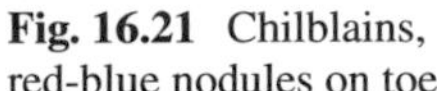
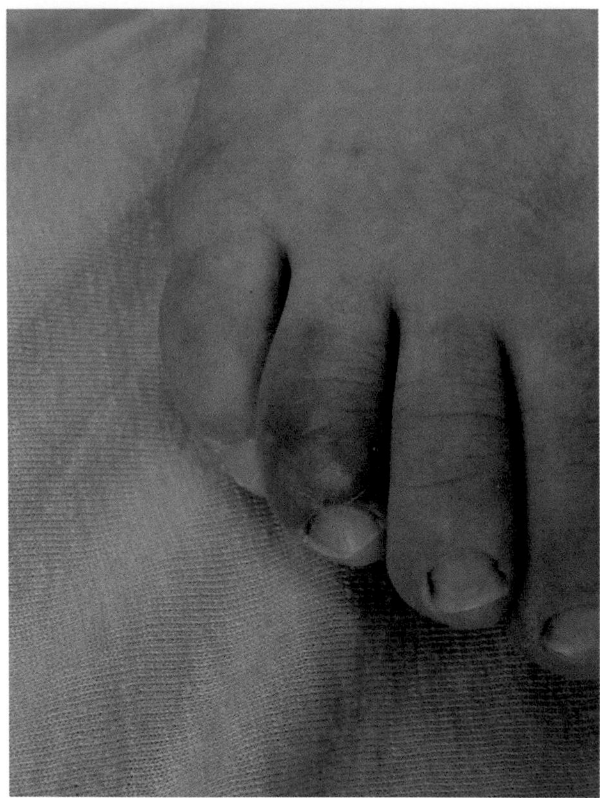

Fig. 16.21 Chilblains, red-blue nodules on toe

Localized heat

Erythema ab igne Those who rely on localized heating such as hot water bottles and space heaters are at risk for developing erythema ab igne. In this condition, the skin in the area of exposure to the heat develops reticulate purple-brown coloration. The skin changes resolve once the contact with the head source is discontinued (Fig. 16.22).

Skin Signs of Drug Use/Abuse

Drug use and abuse can be reflected in the skin by the traumatic effect of delivering the drug, by the effects of the drug itself, or by the effects of contaminants that are included in the drug [10].

- Acute changes of flushing and facial redness occur with alcohol use. The facial redness can become permanent over time, and in chronic use, liver damage may lead to formation of telangiectasias and spider angiomas, jaundice, and nail changes.

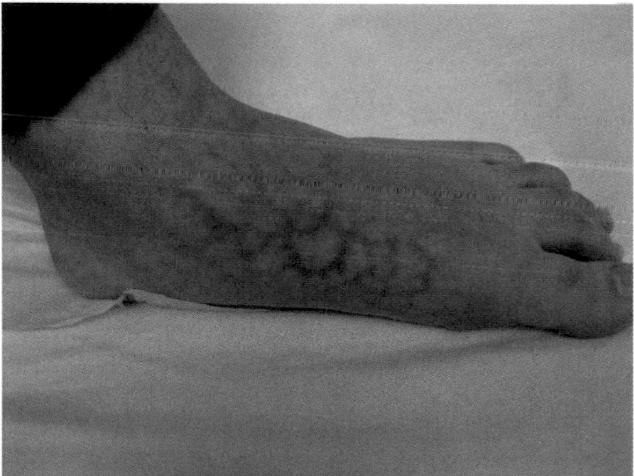

Fig. 16.22 Erythema ab igne from contact heat showing reticulate hyperpigmentation

- Formication is skin picking secondary to the delusion of sensing bugs moving under the skin. It can be seen in cocaine and methamphetamine users.
- Scars are common signs of drug abuse; they can be linear pigmentation at frequent injection sites or circular and depressed from "skin popping."
- Granulomatous reactions and/or skin necrosis can occur at the sites of extravasation of injected drugs.
- Recurrent skin infections including cellulitis, abscess, and necrotizing fasciitis can complicate drug use; they can be difficult to treat and lead to systemic involvement, e.g., endocarditis.
- Vasculopathy (vascular occlusion) and vasculitis can occur after use of adulterated cocaine with levamisole. It presents with a netlike purpura that involves the ears, nose, and other acral surfaces.

Tattoos and Piercings

Tattoo Reactions

Tattooing is increasing in incidence among adolescents. It is estimated that 20–25% of teens have tattoos. They are used by people from all socioeconomic backgrounds. Skin reactions to tattoos do occur and depend on the method of delivery, the media or ink used, and the patient reaction patterns.

- Acute inflammatory reaction: An acute inflammatory reaction to the breach of the skin barrier and the introduction of dye occurs following tattooing. This usually improves after 2–3 weeks and is expected in the course of tattooing. Wound care during this phase includes prevention of infection through keeping the area clean and covered.
- Infections: Infection can be transmitted through the use of unclean needles. Tattoos can be a source of blood-borne disease including hepatitis and HIV. Skin

infections can also be transmitted including folliculitis, abscess, warts, and atypical mycobacterial infections.
- Koebnerization: The Koebner phenomenon describes the tendency of some skin diseases (such as vitiligo, psoriasis, lichen planus, and sarcoidosis) to appear following trauma and has been described following tattooing.
- Allergic reactions: Eczematous reactions develop in response to allergens in the ink. Red dyes are the most common to cause allergic reactions. Henna temporary tattoos may also result in allergic contact dermatitis at the site of application.
- Photosensitive reactions: Certain pigments can react with sunlight and induce a reaction with redness and swelling. Yellow dye (cadmium sulfate) is most likely to cause photosensitive reactions.
- Granulomatous reactions: The normal response to a foreign body in the skin is the development of foreign body granulomas. Such reactions can occur in response to any pigment in the skin and lead to red-purple nodules as the site of the ink.

Tattoo removal Tattoo removal is by laser therapy in which the wavelength of the laser light is matched with the color of the tattoo ink to be removed. Complications include scarring, hypersensitivity response, immediate and permanent darkening of certain tattoo inks, and spread of previously localized allergic reactions.

Piercings

Like tattooing, body piercing has become more popular in recent decades. Common sites for piercing have expanded to include the tongue, lips, navel, nose, eyebrows, upper helix, nipples, and genitals. Complications of piercings include infection, allergic reactions to the metals used, poor cosmetic outcome, keloid scar formation, and Koebnerization of skin diseases (as above). Removal of the jewelry is often recommended when complications arise. Certain sites are particularly prone to complications.

- Ear lobes: Keloid scar formation. Treatment is with intralesional triamcinolone injection or surgical removal of the keloid.
- Traumatic tearing of the lobe. Repair is surgical.
- Upper ears: Auricular perichondritis. Fluoroquinolone antibiotics are recommended due to their coverage of pseudomonas infections.
- Tongue: Chipping of teeth.
- Nipples, navel, and genitals: Prolonged healing time.
- Genitals: Infection, compromise of contraception, tears, paraphimosis, priapism.

Nonaccidental Injury

Nonaccidental injury generally refers to injury secondary to abuse, and this is a risk that homeless, runaway, and refugee youth certainly face. Skin changes can also be self-induced and result from nonsuicidal self-injury, *dermatitis artefacta* or as part of social media challenges.

Skin Signs of Abuse and Maltreatment

Skin signs are recognized in up to 90% of cases of abuse.

- Bruising: Bruising is the most common form of nonaccidental injury. The location, size, shape, and number of bruises may make them suspicious. Bruises that occur due to everyday bumps usually occur over bony prominences, so bruising on softer skin such as the abdomen, ears, and buttocks is concerning. Large bruises and those with characteristic shapes may indicate the source of the bruise as sometimes the pattern of a hand, belt-buckle, or whip can be seen in the bruise. Concern should be raised for those who present with more than three bruises at one time [11].
- Burns: Burns take the shape of the object that causes the burn. Cigarette and cigar burns are small and round. Iron burns will have a sharp edge and may have islands of spared corresponding to depressions in the iron surface. Other metal objects such as forks and buckles will leave a characteristic pattern. Scald burns are often seen in a glove/sock distribution or over the buttock [11].
- Bites: Bites have a characteristic half-moon shape. Human bites cause crush injury more frequently than pierce injury. Toddler bites can be distinguished from those caused by adults by their small size. If the bite does break the skin, antibiotics are recommended [11].
- Sexual abuse: Sexual abuse can be perpetrated on both males and females, but females are more commonly the victims. 90% of perpetrators are men and most are relatives or acquaintances. Anal tears, sphincter dilation, genital bruising, and STIs all can be indications of abuse [12]. All cases of suspected child sexual abuse must be reported to Child Protective Services or police.
- When child abuse is suspect, prompt reporting to child protective services or police is mandatory to assure the safety of the child.
- Adolescents or young adults who present with injuries suspicious of battery may raise the concern about being sex or labor trafficked. All patients with injuries suspicious for battery must be interviewed privately and, depending on local legislation, law enforcement may need to be notified.

Mimickers of abuse: Several dermatologic conditions frequent raise alarm about the potential for abuse and should be considered in the differential diagnosis when evaluating for potential abuse.

- Dermal melanosis (Mongolian spots): Congenital gray-blue pigment, usually in the sacrum but often seen at remote sites. May be mistaken for bruising.
- Post-inflammatory pigmentation: Particularly when following localized eczema, post-inflammatory pigmentation can be mistaken for bruising.
- Phytophotodermatitis and lichen striatus: Both of these conditions present with linear lesions and may have bizarre patterns that raise the concern of a whip-mark or contact with a toxic chemical such as acid.
- Vasculitis: Deep purple bruise-like papules and nodules. Usually found in dependent areas.
- Staphylococcal impetigo, ecthyma, and staph-scalded skin syndrome. Toxins released from *S. aureus* can cleave the skin leaving superficial blisters that resemble burns.
- Lichen sclerosis: Scarring, porcelain-white pigment change, erosions, petechiae, and pain of the vulva can all occur in the setting of lichen sclerosis and may be

quite concerning for sexual abuse. An hour-glass shape to the pigment is a characteristic for the changes seen in lichen sclerosis. Extragenital involvement, when present, may be a clue to the diagnosis of lichen sclerosis.
- Acute genital ulceration: Acute genital ulceration also known as "Lipschutz" ulcer is a nonsexually transmitted condition seen most commonly in adolescent girls. It is most commonly, but not always, associated with EBV infection. It presents with single or multiple deep painful genital ulcerations and often occurs in the absence of any sexual contact. It follows an acute course with rapid onset and healing within approximately 6 weeks. Diagnosis is clinical and is made when other infections have been excluded.

Nonsuicidal Self-Injury

Nonsuicidal self-injury is common during adolescence and is estimated to occur in up to 25% of teens. It usually first emerges during early adolescence and is associated with depression, anxiety, eating disorders, and substance abuse. Methods of self-harm most commonly utilized are banging the skin, cutting, and biting. Often more than one type of injury can be seen. Many teens who self-injure have friends who also do so. When asked, teens report a variety of reasons for causing self-harm including the following: "get rid of bad feelings," "get control of a situation," "relieve negative emotion," and "feel something even if it is pain." Complications of self-injury can include infection and scar formation at the sites of cutting or scratching. Intralesional injections of triamcinolone (10–40 mg/ml) into hypertrophic or keloid scars can help to minimize the itch, elevation, and tenderness [13].

Dermatitis Artefacta

Dermatitis artefacta differs from nonsuicidal self-injury in that persons affected do not readily admit to causing the lesions [1]. It is most commonly seen in females, is most prevalent in teens and young adults, and may be a call for help. Skin changes often result from repetitive trauma, application of toxic substances, scratching with sharp objects, or even painted on with dye, nail polish, or lipstick. *Dermatitis artefacta* can be recognized as bizarre skin lesions that appear in an instant and are clustered in areas that can be reached by the affected individual. Direct confrontation is best avoided initially until a strong therapeutic relationship has formed. Referral to mental health is helpful though is often declined.

Social Media Fads

With the advent of social media, trends can travel quickly and potentially harmful activities catch on in friend groups and can lead to clusters of injuries. A few social media fads with dermatologic consequences have circulated recently.

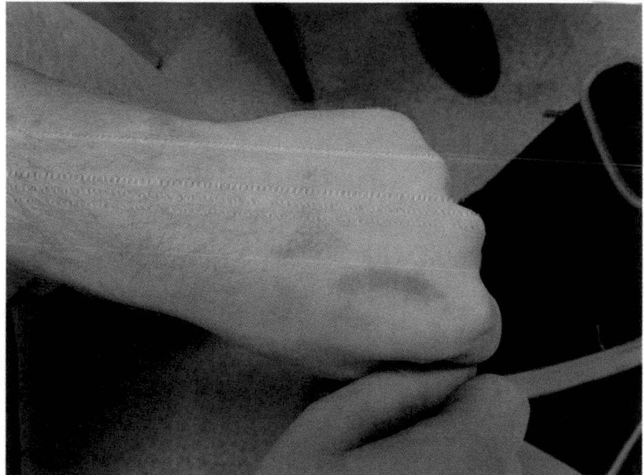

Fig. 16.23 Eraser challenge

- Salt-ice challenge: In this challenge, salt is placed on the skin and then ice is held in contact with the salt. This contact caused localized decrease in skin temperature below the freezing point and can lead to localized frostbite at the site of application.
- Fire challenge: In the fire challenge, a highly flammable liquid such as rubbing alcohol is poured onto the skin and then lit. The premise is that the liquid will flash burn and the fire will be out before the skin is burned. It puts participants at risk for severe burns.
- Eraser challenge: During the eraser challenge, the skin is rubbed with an eraser for a set duration of time, often long enough to sing the ABCs. The result is a friction burn at the site of rubbing (Fig. 16.23).
- Slime challenge: There are several variations to the slime challenge including speed-making of slime and attempts to make slime out of a variety of household chemicals. Several cases of irritant contact dermatitis have been reported in those with frequent exposure to slime.

Useful Resources Free online general dermatology resource

  - www.dermnetnz.org

- Skin infections
  - https://www.aad.org/public/diseases/contagious-skin-diseases
- Atopic dermatitis
  - https://www.aad.org/practicecenter/quality/clinical-guidelines/atopic-dermatitis/topical-therapy/topical-corticosteroids-recommendations
  - https://eczemahelp.ca/wp-content/uploads/2016/11/ESC-Atopic-Dermatitis-Practical-HCP-Guide-2nd-Ed-2016.pdf

- Bedbugs
  - https://www.cdc.gov/parasites/bedbugs/health_professionals/index.html
- Scabies
  - https://www.cdc.gov/parasites/lice/

References

1. Stratigos AJ, Stern R, Gonzalez E, Johnson RA, O'Connell J, Dover JS. Prevalence of skin disease in a cohort of shelter-based homeless men. J Am Acad Dermatol. 1999;41(2 Pt 1): 197–202.
2. Eichenfield LF, Tom WL, Berger TG, Krol A, Paller AS, Schwarzenberger K, et al. Guidelines of care for the management of atopic dermatitis: section 2. Management and treatment of atopic dermatitis with topical therapies. J Am Acad Dermatol. 2014;71(1):116–32.
3. Sidbury R, Davis DM, Cohen DE, Cordoro KM, Berger TG, Bergman JN, et al. Guidelines of care for the management of atopic dermatitis: section 3. Management and treatment with phototherapy and systemic agents. J Am Acad Dermatol. 2014;71(2):327–49.
4. Saary J, Qureshi R, Palda V, DeKoven J, Pratt M, Skotnicki-Grant S, et al. A systematic review of contact dermatitis treatment and prevention. J Am Acad Dermatol. 2005;53(5):845.
5. Eichenfield LF, Krakowski AC, Piggott C, et al. Evidence-based recommendations for the diagnosis and treatment of pediatric acne. Pediatrics. 2013;131(suppl 3):S163–86.
6. Steen CJ, Carbonaro PA, Schwartz RA. Arthropods in dermatology. J Am Acad Dermatol. 2004;50(6):819–42, quiz 42–4
7. Leung V, Miller M. Detection of scabies: a systematic review of diagnostic methods. Can J Infect Dis Med Microbiol. 2011;22(4):143–6.
8. Thomas I, Kihiczak GG, Schwartz RA. Bedbug bites: a review. Int J Dermatol. 2004;43(6):430–3.
9. Goette DK. Chilblains (perniosis). J Am Acad Dermatol. 1990;23(2 Pt 1):257–62.
10. Fink B, Landthaler M, Hafner C. Skin alterations due to abuse of illegal drugs. JDDG. 2011;9:633–9.
11. Jinna S, Livingston N, Moles R. Cutaneous signs of abuse: Kids are not just little people. Clin Dermatol. 2017;35:504–11.
12. Moy JA, Sanchez MR. The cutaneous manifestations of violence and poverty. Arch Dermatol. 1992;128(6):829–39.
13. Lloyd-Richardson EE, Perrine N, Dierker L, Kelley ML. Characteristics and functions of non-suicidal self-injury in a community sample of adolescents. Psychol Moed. 2007;387(8):1183–92.

Chapter 17
Challenges Faced by International Migrants and Refugees to the Health, Development, and Well-Being of Adolescents and Youth

Curren Warf, Evelyn Eisenstein, Abdul Karim AlMakadma, John Howard, Diana Birch, Irene Jillson, and Grant Charles

Part 1: The Scope of Displacement and the Rights of Refugees Under International Agreements

Introduction: The Scope of Displacement

The World Health Organization estimates that globally there are currently 272 million international migrants (up from 150 million in 2000), of whom 25.9 million are refugees (up from 14 million in 2000) and 763 million internal migrants. This represents 3.5% or one in seven of the world's population. There has been an

C. Warf (✉)
Department of Pediatrics (Retired), Division of Adolescent Health and Medicine, British Columbia Children's Hospital, University of British Columbia, Vancouver, BC, Canada

E. Eisenstein
University of the State of Rio de Janeiro, Rio de Janeiro, Brazil

A. K. AlMakadma
College of Medicine, Alfaisal University, Riyadh, Saudi Arabia
e-mail: abalmakadma@alfaisal.edu

J. Howard
National Drug and Alcohol Research Centre, UNSW Medicine | Faculty of Medicine, University of New South Wales – Sydney, Sydney, NSW, Australia

D. Birch
Youth Support, London, UK
e-mail: drdbirch@youthsupport.net

I. Jillson
Department of Family Medicine, Georgetown University School of Medicine, Washington, DC, USA

G. Charles
School of Social Work, University of British Columbia, Vancouver, BC, Canada

C. Warf, G. Charles (eds.), *Clinical Care for Homeless, Runaway and Refugee Youth*, https://doi.org/10.1007/978-3-030-40675-2_17

almost 50% increase since 2000 and a higher number than ever in human history. About 86% of these people are now hosted by developing countries. There were 41.3 million internally displaced people in 125 countries in 2019 (up from 21 million in 2000). These people were displaced primarily by disasters (24.2 million) or conflict and violence (6.9 million in 37 countries). There are about 13 million child refugees, 936,000 asylum-seeking children, and 17 million children who have been forcibly displaced inside their own countries. This is a doubling of numbers since 2000 [1].

The majority of international migrants leave for work or education or to rejoin family. Of international migrants, 65 million have been forcibly displaced [2]. The largest number of displaced people were hosted by Asia (14.7 million), followed by Africa (6.3 million), Europe (3.5 million), North America (970,000), and Latin America and the Caribbean (420,000). According to the International Organization of Migration [3], by the end of 2016, there were a total of 22.5 million refugees with 20.4 million under the auspices of the United Nations High Commissioner on Refugees (UNHCR) mandate. Additionally, there are 5.5 million refugees registered by the United Nations Relief and Works Agency (UNRWA) for Palestinian Refugees in the Near East, marking the highest number of refugees on record. The crisis of refugees has rapidly expanded with the rapid growth of the conflicts in the Middle East and the state sponsored genocide of the Rohingya in Myanmar.

A large portion of global migrants and refugees are children, recently estimated to be about 31 million, of whom 13 million are child refugees, 936,000 asylum-seeking children, and 17 million who had been forcibly displaced within their country of origin [3–5]. An estimated 75,000 unaccompanied and separated children lodged an individual asylum application in 70 countries in 2016. This is thought to be an underestimation of the true number of unaccompanied and separated children [6].

A special subcategory within the overall population are irregular (undocumented) migrants and refugees; these are individuals who leave their home displaced by violence, persecution, environmental catastrophe, or poverty or for other reasons to enter a country without legal documents or permission. The exact numbers of people within this category are notoriously difficult to determine and are not known given that they operate out of official sight [7].

The only existing database on global migrant fatalities is the International Organization for Migration's Missing Migrants Project [7]. Refugees are the migrant population most likely to be victims of human trafficking [8]. They are also most likely to die while attempting to migrate. Commonly, bodies are lost in the desert at the US-Mexico border, in the Mediterranean Sea in attempted passage from North Africa to Europe, and in other situations. Data about deaths is not aggregated according to migration status, adolescents are confounded with adults, and child deaths are often not recorded [7]. Frequently what one is left with are news reports of disturbing tragedies.

International refugees and migrants face grave barriers in obtaining basic healthcare. These barriers vary according to migration status. Irregular or undocumented migrants frequently arrive without legal documents or permits, are subject to detention and deportation, are most excluded, and face the greatest barriers to access healthcare [9, 10]. They may only be able to access care if they pay the entire cost of care or in emergency circumstances. These barriers inherently exclude them from preventive services or primary care and force children, youth, and their families to wait until medical conditions are more advanced and expensive to treat if they access health services at all.

Migrants' access to healthcare demands urgent attention. According to the World Health Organization, and in accordance with international human rights frameworks, all WHO member states, including Canada, the United States, and other developed countries, should commit to protecting the right to health and the right to access health services for migrants, refugees, and asylum seekers regardless of migration status [11, 12].

Factors Driving Migration

There are five major factors that drive large-scale migration including (1) poverty and economic insecurity, (2) social violence in the country of origin, (3) extreme ethnic persecution, (4) active warfare, and (5) climate and environmental change. While there is, unfortunately, an almost endless list of examples within each category, the following provides an overview of the current state of affairs.

Poverty and Economic Insecurity

Poverty and economic insecurity have traditionally played the major role in motivating migration. This remains the case in much of the world, though paradoxically migrants may move to a situation where they are even more economically marginalized and insecure and are no better off than where they had left. However, the drive for more opportunities, especially for one's children, is strong and persistent. It is important to remember that poverty and economic stagnation in the developing world is commonly the historic and ongoing colonial legacy of economic and political exploitation.

Social Violence

A second driver of migration is social violence in the country of origin. This has been a particularly significant factor for those migrants to the United States from Central America and recently from Mexico. The violence originates from gangs, police or the military, ethnic persecution, or interpersonal violence and in particular violence directed against women and sexual minorities [13]. While data in this area is sparse, the persecution of LGBT adults and youth clearly plays a major role, sometimes under the guise of "moral cleansing" [14].

Ethnic Persecution

A third factor is extreme ethnic persecution which creates situations from which people flee in mass. Extreme ethnic persecution forced the Rohingya population to leave Myanmar in 2017. Their only crime seems to be living as a discernible Islamic and ethnic minority in a predominantly Buddhist country. They were driven without possessions from their land to Bangladesh; in Bangladesh they became "stateless persons" as well as displaced refugees [1]. Similarly, peoples such as those of the Yazidi religious faith have been forced to flee Syria, and indigenous peoples forced to flee Guatemala. There are many other examples.

Active Warfare

A fourth cause of migration is active warfare involving the military of various countries that has created intolerable conditions for children and families. This commonly results in the destruction of the healthcare and educational systems. Highly destructive weapons including cluster bombs, targeted aerial bombings of hospitals, and other social infrastructure commonly occur. There are many examples of this including Yemen, Iraq, Afghanistan, and Syria. Most of these wars can be understood as attempts by outside powers to extend their influence or carry out purportedly strategic maneuvers, with no meaningful regard for the well-being of the local people. With the destruction of the health infrastructure, potable water supplies, and sewage systems, infectious diseases become major threats; as an example, Yemen is currently experiencing the largest cholera epidemic in recorded human history. An estimated 41.3 million people were displaced by conflict and violence in 2018, the highest on record since monitoring was initiated by the Internal Displacement Monitoring Centre in 1998 [1].

Climate Change

The fifth and a growing cause of migration is climate and environmental change. This is perhaps the least understood of the factors driving migration and, as such, requires additional attention in this chapter. Climate change plays a significant and growing role in the displacement of populations. In 2018 approximately 61% or 17.2 million of the world's internally displaced population was caused by natural disasters. Although being seen throughout the world, the Western Pacific is particularly prone to extreme weather events with floods, droughts, rising sea levels, and storm surges including tsunamis, cyclones, and typhoons that are expected to become more frequent and more severe due to the impact of global warming and climate change [15, 16].

A prime example of the health impact of climate change occurred in March 2019, when two subsequent cyclones, driven by global warming, devastated Mozambique, Zimbabwe, and Malawi, destroying the homes and crops of some 2 million people [17]. This destruction was shortly followed by an epidemic of cholera, with the expectation that malaria, dengue fever, and measles will soon become widespread. HIV treatment has been interrupted. Starvation is emerging as a significant threat [18].

Global warming is also having an escalating effect in the Americas, with more frequent and more powerful hurricanes affecting the environment of Caribbean island nations and on indigenous communities in South America. Low-lying densely populated urban areas in many countries are threatened, for example, New Orleans in Louisiana, USA, and Jakarta, Indonesia, are increasingly subjected to widespread flooding.

Migration and human displacement from rural to urban areas, and between countries and continents driven by climate change-related drought, crop failure, and food shortages, as well as outbreaks of infectious diseases including cholera outbreaks and measles among unvaccinated migrants and refugees, will be significant [19].

Climate change is also an emerging factor in driving migration from Central America and Mexico to North America. Rising temperatures and drought have affected food production, wiping out harvests and leaving families destitute. A large proportion of people in Central America live in rural areas and are especially vulnerable to climate change and drought. An estimated 82% of maize and bean crops were lost in Honduras due to drought conditions in Central America that put about 3 million people at risk for food insecurity [1]. The World Bank concluded that over the next three decades, 1.4 million people could be driven to leave their homes in Mexico and Central America due to climate change [20].

In addition to the extreme weather events mentioned above, much of the world's population will be subject to extreme recurrent heat waves profoundly affecting agriculture, food production and supplies, and availability of potable water, with flooding of coastal and low-lying areas of the world. This will force widespread migration disrupting core public health infrastructure and overwhelm health services. Lower-income communities and marginalized populations, with lower capacity to prepare for and cope with extreme weather and climate-related events, are expected to experience greater impacts.

Climate change increasingly threatens indigenous communities' livelihoods, economies, health, and cultural identities by disrupting social, physical, and ecological systems [21]. These effects will take place worldwide in the coming years in North America, Latin America, Asia, sub-Saharan Africa, and the Middle East. Climate change is truly a global crisis that will continue to escalate and unfold, inevitably give rise to increased forced migration, and threaten the world of future generations for the foreseeable future. With the effects of global warming expected to increase, the number of environmental migrants is expected to reach from 200 million to 1 billion people by 2050 [22].

The 2018 report from Lancet *Countdown on health and climate change: shaping the health of nations for centuries to come* [23], *the Fourth National Climate Assessment* [24] released in 2018, and the 2018 *IPCC Special Report, Global Warming of 1.5 C; Summary for Policymakers* [25] provide overwhelming scientific evidence for the advance of global warming and impending disastrous effects on human health with inevitable widespread migration.

New Factors Enabling Migration and the "Healthy Immigrant Effect"

In addition to the aforementioned core factors, there are a number of influences that make migration more accessible including the digital revolution, lower travel costs, and improved technology and feasibility of travel. Another influence is the desire to access health services.

It is important to appreciate that migration does not always have a negative impact and may open opportunities for the future of the individual, the family and, significantly, the receiving country. Immigrant populations frequently experience better health than native populations [26]. This "healthy immigrant effect" may be due to self-selection of voluntary immigrants with educated, wealthy, and healthy people being more likely to have opportunities to immigrate and the exclusion of poorly resourced and less healthy migrants at immigration pre-screening.

The "healthy immigrant effect" does not exist for forced migrant populations who flee armed conflict or ethnic persecution, as forced migration is involuntary, occurs on short notice, and impacts all classes of the community [27]. Even within situations of migration for economic opportunities, there can be detrimental consequences. Parents who migrate for economic opportunities, whether internally or internationally, commonly leave young children and adolescents behind for extended periods. This loss of primary consistent attachment figure is known to have pernicious negative effects on the emotional well-being and development of children and youth.

International Agreements on the Right to Health for Migrants and Refugees

The right to health is a fundamental, internationally recognized, and ratified human right. The right to health is recognized in the inherent dignity of the equal and inalienable rights of all members of the human family by the United Nations Universal Declaration of Human Rights signed in 1948 by all countries which states that:

> Everyone has the right to a standard of living adequate for the health and well-being of himself and of his family [28]

The International Covenant on Economic, Social and Cultural Rights clearly expresses that the right to health obligates governments to ensure that:

> Health facilities, goods and services are accessible to all, especially the most vulnerable or marginalized sections of the population in law and in fact, without discrimination on any of the prohibited grounds [29].

The right to health for refugees and migrants is recognized in the International Framework of Human Rights elaborated by the Member States of the United Nations and is upheld by international human rights law [30]. These rights are further affirmed by the United Nations High Commissioner for Refugees (UNHCR) Convention Relating to the Status of Refugees [31, 32].

The World Health Organization Constitution affirms that "the highest attainable standard of health is one of the fundamental rights of every human being" [33].

Basic principles advocated by the World Health Organization include [34]:

1. Promoting universal health coverage
2. Reducing mortality and morbidity among refugees and migrants through public health interventions
3. Protecting and improving the health and well-being of women and girls
4. Promoting continuity of care
5. Promoting gender equality and empowering women and girls
6. Improving communication and countering xenophobia
7. Strengthening partnerships, coordination, and collaboration

Accessibility of Healthcare

The UN Committee on Economic, Social and Cultural Rights comments that implementing the International Covenant on Economic, Social and Cultural Rights entails "being able to receive care which is available, accessible, acceptable and of good quality." Accessibility is described in four dimensions: non-discrimination, physical accessibility, economic accessibility and information accessibility [35].

Nutrition, Water, Housing, and Sanitation

The UN Committee on Economic, Social and Cultural Rights states that the right to health must be interpreted broadly to embrace key socioeconomic factors that promote conditions in which people can lead a healthy life. These include "food and nutrition, housing, access to safe and potable water and adequate sanitation, safe and healthy working conditions, and a healthy environment" [36].

Attaining Health Equity for Migrants and Refugees

In addition to the universal right to healthcare, the special needs of migrants and refugees have to be taken into account. The United Nations High Commissioner on Refugees (UNHCR) holds that ensuring the health of refugees and other forcibly displaced people is a key priority and advocates:

1. Cost-free essential primary healthcare and emergency services during an emergency
2. Childhood vaccinations
3. Prenatal and delivery care
4. Communicable disease control

The World Health Organization holds that universal health coverage is a key aspect of the right to health [37] and is defined as:

> Ensuring that all people have access to needed promotive, preventative, curative, and rehabilitative health services, of sufficient quality to be effective, while also ensuring that people do not suffer financial hardship when paying for these services [38].

The "WHO Rapid Review: Addressing the Health Needs of Refugees and Migrants" states:

> The inclusion of migrants, refugees and asylum seekers in Universal Health Care policies and financial protection is imperative to uphold the right to health and access to health services for these populations. States should consider linking Universal Health Care for migrants and refugees to the entitlements of the local population.... Reforms to include migrants, refugees and asylum seekers in universal health coverage schemes will require strong political decisions from agencies outside the health sector that govern migration and labor policies [39].

Inclusion of migrants and refugees in Universal Health Care is a human rights imperative because they may be vulnerable to discrimination and exploitation and their access to healthcare may be hampered by political, legal, economic, cultural, and practical barriers [40]. The location of refugees and migrants can vary widely, whether they reside in urban areas, refugee camps, or urban areas, whether in poor or wealthy nations; all need access to healthcare.

Health status and health equity for immigrants, in particular children and youth, is not solely the result of health policy or health services but requires a willingness of policy makers as well as clinicians and public health officials to address political and socioeconomic factors and institutions that affect migrant and refugee health. Their health depends on sectors other than healthcare including education, employment, food access, housing, water, sanitation, family cohesion, transportation, and more. In addressing challenges to the health of refugees and migrants, including children and adolescents, it is important to grasp the complexity of the challenges they face [41].

The health of migrant and refugee communities can be affected positively or negatively by social policy changes. For example, reduction of funding for welfare, housing, hospitals, and community agencies can result in reduced access to healthcare, housing instability, homelessness, lack of employment, increased social isolation, deterioration of mental health, and increase in family violence [41] with profound and lasting impact on the physical and mental health of children and youth.

Examples of Existing Models of Provision of Universal Health Coverage for Migrants

A number of European Union countries provide irregular (or undocumented) migrants with insurance coverage in the national health system, even without financial contributions [40]. In 2010, France, Italy, Netherlands, Portugal, and Spain gave "undocumented migrants access to virtually the same range of services as nationals of that country" [42]. These serve as model approaches of what can be accomplished.

Each member country of the Association of Southeast Asian Nations (ASEAN) – including Indonesia, Malaysia, the Philippines, Singapore, and Thailand – provides a system of Migrant Inclusion Health Insurance, each unique to the country [43].

In 2014, the 53rd Directing Council of the Pan American Health Organization the Member States approved the Strategy for Universal Access to Health and Universal Health Coverage as the overarching framework for health system action to protect the health and well-being of migrants. In April 2017, the ministers of health and health authorities of Latin American countries signed the Ministerial Declaration on Migration and Health in Mesoamerica which recognizes the commitment to improve the health of migrants. In November 2017, the South American Conference on Migration highlighted the importance of inclusive public policies on migration that consider migrants to be "under the same conditions as nationals in the host country regardless of their origin, nationality, or immigration status."

Education for Migrant Children and Young People: A Key Determinant of Health

Education is a key determinant of health, and schools are common points of access for nutrition, health education, healthcare, and counseling for children and youth. Education is integral to the improvement of population health. Refugee and migrant children commonly have challenges in accessing education related to lack of fluency in the language of their new home, prior interruption of education for months or years, and commonly a need to catch up with peers; they may also struggle in school because of post-traumatic repercussions and learning disabilities.

For children and youth who have missed out on their education due to circumstances they had no control over, there may be accelerated learning programs available to complete primary education in a shorter period of time providing certification and allowing continuation in formal post primary education.

Education is essential for refugee and migrant children, youth, and adults to fully participate in their new society and can play a signal role in enabling economically and socially marginalized children and adults to leave poverty.

Indigenous people who are refugees and migrants, including children and adolescents, face additional barriers when migrating. They have commonly been traumatized by military persecution prior to leaving and do not speak the dominant language – for example, indigenous refugees fleeing persecution in Guatemala who arrive in the United States commonly speak neither English nor Spanish, have poor educational background, and face significant barriers in integrating into the host society, including accessing education, housing, and healthcare.

The process of immigration can take months or years. During this period refugee children and youth may languish in refugee camps, not attend school, or live in areas where their native language is not spoken. They may not have opportunities to develop job skills; participate in healthy opportunities of leisure, sports, or recreation; and at times be further traumatized. It is essential that in environments where children and youth are held, including refugee camps and temporary shelters, their educational needs be prioritized to prepare them for social integration and employment at the earliest opportunity.

In the United States, all children are entitled to free public education and specialized educational services regardless of immigration status [44].

All migrants and refugees have the right to education as articulated by the Universal Declaration of Human Rights, the UN Conventions on the Rights of the Child, and multiple other international agreements [45].

Reducing Morbidity and Mortality Through Public Health Interventions

Prevention of Communicable Diseases

One of the key priorities of the World Health Organization is the provision of vaccinations for vaccine preventable diseases [46]. Key infectious diseases such as measles, mumps, rubella, polio, and hepatitis B are high-priority targets for vaccination, particularly in migrant communities [47]. Many migrants and refugees may not have had access to vaccines or may not understand local vaccination programs; in addition, there have been high rates of dropout from universal vaccination programs, and records remain incomplete or lost, so that many migrant children either have lack of vaccination or the status is unknown [48].

It is important to make available written material about immunizations and other health interventions in the first language of the recipients of care whenever possible. There is evidence that written material in the patient's language is associated with improved trust in the healthcare provider and lead to improved vaccination rates [49].

Current guidelines recommend catchup immunizations for migrant children with incomplete or absent vaccination records, which has been shown to be effective [50]. Under conditions when vaccination records are not available among displaced persons and refugees, there is some evidence that mass vaccination for measles can be cost-effective and more effective than targeted immunization [51]. It is essential that all children and youth be screened for tuberculosis with evaluation, treatment, and monitoring.

Immunizations

For families in refugee camps, in addition to the common childhood vaccines, other vaccines may be indicated such as oral cholera vaccine as had been utilized in refugee and internally displaced person camps in Iraq [52]. Promotion of regular handwashing with access to clean water has been shown to be effective in reducing transmission of cholera.

During periods of emergency displacement of people, there are commonly outbreaks of HIV and TB, as well as outbreaks of malaria in specific areas of Africa and Asia. It is important to continually evaluate trends of these conditions and respond effectively [53].

Potable Water

Armed conflict and climate disasters related to global warming both threaten availability of potable water to large populations threatening large populations. In particular, cholera, once thought to have been relegated to history, has had repeated grave outbreaks. In 2018 cyclones devastated Mozambique and cholera emerged as a major threat to the population. In 2010, a historic outbreak of cholera took place in Haiti following devastation of an earthquake with flooding and contamination of the water supply. Cholera remains a problem in Haiti.

The comparative incidence of cholera in Haiti has been far exceeded by the continuing catastrophe in Yemen where cholera remains at unprecedented epidemic proportions since 2016–2017; the World Health Organization has stated that, with over one million cases, this is among the worst epidemics of cholera in recorded human history. This epidemic is directly related to the systematic destruction of the sanitation system and water supplies through aerial bombing by Saudi Arabia.

Consequences of Malnutrition

Prior to migration, children and youth may have experienced significant malnutrition over an extended period of time at early developmental stages which can lead to pernicious learning disabilities in addition to pubertal delay for adolescents and other signs of malnutrition. It is essential in the course of stabilization that particular effort be made to assure regular and reliable access to adequate food and nutrition, housing, water, and toilet and bathing facilities.

Protecting and Improving the Health and Well-Being of Girls and Young Women

The WHO recognizes that "gender equality is not simply a female issue and can only be achieved through partnership between women and men and girls and boys… (it) implies that the interests, needs and priorities of both women and men are taken into consideration" [54] and that "Capacity building programmes for women migrants and refugees, and strategies for strengthening women's participation and leadership can be adapted for different cultures and local contexts" [55]. "Extensive research indicates that a gendered divide exists for equal opportunity in many societies globally. Whilst discrimination affects all women, a disproportionate effect is evident for those further marginalised by refugee or migrant status" [56]. "Informed by age, religion, race, ethnicity, disability, displaced women and children are at higher risk of sexual and gender-based violence and harassment and humiliation. Migration can challenge traditional gender-roles and compromise accessibility to services" [57].

Reproductive Health

Across the spectrum of sexual and reproductive health, it is essential to acknowledge the heterogeneity of women's beliefs and the influence these beliefs have on how, when, and why women access sexual and reproductive health services [58]. Migrant women and girls are an exceedingly diverse group, and sexual and reproductive health is shaped by economic and migration status, ethnicity, culture, religion, gender, and family and personal experiences [59].

Migrant and refugee women, particularly those under age 20, who have limited language proficiency and education, single, and/or have an unplanned pregnancy are most vulnerable to not seeking care [60]. Young women who are pregnant and seeking asylum may avoid prenatal care for fear of facing deportation or due to perceived lack of service eligibility and fears related to registering with the authorities that may lead to deportation [61]. This may be further complicated by local clinical service providers and others in the healthcare workforce lack of familiarity with eligibility qualifications and policies [61].

Though highly diverse, young migrant women and girls commonly come from backgrounds of economic hardship, have limited knowledge of how to access the existing healthcare system, and have few resources. When they seek work in a new country, they are often paid extremely low wages and are unable to afford decent housing accommodation, or they might have to travel extensive distances for work, putting further strain on limited resources and reducing accessibility to civil and health services. Women's lack of access to the labor market leads to lower-paying and less regulated jobs, including domestic work. This may expose women to exploitation and human trafficking. A new Counter Trafficking Data Collaborative (CTDC) providing the first data on global human trafficking has identified over 40,000 registrants from 107 countries, 54% women, 20% girls, 22% men, and 5% boys. There were regional differences in the types of trafficking with the Americas predominately sex trafficking, Europe predominately labor trafficking, and Asia and Africa with relatively similar proportions [62].

Housing is a potential area of disadvantage and inequality for women, especially where women are seeking refuge from a violent partner. Women, unable to find work, may be at greater risk for physical or sexual exploitation causing inequalities to become further entrenched [63]. They commonly also have linguistic barriers that can significantly impair access to healthcare and health education [59]. They may have little idea of their rights and what resources are (or are not) available. Whatever access they may have had to family planning or contraception has likely been interrupted and discontinued during the migration process [64].

The Columbia University Mailman School of Public Health has developed "The Reproductive Health Access, Information and Services in Emergencies" (RAISE) model of ensuring good quality comprehensive reproductive health services in emergency situations [65]. The five main areas of focus for RAISE are:

1. Basic and comprehensive emergency obstetric care, including post-abortion care
2. All family planning methods and emergency contraception
3. Sexually transmitted infection prevention and treatment
4. HIV prevention, including voluntary counseling and testing, prevention of mother to child transmission, and referral and medical response
5. Referral for gender-based violence

Since 2011, the RAISE initiative has had a more intensive focus on contraceptive services and abortion-related services in humanitarian settings to address significant gaps in service [66].

Challenges to Mental Health

There are many factors associated with becoming a migrant or refugee associated with severe challenges to mental illness including personal experience of trauma, loss of loved ones (especially parents and siblings), social isolation, barriers to access to care, experiencing ethnic, gender or religious discrimination, and erratic access to and utilization of services. All of these can precipitate negative mental health outcomes [67].

Many refugees and asylum seekers, in particular children and youth, have survived significant traumatic experiences. The mental health impact of these experiences varies according to the developmental level of the child or youth. The strongest protection that children have to protect them from these exceedingly difficult and critical experiences is the consistent support and presence of their parent or consistent caregiver, usually their mother and/or father. Forced separation from parents, loss of parents, or incapacity of parents because of their own trauma can be developmentally devastating for children. This is particularly so under circumstances of migration when the past community has been lost, contact with grandparents and extended family members and friends is impossible, and there has been a disruption of relationships with familiar friends and peers.

Policies that result in the involuntary and unjustified separation of children and youth from parents or caregivers, particularly for prolonged periods, lead to significant psychological trauma and reduce resiliency. In working to attain health equity, it is of high importance to consider the cultural and language barriers and maximize efforts to recruit health personnel who are aware and culturally competent to address these barriers.

The UN Conventions on the Rights of the Child Article 9 states that:

> States Parties shall ensure that a child shall not be separated from his or her parents against their will, except when competent authorities subject to judicial review determine, in accordance with applicable law and procedure, that such separation is necessary for the best interests of the child...such as one involving abuse or neglect of the child by the parents, or one where the parents are living separately and a decision must be made as to the child's place of residence [68].

The Society for Adolescent Health and Medicine issued a Statement on Forced Family Separation stating:

> It is deeply and profoundly damaging to the emotional development and health of any child or adolescent to be involuntarily separated from their mother or father and this separation can affect their emotional and physical health and development for their entire lives. This inhumane approach conflicts with our society's, our families' and our profession's most fundamental responsibility to protect children and adolescents [69].

In addition, children and youth in the course of migration or when encountering the new society may experience assault or trauma, including sexual assault and/or exploitation. Some may have been involved in survival sex or coerced into prostitution. Under some circumstances, youth may have been forced to participate as child soldiers. All of these experiences greatly endanger the mental health and well-being of the child and youth. Under the most grave circumstance, children and youth may have survived war, lost family members, survived significant injuries, or even experienced torture. Displacement, loss of family and loved ones, survival of war, and postmigration detention put them at higher risk for morbidity from mental health conditions [70].

The result of severe trauma may lead to multiple mental health diagnoses. It is essential to keep in mind that the spectrum and complexity of children and youth's response to trauma and loss of loved ones can have varied and pernicious effects. The diagnostic label is less important than finding stability and reconciliation.

Refugee women and girls may have survived armed conflict and experienced significant trauma and loss, including sexual assault, intimate partner violence, or loss of offspring or male partner. Under some circumstances, young refugee women may have participated in sex work or survival sex and carry a high risk for sexually transmitted infection, including HIV [71].

Migration factors that affect mental health

Premigration	Migration	Postmigration
Adult		
Economic, educational, and occupational status in country of origin	Trajectory (route, duration)	Uncertainty about immigration or refugee status
Disruption of social support, roles, and network	Exposure to harsh living conditions (e.g., refugee camps)	Unemployment or underemployment
Trauma (type, severity, perceived level of threat, number of episodes)	Exposure to violence	Loss of social status
Political involvement (commitment to a cause)	Disruption of family and community networks Uncertainty about outcome of migration	Loss of family and community social supports. Concern about family members left behind and possibility for reunification Difficulties in language learning, acculturation, and adaptation (e.g., change in sex roles)
Child		
Age and developmental stage at migration	Separation from parent/caregiver/community/extended family	Separation from parent/caregiver Stresses related to family's adaptation Security of housing and food
Disruption of education	Exposure to violence	Difficulties with education in new language
Separation from extended family and peer networks	Exposure to harsh living conditions (e.g., refugee camps) Poor nutrition	Acculturation (e.g., ethnic and religious identity; sex role conflicts; intergenerational conflict within family) Discrimination and social exclusion (at school or with peers)

Kirmayer, L. J., Narasiah, L., Munoz, M., Rashid, M., Ryder, A. G., Guzder, J., Hassan, G., Rousseau, C., Pottie, K., Canadian Collaboration for Immigrant and Refugee Health (CCIRH) (2011). Common mental health problems in immigrants and refugees: general approach in primary care. *CMAJ*: *Canadian Medical Association journal = journal de l'Association medicale canadienne*, *183*(12), E959–67

Fostering Recovery

Critical in their recovery is security of home; presence of familiar and loved adults, especially parents and siblings; and reliable access to food and nutrition. The immigration process in the accepting country can foster resiliency either by respecting and maintaining these critical relationships, promoting safety, food security, housing, and education, or may complicate the child or youth's trauma by separating him or her from their mother and father and put them in postmigration detention disrupting their core relationships. These practices are destined to complicate the mental health of youth as they mature.

Valuing Resiliency

It is critical that those who care for children who have survived these traumatic experiences be aware that children and youth are frequently capable of great resilience despite traumatic beginnings, provided that they are given stability, love, education, and opportunities to develop skills and a sense of self. Understanding the cultural assets that migrant children, youth, and families bring and facilitating dialog that supports these families as valuable resources to society can support integration and foster resilience [44]. Management of children and youth does not only need multidisciplinary experts but the involvement of experts or trained persons from within the same culture fluent in the same language.

Mental Health Assessment and Human Rights Violations

Clinicians need to consider the intersection of mental health assessment and treatment with human rights violations, and the impact of restrictive immigration policies on asylum seekers and refugees, and also on clinicians, clinical practice, and professional ethics.

There needs to be routine screening and ongoing assessment that includes use of child- and adolescent-specific, recognized valid, culturally appropriate clinical diagnostic and treatment tools and clinician ratings.

Unaccompanied Children and Youth

Unaccompanied children have specific needs – age and vulnerability place them at particular risk for exploitation and abuse, violence, forced labor, and denial of education and basic services, including health. Their specific circumstances need to be recognized and their needs provided for like adequate nutrition, sleeping conditions, and vaccinations. Unaccompanied children and youth need stabilization, recognition, and acknowledgement of their language and cultural background; engagement in education, sports, arts, and skill building; and the opportunity to develop consistent relationships with caring adults.

Unhindered and prompt referrals for health professionals need to be responded to in a timely manner with efficient non-bureaucratic processes in place for evacuation and transfer to the most appropriate specialist care.

Avoidance of Bias

Healthcare providers bring their own personal cultural biases that can implicitly or explicitly affect the provision of care [44]. It is essential that providers bring both a sense of cultural humility (the concept of openness and respect for differences) and cultural safety (the recognition of the power differences and inequities in health and the clinical encounter that result from social, historical, economic, and political circumstances). Cultural humility and safety are demonstrated through the values of empathy, curiosity, and respect [44]. The use of disparaging language requires particular attention. Terms such as "boat people," "illegals," "queue jumpers," and equating asylum seekers, refugees, and unauthorized arrivals with "criminals" create unwarranted fear among citizens of what will happen if they are released into the community. The exaggeration of any crime committed by a few and racial profiling feed into this. Harsh political rhetoric with nativist and racist themes characterizing migrants as criminals or with other slurs need to be challenged and exposed. Terms that obscure their plight and status and deny political responsibilities under international treaties and conventions need to be challenged.

Lessons Learned, Program Models, Best Practices, Policy Directions

Effective program models include training and motivating young people to participate in all the daily activities and needs. Youth can work as teachers for the youngest, paramedics, nursing assistants, sanitation workers, sports coaches, and mentors and in other areas; through this participation, they not only contribute to the betterment of the conditions of children and youth but also develop meaningful education and practical skills that can play a significant role in their own recovery. Effective programs allow and encourage capable young people to be productive and to participate in jobs and activities that help their communities, to improve their physical and living environments – including camps – and to become strong, clean, fun, and optimistic; they should not be encouraged to be totally dependent on others, but to be productive and develop skills and make a contribution. Many can do well in teaching, development of sanitation, cooking and food preparation, first aid and clinical assistance, marketing, selling, and even peer counselling with mentorship.

Part 2: The Health and Treatment of Child and Adolescent Refugees and Migrants in Host Countries

....

Migrant and Refugee Children and Adolescents in the United States

The New Colossus
by Emma Lazarus, November 2, 1883
Poem of the Statue of Liberty in New York Harbor welcoming immigrants to America

Keep, ancient lands, your storied pomp!" cries she
With silent lips. "Give me your tired, your poor,
Your huddled masses yearning to be free,
The wretched refuse of your teeming shore.
Send these, the homeless, tempest-tost to me,
I lift my lamp beside the golden door!

The United States can be fairly described as a "nation of immigrants" and their descendants (with the notable exceptions of indigenous peoples and the descendants of enslaved people brought forcibly from Africa over the initial 400 years of European settlement). New waves of immigrants have frequently faced harsh and continuing discrimination in becoming integrated into society.

The challenges migrants and refugees from Mexico and Latin America face who enter and survive in the United States go back many decades. Immigrants have come to the United States for many decades as agricultural workers and other laborers, some starting new businesses and contributing greatly to the growth of the US economy. Many immigrants stayed, raised children and grandchildren. Immigrants and their descendants joined various professions, served in the military, and became health professionals.

Separation of Migrant Children and Adolescents from Their Parents

Beginning in 2017 and continuing through 2019 and beyond, the treatment of migrants has undergone qualitative changes with the growth of xenophobia in the United States. In the spring of 2018, the US administration proclaimed a "zero tolerance" immigration policy requiring the separation of all children, including infants through adolescents, from their parents. As of December 2018, 2737 children who had been involuntarily separated from their parents were identified. However, documentation was found that the separations had actually begun over 6 months earlier, in 2017, than had initially been reported and that over 700, and likely over 2000, additional migrant children had been taken [72]. This action took place in the absence of a coordinated formal tracking system between the relevant federal agencies of the Department of Homeland Security (DHS), which separated the children from their parents, and the Office of Refugee Resettlement, Health and Human Services, which took the children, so that many were not able to be located for reunification with parents. The government's own lawyer acknowledged that the executive order contained no procedure to reunify the children *and* allowed the government to continue separating families. By its own admission, the government had lost track of 40 parents and deported 400 others without their children. Spokespeople for the government then declared that they were not responsible for the reunification of families but advised using a network of volunteers and non-profit organizations to do so [73].

In January 2019 about 1500 unaccompanied and undocumented teenagers aged 13–17 years were held in the Tornillo single tent encampment in the Texas desert; the camp had an initial capacity of 360 but had been rapidly expanded. This shelter is on federal property and is not licensed by Texas child welfare officials so that it does not have to adhere to the same standards and regulations of other migrant youth shelters. There is an additional migrant youth shelter at a former Walmart Supercenter in Brownsville, Texas, with a capacity of 1401 youth. As of October 2, 2018, there were 13,289 migrant children held according to federal data [74]. Officials of the Customs and Border Protection, the Department of Homeland Security agency responsible for separating families, estimated in November 2019 that they anticipated separating 26,000 children without plans or means to reunify them with their parents [75].

The policy of taking children was portrayed by the administration as a key effort to deter migrant families from trying to enter the United States from the Southwest border, the common area of migration for those fleeing violence and deep poverty in Central America. Involuntary separation of children from parents was highly traumatizing for both children and parents, in many cases leaving parents without any idea of where their children were and placing children in foster care facilities hundreds or thousands of miles away from where their parents were held. Additional policies prevented placing children with relatives. Children were transported to scattered facilities throughout the United States, while parents were generally held in facilities at the border [72]. Adolescents were removed from federal shelters on their 18th birthday, when they became legal adults, and transported in ankle chains to adult detention facilities [76]. The border was effectively militarized with tear gas assaults carried out on parents and children waiting at the border [77].

The American Academy of Pediatrics released a statement strongly condemning these practices on June 15, 2018 [78], stating "Separating children from their parents contradicts everything we stand for as pediatricians-protecting and promoting children's health. We know that family separation causes irreparable harm to children." The AAP also stated in September 2019 that "Both the separation of children from their parents and the detention of children with parents as a tool of law enforcement are inhumane, counterproductive, and threatening to short- and long-term health. Immigration authorities should not separate children from their parents nor place children in detention" [44].

The Society for Adolescent Health and Medicine also issued a Statement on Forced Family Separation stating:

> "It is deeply and profoundly damaging to the emotional development and health of any child or adolescent to be involuntarily separated from their mother or father and this separation can affect their emotional and physical health and development for their entire lives.

This inhumane approach conflicts with our society's, our families' and our profession's most fundamental responsibility to protect children and adolescents" [69].

The situation continues to unfold with family groups of migrants leaving home after experiencing extraordinary levels of violence and economic stagnation, walking thousands of miles from Honduras and Guatemala to find more stability and a promising future in the United States. On March 9, 2019, the New York Times reported that for the prior 9 months, the US administration continued to separate migrant families even after retracting its policy to do so, taking over 200 children from their parents or relatives and putting them in institutional care. Some children ended up staying months in foster care or shelters separated from their parents by hundreds or even thousands of miles [79].

On March 30, 2019, the New York Times graphically described children who had been detained in a makeshift encampment with military tents, four times over its planned capacity, under a bridge in El Paso. The children covered their faces with their hands to protect themselves from blowing dust. Families sat on gravel with trash, ripped Mylar blankets and debris behind razor wire. An American veteran who had come out to provide support for the migrant families described the place as looking like a concentration camp. There were other similar situations developing along the US-Mexican border that stretched for over 1900 miles [80].

It should also be noted that religious minorities, in particular Muslims, have been subjected to higher levels of discrimination and xenophobic rhetoric. This has included an unprecedented discriminatory attempt to completely ban granting immigration and asylum for Muslim refugees, from powerful political voices in the United States.

Conditions of Migrant Workers in the United States

Migrants in the United States work in some of the riskiest industries in their destination communities, including agriculture and construction, which have higher injury and fatality rates than other sectors [81]. About 10,000 to 20,000 pesticide injuries are medically treated each year in the United States with migrant farmworkers incurring the most risks of pesticide exposure and associated health risks including risks to fetal development and health of young children [82]. Their housing tends to be characterized by unsafe drinking water; crowding, substandard, and unsafe heating, cooking, and electrical systems; poor sanitation; dilapidated structures; and food insecurity. For example, it is estimated that more than half of the migrant farmworker households in the United States suffer from food insecurity due to their limited access to transportation, food storage, and cooking facilities [83]. These factors are immediately relevant to the physical health, nutrition, and psychological health of children and youth, as well as access to education.

Notwithstanding the grave economic hardship that many migrant workers must endure, many are able to send remittances home to their families in their countries of origin from their earnings in North America that can improve the economic conditions of their families. These remittances have had a positive effect on health and well-being of children and youth as these houscholds have better human development outcomes, less crime, better education, and greater access to health services. For example, a study in Nicaragua found that about 48% of remittances were used to pay for health services, 27% for home improvements, 15% for education, and 10% for savings. There is estimated to have been a total outflow of $68 billion remittances from the United States in 2017 [84]. However, family separation may have a negative impact on health and well-being, including psychological trauma, material hardship, residential instability, and family dissolution [85].

Migrants' motives for leaving their countries of origin include the lack of employment and education opportunities, to escape from conflict and discrimination and the desire to raise families in economically and politically stable and safer environments. In some cases, immigrants may be healthier than the general population when they arrive and have a high level of motivation, but their health may deteriorate after settlement due to unfamiliar social conditions and/or restricted access to health services [41].

Life Conditions of Migrants and Refugees in Europe

Europe hosted 75 million migrants in 2015 or about 31% of the world's migrants [86]. Turkey has accepted 4 million refugees as of 2018, the world's largest number for a single country, of whom 1 million are age 15–24 and over 3.5 million are from Syria [87].

Unaccompanied Asylum-Seeking Children (Under 18 Years of Age)

Globally, the record number of applications from unaccompanied asylum-seeking minors exceeded 98,000 in 2015 at which time Sweden and Germany received the highest number (over 35,000) [88].

In the year preceding March 2018, there were 2307 asylum applications in the United Kingdom from unaccompanied minors, 25% down from 2017 after two consecutively high years. Of these applications, 30% were from Sudan and Eritrea with 11% each from Vietnam and Iraq. Only 56% of these applicants were granted asylum, and an additional 17% were refused asylum but allowed temporary leave to remain[1,2]. Those refused were rejected due to a determination that their countries of origin were "safe" and were deemed to be over 18 years old.

There are serious concerns that many young people are being erroneously categorized as over 18 years old by border officials and social workers who are untrained in age assessment and adolescent health and development. The question of age assessment has been the subject of interagency and international discussion [89–91] and research [92–94]. The highest number of age disputed cases and refusals based

[1] User Guide to Home Office Immigration Statistics; https://www.gov.uk/government/uploads/system/uploads/attachment_data/file/232217/user-guide-immig-statistics.pdf

[2] National Statistics, Immigration statistics, year ending September 2018: data tables; https://www.gov.uk/government/statistics/immigration-statistics-year-ending-september-2018-data-tables

on age were from Afghanistan with 125 and Vietnam with 56. Errors in age assessment do not only cause asylum claims to be denied but also lead to minors being placed in adult detention, minors being denied essential health services, and minors being excluded from education.

The official UK Home Office Statistics show that in 2017 there were a total of 1998 unaccompanied asylum seekers under the age of 18, of which 380 were from Afghanistan, representing a 34% reduction in the 10 years since 2007; the peak number of Afghan minors seeking asylum occurred in 2009 when Afghan minors (1438) represented 50% of all asylum-seeking children (2800). There are shifts in the numbers arriving from various countries dependent on the political situation, warfare, and level of danger in the area. Changes are also affected by authorities clamping down on routes of travel, increased security, and variable availability of assistance.

Closure of "The Jungle"

As a significant example, the closure of the "Jungle," the infamous camp near Calais, France, caused increased hardship for many groups. The camp was reported as being operational between 2015 and October 2016, but immigrants had previously congregated in the area for a number of years; 1500 refugees from Eritrea, Sudan, Ethiopia, and Afghanistan continue to create shelter in makeshift tents and anything else which can cover them, given the absence of adequate shelter, food, water, and sanitation. In October 2016, fearing that many would be evicted from their homes in the midst of winter, Help Refugees and L'Auberge Des Migrants took the first census of the Calais camp and found numbers far in excess of the official estimates: 5497 total residents of whom 651 were children, and of these children 423 were unaccompanied.[3] The numbers fluctuate as more arrive each week.

Following the closure of the camps in Calais, there was an operation to transfer children to the United Kingdom. Between October 1, 2016, and July 15, 2017, a total of 769 children were transferred to the United Kingdom from Calais, including 227 children from Afghanistan, 211 from Sudan, 208 from Eritrea, and 89 from Ethiopia [95].

Subsequently, children have been encountered in night raids by police who have torn down their tents, fired tear gas directly at minors, and subjected them to violence. Restrictions over travel from France to the United Kingdom reduced the numbers reaching the United Kingdom but increased the level of danger young people confront, as asylum seekers spend months or years repeatedly attempting to cross the Channel in containers, lorries, or the Eurotunnel train, sometimes with fatal consequences. Adolescents have been frozen to death in refrigerated compartments, been suffocated in empty tankers, been crushed by lorry axles, and have perished or been seriously injured on other phases of the journey. Many deaths are unreported. A concerning development has been the increased use of boats to

[3] Calais Camp – Total number of residents revealed for the first time – 423 unaccompanied minors; https://helprefugees.org/news/calais-camp-total-number-of-residents-revealed-for-the-first-time-423-unaccompanied-minors/

attempt the Channel crossing; 539 people made the attempt in 2018, 80% of whom since October 2018 [96].

During December 2018 in the Calais area of northern France, there were 972 reported incidents of disproportionate physical violence including three boys sleeping under a bridge who were violently woken by police and sprayed with a noxious chemical agent, struck with batons, handcuffed, and arrested without explanation; youths beaten to the point of losing consciousness; and people tear gassed in the mouth. During a violent raid by French riot police, Compagnies Républicaines de Sécurité (CRS), teargas was fired at refugees to disperse them as officers cleared out the sleeping areas. A rubber bullet was fired by a police officer striking a 16-year-old Eritrean boy in his face; he lost his eye, sense of smell, and hearing in one ear. A British aid worker who witnessed the incident said "… I saw through the smoke a boy being carried by his friends, covered in blood. He had been hit in the eye and they had no way of getting him to hospital… His friends were crying; it was a group of minors and the boy himself was 16" [97].

Children can be caught in the wasteland of illegal camps with no recourse for support and at the mercy of traffickers, violent gangs, and overzealous security forces.

Australia and the South Pacific

Detention is a dangerous place Children and adolescents in Australian immigration detention centers and mental health outcomes.

Australia is a nation of immigrants, with almost 50% of the population either born overseas or having at least one parent born overseas. Most migrants and refugees who come via the UN High Commissioner on Refugees camps settle well and have productive lives with access to necessary services, education, health, and social security.

All nations use some restrictive immigration practices to regulate migration and for political purposes, national security, deterrence, and border control. For almost 30 years, Australia has indefinitely detained all asylum seekers arriving without authorized travel documents in onshore and offshore secure facilities until claims are resolved, or they are deported. Mandatory Detention was introduced in 1994, with the aim to deter "unauthorized arrivals," who mostly arrived by boat. Recent Australian governments, from both major political parties, have enacted laws to "turn back the boats" that were dangerously overcrowded with asylum seekers who could or would not wait in what have been euphemistically referred to as "orderly queues" in UNHCR facilities. The "Detention" of children is a "last resort" directive in the Australian Migration Act of 1958 (as amended), which is ignored in this approach [98–101].

There have been three waves of "boat arrivals" into Australian territorial waters: 1976 to 1981 Vietnamese refugees; 1989 to 1998 Indochinese asylum seekers; and from 1999 people of Middle Eastern origin, mainly Afghanistan (primarily of Hazara ethnicity), Iran, and Iraq being transported by people smugglers [102, 103]. Most departed from southern Java in Indonesia where many refugees from the Middle East and East Africa "wait." Australia was regarded as a preferred destination for thousands of refugees seeking asylum and fleeing dire situations of civil unrest, war and persecution, and for others the hope of a better life and economic prosperity. Most made for Christmas Island (an Australian territory), about 2700 kms from Darwin or Perth on the western coast of Australia, but only 600 kms from southern Indonesia.

The "Pacific Solution"

In 2001 the "Pacific Solution" was introduced for detention outside Australia in Papua New Guinea (PNG) and Nauru, with offshore processing of refugees. The policy was strongly criticized, and it ceased in 2007, only to be reinstated in 2012 after a number of unseaworthy vessels sank or ran aground, with a significant number of asylum seekers and migrants drowning at sea [100, 101]. These often unseaworthy vessels had poorly skilled crews navigating through dangerous seas and weather.

Map 1 illustrates the locations of on- and offshore immigration detention facilities.

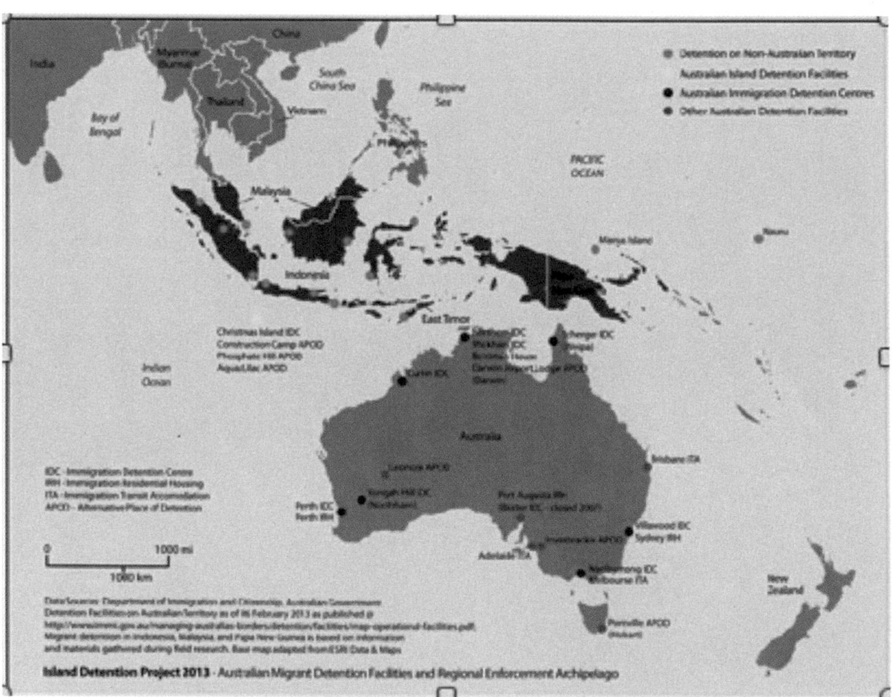

Locations of Australian immigration detention facilities. (Source [104])

The enacted laws have virtually stopped all "unauthorized maritime arrivals," and those who arrived or were intercepted in Australian waters prior to the "strengthening of Australia's borders" were transferred to Manus Island, Papua New Guinea, or Nauru, rather than remaining on Christmas Island. The majority of these "unauthorized maritime arrivals" detained offshore have been assessed as genuine refugees and subject to the relevant international treaties and conventions. However, the health outcomes for those detained in the offshore facilities have been significantly negative, especially for mental health, and most particularly for children and adolescents.

This lack of fully accessible, efficient, and appropriate comprehensive health facilities and specialist services on these remote islands; bureaucratic processes imposed by the governments of Australia, PNG, and Nauru; delays in requests for transfers for medical treatment; bureaucrats (not medical officers) making the decisions, who often reject opinions of requesting medical officers; and travel times to mainland cities with required services have exacerbated preventable serious medical deterioration in many cases [98–101, 105–113].

Adequate scrutiny of facilities and the health condition of detainees has been restricted by the remoteness of the centers, many experienced professionals banned, and media access severely limited.

As of late 2019, most of the children have been relocated to the mainland but are not able to settle in Australia; they are required to go to a third country that will accept them or return to their country of origin. What has been regarded as "cruel and inhumane" treatment has led to physical and mental health deterioration among these young people, including psychosis, severe depression, self-harm, and suicides. Medical and other organizations have condemned the approach, as have UN agencies [98–101].

Mental Health Outcomes for Child and Adolescent Refugees and Migrants in Australia

Child and adolescent development occur within the context of caregiving relationships, usually in the family. War, political upheaval, persecution, trauma, and forced migration impose considerable stress on parents and their capacity to be effective parents and meet the needs of their children and adolescents. Parental mental health suffers, as does that of their offspring, with some parents too unwell to provide adequate care and parenting.

Physical health issues among children and adolescents both in offshore and onshore detention are often exacerbated by, or exacerbate, mental health concerns. Somatic symptoms (sleep, eating, and pain) are common. Detainees live in a tropical climate, and witness hunger strikes, lip sewing, jumping off heights, self-immolation with petrol, and violent assaults perpetrated by other detainees, guards, and locals.

There is extensive Australian research on the impact of such incarceration that reveals high levels of psychiatric impairment, evident even after short periods of detention, and which increases with the length of the detention. Depression, post-traumatic stress disorder (PTSD), self-harm, voluntary starvation, suicide attempts and suicide, psychotic disorders, and complex mental health problems are all found. In addition, developmental delay and regression, attachment disorders, and emotional and behavioral disturbances are evident.

Indefinite Detention of Refugee Children and Youth

The uncertainty related to indefinite detention, despair, loss, displacement, excessive surveillance, control of movement, exposure to trauma and unrest, riots, and violence within detention facilities all escalate the negative impacts. Hope and optimism are crushed, and resilience worn down or erased in closed systems, within the walls of secrecy.

The experience of indefinite immigration detention on child and adolescent refugees has been described as breaking minds, breaking the children, breaking up families, breaking women, breaking bodies, and obstructing medical care [111].

The Submission by the United Nations High Commissioner for Refugees on the "Inquiry into serious allegations of abuse, self-harm and neglect of asylum seekers in relation to the Nauru Regional Processing Centre, and any like allegations in relation to the Manus Island Regional Processing Centre" [101] highlights the indefinite detention in punitive conditions and highly securitized environment the migrant and refugee youth are exposed to. They experience a lack of long-term viable solutions, continuing exposure to violence and trauma, family separation in some cases, and loss and impairment of identity and culture. They live with a fear of persecution, imprisonment, torture, and death if returned to country of origin. These factors result in predictable and preventable mental health deterioration. This is particularly so for LGBT youth, for torture and trauma survivors, and for those who were child soldiers.

Traumatic Withdrawal Syndrome

A "traumatic withdrawal syndrome" has been observed in refugee children and adolescents transferred from Australia to the Nauru Regional Processing Centre. They are exposed to ongoing trauma, feel hopeless and helpless, and give up on engagement with the world. This is expressed through partial or complete withdrawal in three or more of the following domains: eating, mobilization, speech, and attention to personal care (including self-toileting). Active resistance or non-response to acts of care and encouragement and social withdrawal are evident, as well as increased prevalence of the "freeze-isolate-withdrawal" response, including pervasive uncertainty and ongoing re-traumatizing experiences [100].

The 2014 report of the Australian Human Rights Commission national inquiry into children in immigration detention data on children and adolescents in detention assessed as having a mental health disorder/illness was presented [98] and is presented in Table 17.1, illustrating the types of mental health presentations found in this group of children and youth on a single day: 10 July 2014.

Table 17.1 Children and adolescents in detention in Australia assessed as having a mental health disorder/illness July 10, 2014

Age of child	Nature of mental health disorder	Months in detention at July 2014
2	Childhood attachment disorder	11
3	Depression	11
7	Adjustment disorder; mixed anxiety disorder of social functioning; attachment disorder	9
7	Adjustment disorder; depressive disorder	11
7	Adjustment disorder	11
7	Anxiety disorder; post-traumatic disorder	11
8	Anxiety disorder; personality disorder (post-injury)	11
8	Anxiety disorder; major depressive disorder	16
9	Depressive disorder	12
9	Mixed anxiety and depressive disorder; post-traumatic stress disorder	11
9	Adjustment disorder; mixed anxiety and depressive disorder; post-traumatic stress disorder	11
9	Adjustment disorder; mixed anxiety; and depressive disorder	12
9	Anxiety disorder	15
10	Post-traumatic stress disorder	12
10	Anxiety disorder; post-traumatic stress disorder	11
11	Depression	11
11	Depressive disorder	11
12	Post-traumatic stress disorder	12
12	Adjustment disorder; depressive disorder	11
13	Depression – psychotic; mixed anxiety and depressive disorder; post-traumatic stress disorder	11
13	Post-traumatic stress disorder	7
14	Depression; adjustment disorder	12
14	Adjustment disorder; anxiety disorder; depressive disorder; post-traumatic stress disorder	11
14	Depressive disorder; mixed anxiety and depressive disorder	11
15	Adjustment disorder; depressive disorder	11
15	Anxiety disorder; depressive disorder; personality disorder; post-traumatic stress disorder	11
15	Mixed anxiety and depressive disorder	11
15	Depressive disorder	11
16	Adjustment disorder; mixed anxiety and depressive disorder	11
16	Post-traumatic stress disorder	7
16	Depression	14
16	Post-traumatic stress disorder	8
16	Mixed anxiety and depressive disorder; post-traumatic stress disorder	12
17	Adjustment disorder; post-traumatic stress disorder	10

(continued)

Table 17.1 (continued)

Age of child	Nature of mental health disorder	Months in detention at July 2014
17	Anxiety with depression; bipolar disorder; mood disorder; depressed mood	11
17	Depression; bipolar disorder; adjustment disorder; attention deficit hyperactivity disorder	11

About 95% of children and adolescents in detention surveyed in a Darwin detention center in 2015 were in the clinical range for PTSD, trauma, and hopelessness and despair [108]. Statements made by their parents (p.19) included:

> She has no friends. She cries all the time and says I want to go from here. She has cut herself with a razor on her chin, face, chest. She eats poorly, has daily headache and tummy pain …. Every night she wakes up and screams that someone is coming to take her back to Nauru. Mother of girl aged 7

> He is depressed, scratches himself till he bleeds. Bites his nails. Doesn't associate with anyone including family. He saw the mental health team once and was told that he is in need of "big attention" but he has seen no one yet. Mother of boy aged 16

A study of the mental health of children, adolescents, and parents detained on Christmas Island [107] revealed comorbid depression in 86% of adolescents, and 7 and 6% of children had a high probability of psychiatric disorder.

Impact of Indefinite Immigration Detention

Incidents of mental health presentations reported in public domain from data available from the Australian Department of Immigration and Border Protection for February to August 2018 for transfers to the mainland for specialized services from Nauru, often after court intervention, include:

- 10-year-old boy, attempted suicide three times and needed surgery.
- Young girl, not yet a teenager, attempted suicide three times.
- 14-year-old girl, been on Nauru for nearly 5 years, doused herself in petrol and tried to set herself alight – then immigration minister refused transfer to mainland for specialist care, until case taken to court.
- 17-year-old boy acutely unwell and suffering psychosis, rarely ate, and did not go to school.
- Adolescent girl suffering a severe major depressive disorder and "trauma withdrawal syndrome."
- 12-year-old boy on Nauru for 5 years, refusing food and fluids for nearly 2 weeks, suffering from "resignation syndrome." He weighed 36 kg and could not stand when transferred to mainland for specialist care – mother and sister transferred with him, but placed in detention on the mainland.

- 17-year-old girl, once dreaming of becoming a doctor, diagnosed with "resignation syndrome" and is refusing all food and fluid.
- 12-year-old girl who made several suicide attempts, tried to set herself on fire.
- 14-year-old boy, suffering a major depressive disorder and severe muscle wastage after not getting out of bed for 4 months [114].

It is clear that immigration detention is dangerous for children and adolescents, and their parents, and is not in their "best interests," especially in relation to mental health and psychosocial development.

Part 3: Regional Conditions That Drive Refugees and Migrants to Leave

To appreciate the challenges faced by refugees and migrants, in particular irregular (or undocumented) migrants, it is critical to understand the conditions from which they are fleeing. The global refugee population stood at 25.9 million people at the end of 2018 with 5.5 million Palestinian refugees under the mandate of the UN Refugee Works Agency and 20.4 million refugees under the mandate of the UN High Commissioner on Refugees [115]. Below is an exploration of the scope of the problem and the conditions from which young people leave in Latin America, the Middle East, and North Africa with very brief recent history to put the development of such dire conditions into context. Common challenges include fleeing political and social violence or warfare, ethnic or religious persecution and displacement, fleeing natural disasters that have led to drought, crop failure and hunger, and prolonged, even multi-generational stagnation in refugee camps with a loss of hope for the future of oneself and one's children. This is not meant to be a comprehensive history or description of conditions, but to highlight major examples and factors in contemporary situations. It is important to recognize that the drivers for forced migration are shaped by the legacy of historic forces, social biases, climate change, and other factors that are beyond the ability of individuals and their families to address.

According to official government statistics provided by the UN High Commissioner on Refugees in 2018, 92,400 refugees were resettled in 25 countries: Canada admitted the largest number (28,100), the United States admitted the second highest (22,900), Australia settled 12,700, and the United Kingdom 5800. Unfortunately, UNHCR estimated that 1.4 million refugees were in need of resettlement and a gap of over 90% exists between the needs and actual resettlement [115].

Latin America, the Caribbean, and North America

North America hosted 54 million or about 22% of international migrants in 2015 [116] with the United States being the destination for 46.6 million in 2015 [116]. Of those in the United States, about 11.1 million are irregular (or undocumented) migrants [116].

Key Findings of the World Health Organization on Refugees and Migrants

In 2017, Latin America and the Caribbean contributed 10 million international migrants to a worldwide total of 258 million international migrants. The large majority of international migrants in South America move within the region [1]. About 15.2% of the total population of North America are international migrants. In the Americas, the number of people migrating across international borders has surged by 36% in the last 15 years, reaching 63.7 million in 2015; of these migrants, 808,000 were defined as refugees.

The World Health Organization (WHO) report on *the Health of refugees and migrants, WHO Region of Americas 2018*, found that migration in the Americas exhibits four trends [117]:

1. A steady flow of returnees due to economic crises and inhospitable social settings in high income countries
2. The receipt of remittances from migrants living in high-income countries as an important source of income for several Latin American and Caribbean countries
3. Human trafficking and the smuggling of migrants
4. The contribution of Latin American and Caribbean communities in the United States, Canada, and Europe to the development of cultural, economic, and social ties with their countries and communities of origin

Social conditions in many countries, particularly in the Central American nations of Honduras, Guatemala, and El Salvador, are exceedingly dangerous, and residents are subject to among the highest homicide rates in the world, kidnapping for ransom, economic stagnation, governmental corruption, and widespread organized crime. Tens of thousands of people flee these conditions with their children, leaving home for the promise of a better life, willing to confront the grave dangers that lay in wait for the long and dangerous journey north.

In Guatemala in particular, there is a long history of persecution of indigenous peoples, with destruction of villages and the forced displacement and killing of populations. These factors drive indigenous people from their historic homes to migrate north, for them, to the unknown; these refugees commonly do not speak either Spanish or English and the children have commonly been denied basic education. Guatemala has a long history of military dictatorship dating back to 1954 when the last democratically elected government was overthrown through a US CIA coup d'état [118]. Guatemala has a large number of indigenous non-Spanish-speaking people who have been targeted and subjected to massacres and other atrocities and driven off their lands. These people commonly migrate north to the United States with their children. El Salvador had been involved in a long and complex civil war [119] and now has an unstable military and police force and gangs emboldened by the drug trade who exert powerful influences. Honduras' last democratically elected government was overthrown by a military coup in 2009 [120], and since there has been an eruption of social violence, gangs, and a corrupt police force. All of these countries have very high levels of unemployment.

There is a long and tragic history of military intervention by the United States in Central America and other areas of Latin America that is beyond the scope of this chapter but is critically pertinent in that it has laid the groundwork for the current dire situation from which so many migrants feel forced to leave with their children.

For many from Latin America, irregular (undocumented) migrants experience a perilous journey north, traveling under dangerous, even life-threatening conditions. Migrants from Central America often ride on moving cargo trains, colloquially known as La Bestia (or The Beast), on their journey across Mexico to the United States. At other times, migrants walk hundreds or even thousands of miles with children, encountering deprivation and hunger, as well as the generosity of others, on their way north. Along the way they face physical perils including death. They are also subject to extortion and violence at the hands of gangs affiliated with organized crime [85]. The Institute of Migration estimates that in the period 2014 through 2018 there were 2970 known deaths of migrants, including 127 children; this is thought to be a significant underestimation as many bodies are found in isolated areas across a border that runs through desert [121]. The leading causes of death at the US-Mexico border were drowning, presumed murder, and unknown. The hope that guides them that they can provide their labor, that their children can have an education and a better life, sustains them through great hardship, as it has prior generations of migrants and refugees who have brought their gifts and talents.

The Middle East and North Africa

The United Nations Economic and Social Commission for West Asia estimates that about 200,000 to 2 million children live on the streets. Instead of proper rehabilitation and stabilization, many of the children are detained in cells with adult criminals and subjected to abuse and maltreatment. The following table shows the number of displaced children by country and primary reason.

Country	Displaced children	Reason(s)
Syria	70,000+	War
Jordan	N/A	Economy/social
Egypt	200,000–3,000,000	Political
Afghanistan	235,000	War
Iraq	100,000+	War

Why People Become Refugees in the Middle East [4]

Like other areas in the world, there are 5 reasons:

1. Religious/national/social/racial/political persecution
2. War

[4] Global citizen - https://www.globalcitizen.org/en/content/reasons-why-people-become-refugees/

3. Experiencing discrimination because of gender/sexual orientation
4. Hunger
5. Climate change

During the second decade of the current century, most of the countries in the Middle East have suffered from institutional instability, violence, economic disruption, and social instability and uncertainty. Many of the governments failed to bring adequate development and growth, failed to maintain minimal human rights, and were characterized by corruption. During the Arab Spring, these failings led to many citizen uprisings that were violently suppressed, and those political movements ended in a failure to achieve any of the promising positive intended goals. Since then, there has been an ongoing failure to respect international human rights and law, with catastrophic results affecting essentially all aspects of life, including areas of health, education, economy, and security. The health consequences for children and youth and their families are incalculable.

Women, children, adolescents, and ethnic and religious minorities have suffered disproportionately. As a result, areas in the Middle East are crowded with millions of refugees, displaced families, and migrants, including children and youth.

Iraq

In 2003, the United States invaded and occupied Iraq. This war resulted in massive casualties, estimated to be from 500,000 to over one million deaths [122, 123]. The destruction of urban centers, displacement of millions, destruction of the healthcare system, and creation of millions of refugees have had dire consequences. This invasion set in motion a series of massive population displacements, extreme polarization of religious groups, and terrible violence that continues to unfold. In late 2015, the UN High Commissioner for Refugees reported that over 4.4 million Iraqis were internally displaced and an additional 264,000 were refugees abroad [124]. The legacy is all the more tragic as the invasion was justified by documented false allegations of Iraqi possession of weapons of mass destruction. It is difficult or impossible to provide an accurate picture of the health consequences of these tragic events, but they are vast and have had a disproportionate impact on children and youth.

Syria

Following the initiation of the Iraq war, there has been increasing religious polarization in Syria, the engagement and intervention of multiple regional and international armed forces in Syrian affairs (including both the United States and Russia), an extremely complex civil war and consequent vast number of non-combatant casualties and displacement of much of the population.

The trauma, injuries, and loss of available clinical services over such a brief period are impossible to calculate, and events continue to unfold. The population of

Syria before this ongoing and evolving crisis was about 22 million, according to the UN Office for the Coordination of Humanitarian Affairs (UNOCH). Well over the majority of the population has been displaced. As of December 2018, UNOCH reported that within Syria itself there were 6.6 million refugees and over 6.1 million internally displaced persons of whom 5.6 million were children; outside of Syria, there were over 6.2 million registered refugees of whom 2.6 million are children [125]. At the end of 2018, Syria had over 2.3 million internally displaced persons [1].

Syria, historically a relatively affluent, highly educated, and well organized society, has suffered a breakdown of the healthcare system to the extent that an unprecedented epidemic of polio emerged. The UN was successful in promoting vaccinations so that the epidemic seems to be contained at this time. Access to potable water, nutrition, and engagement of children in school remain unreliable.

The UN High Commissioner on Refugees has found that about 70,000 Syrian refugee children in Jordan and Lebanon are living without their fathers. Further, about 4000 children are living without either of their parents, who have been killed, imprisoned, or lost [126].

Yemen

The situation in Yemen represents the world's worst ongoing man-made humanitarian catastrophe, not only in the Middle East, but in the world [127]. Yemen has been subjected to an unprecedented level of violence initiated and sustained through about 18,000 airstrikes by Saudi Arabia since 2015 using modern weaponry purchased from the United States and Great Britain [128]. Laser-guided bombs in August 2017 hit a school bus leaving, aside from large numbers of casualties, remnants indicating the bomb had been made in the United States. The physical infrastructure, including effectively all bridges, has been largely destroyed [129].

Of a total population of about 28 million, through war and violence, about 3 million people have been displaced and 2 million left homeless (commonly after homes have been destroyed by bombing). The displaced Yemeni people live in a harsh and poor conditions or in makeshift shelters. Many of those who sought refuge went to neighboring countries like Oman, Saudi Arabia, Somalia, Ethiopia, Sudan, and Djibouti; about 280,000 of the Somali refugees in Yemen have been displaced once again from their place of refuge in Yemen.

Almost 22 million people in Yemen are in need of urgent help and support, including 15 million children and adolescents who are at the edge of starvation[5]. According to the UN Population Fund (UNFPA-the UN's sexual and reproductive health agency), "lack of food, displacement, poor nutrition, disease outbreaks and eroding health care have heavily affected the health and well-being of 1.1 million malnourished pregnant and lactating women, causing numerous cases of premature

[5] USA for UNHCR; the Yemen Crisis; https://www.unrefugees.org/emergencies/yemen/

or low-birth weight babies, severe postpartum bleeding, and extremely life-threatening labor processes," if the situation continues to deteriorate, up to two million mothers could end up being affected [130]. About 8 million people in Yemen, anticipated to grow to 14 million soon (about half of the population), rely on emergency rations; there are about 1.8 million severely malnourished children. This is an ongoing catastrophic man-made famine. The United Nations has stated that it could soon become the "worst famine seen in the world in 100 years" [131]. Famine disproportionately affects infants and small children who are the principal casualties, leading not only to deaths, but destined to leave a legacy of impaired growth, vulnerability to infectious disease, and neurological damage as adolescents and adults. Yemen continues under a strict military air and sea blockade enforced by Saudi Arabia with arms purchased from the United States and Britain, which bars or seriously delays delivery of food and essential medical supplies in what may amount to a war crime [129].

The largest cholera epidemic in the world took place in Yemen, with over 2 million cumulative cases between October 2016 and September 2019 [132], 25% of which were among children that led to extraordinarily high rates of mortality and morbidity following the systematic destruction of the sanitation system and water supply through aerial bombing by Saudi Arabia [133]. Cholera remains a threat in environments where the accessible water has been contaminated through destruction of public health infrastructure and potable water is not readily available. The World Health Organization has stated that, with over one million cases, this is among the worst epidemics of cholera in recorded human history. There has also been the destruction of food supplies so that starvation in 2018 has been at epidemic levels. Children are the principal casualties.

Dengue fever is now prevalent in refugee camps, driven by mosquitoes that breed in stagnant water. Vaccinations have been interrupted, leading to increased prevalence of preventable infectious diseases including measles and diphtheria.

In an interview by a New York Times journalist with Yemen's Health Minister, Dr. Taha Mutawakel, he described an increase in incidence of birth deformities and childhood cancer, in which the Health Minister attributed to toxic residues in the soil and air left by the thousands of bombings. He stated that by November 2018, 85 medical workers had been killed and 231 injured. Drugs for chronic medical conditions have been unavailable so that 250,000 people with insulin-dependent diabetes are in danger of dying as are about 1200 people with kidney disease dependent on dialysis. Most of the health clinics have been demolished by bombs. In August 2018, the only hospital in the city of Al Hudaydah which provides critical neonatal and emergency care was attacked, leaving 90,000 pregnant women and adolescent girls at high risk [130]. All commercial flights are barred, preventing Yemeni children and adults from accessing referrals for urgent medical and surgical treatment outside of Yemen [129].

Though prior to the war there had been a decline in child marriage through the efforts of Yemeni lawyers, educators, and activists, it is now on the rise. A UNICEF official was referred to as saying that child marriage now occurs with about 65% of adolescent, and even preadolescent, girls; the rate tripling since 2015. This is driven by the impossible challenge that parents face in feeding their daughters; child marriage results in being taken out of school, early childbearing, and illiteracy of adolescent and adult women. Boys are picked up as child soldiers and are "visible everywhere" [129].

Education of children and youth has been interrupted; 2 million children were estimated to be out of school as of January 2017. Between March 2015 and November 2017, 256 schools had been destroyed, with 1413 schools partially destroyed through airstrikes and shelling, and an additional 150 schools occupied by military groups [134]. The legacy of the war is destined to play out over the coming decades in the lives of children and youth affected by this conflict.

Displaced Palestinians and Refugees

Palestinians constitute the world's largest refugee population numbering about 5.5 million under the United Nations Refugee Works mandate. Their situation cannot be understood without some appreciation of the history that led to their displacement following the conclusion of World War II. Many of the Palestinians remain refugees, living generation after generation in refugee camps and displaced repeatedly. The prolonged suffering of the Palestinian people is the result of the lack of resolution of the refugee crisis over many decades and multiple generations. Below is a brief summary of the historic events that have shaped the current situation and a description of their current living conditions.

Since the end of World War II, Palestinians have confronted an unprecedented displacement from their homeland that remains unresolved. Millions have become refugees. This mass displacement followed in the wake of an historic genocide focused on the Jewish people, principally in Poland, Germany, and Eastern Europe, led by German Nazis or fascists. This genocide, implemented systematically with mass deportations, concentration camps, gas chambers, and forced labor, resulted in the killing of some six million Jewish people, a million or more Roma people (or gypsies), over 2 million ethnic Poles, tens of thousands of disabled people including disabled children and people with mental illness, tens of thousands of homosexuals, and tens of thousands of the political opposition. Total worldwide deaths from World War II were about 70–85 million (about 3% of the world's population) of whom 50–55 million were civilians. The majority of deaths occurred in the Soviet Union (26.6 million) and China (20 million).

Almost 30 years before the conclusion of World War II, on November 2, 1917, shortly after World War I, the British Government represented by Arthur Balfour had issued a letter stating "His Majesty's Government view with favor the establishment in Palestine of a national home for the Jewish people, ...it being clearly understood that nothing shall be done which may prejudice the civil and religious rights of existing non-Jewish communities in Palestine…" [135] This became known as the Balfour Declaration. This declaration was made without consultation of the people of Palestine.

Following the conclusion of World War II, many Jewish survivors of the Nazi genocide, or Holocaust, relocated to what was then the Palestinian British Protectorate, with purported protections for the rights of the indigenous Palestinian people. Palestinians were a religiously diverse population rooted for many centuries in the Palestinian lands consisting of Muslim, Christian, and Jewish peoples who historically had lived in an integrated social environment. With the creation of Israel, hundreds of thousands of Palestinians were forcibly displaced from their villages and homes and driven into refugee camps.

Political unrest and violence began and escalated and ultimately broke out into open warfare in the fall of 1947. By 1948, the majority of Palestinians, about 700,000 to 800,000 people from 500 to 600 villages, were displaced. They were either [136] expelled or fled from their homes for fear of being killed, as had actually taken place in a number of villages.[6]

Since 1950, the United Nations Refugee Works Agency (UNRWA) has had responsibility for populations in the Gaza Strip and the West Bank. UNRWA defines Palestinian refugees as "persons whose normal place of residence was Palestine during the period 1 June 1946 to 15 May 1948, and who lost both home and means of livelihood as a result of the 1948 conflict." The operations of UNRWA started in 1950, at that time serving about 750,000 Palestinian refugees. Since then, with population growth and increase in members of Palestinian refugee families, the number of refugees registered with UNRWA today exceeds 5 million [137].

There are an additional one million Palestinians who originate from the displacement in 1948 but who could not or did not register with UNRWA for assistance. These individuals live in many countries around the world, including Jordan, Saudi Arabia, Egypt, the Gulf Countries, Chile, and the United States. About 18 percent of the population of historic Palestine remains Palestinian.

As a consequence of the 1967 war with the occupation of the Gaza Strip and the West Bank, almost one million additional Palestinians were displaced from their communities. They represent the second largest group of refugees. UNRWA responded by establishing another 10 refugee camps to accommodate and serve

[6] This forced mass displacement of Palestinians set the stage for commemorating the 15th day of May 1948, known by Palestinians as Nakba, or catastrophe (Nakba means the collapse and disappearance of an entire society) signifying that Palestinian society, which had existed for centuries, had been for the most part destroyed.

None of the Palestinians who fled or were expelled could return, contrary to Palestinian refugees' right to return to the homes as declared by the United Nations' General Assembly Resolution 194 (III) of December 1948, paragraph 11, in which the U.N. General Assembly, Resolves: "that the refugees wishing to return to their homes and live at peace with their neighbors should be permitted to do so at the earliest practicable date, and that compensation should be paid for the property of those choosing not to return and for loss of or damage to property which, under principles of international law or in equity, should be made good by the governments or authorities responsible; Instructs the Conciliation Commission to facilitate the repatriation, resettlement and economic and social rehabilitation of the refugees and the payment of compensation…"

Conclusion on voluntary Repatriation, UNHCR, Executive Committee, No. 40 (XXXVI), 1985

them. A third group of Palestinians are internally displaced refugees who remain within the Israeli or Palestinian territories but not in their original homes [138].

Today, about one-third of Palestinian refugees, or about 1.5 million people, live in 58 refugee camps established by the UNRWA, generally on land leased from local landowners (so that they do not own land themselves) located in Jordan, Lebanon, the Syrian Arab Republic, the Gaza Strip, and the West Bank, including East Jerusalem. Others live in those countries but outside of refugee camps.

The remaining two-thirds of Palestinian refugees reside in and around the cities and towns of the host countries and in the West Bank and the Gaza Strip [137]. About 2 million (40%) live in Jordan, 1 million (20%) in Gaza, 760,000 (16%) in the West Bank, 460,000 in Syria, 420,000 in Lebanon, and 34,000 in Iraq [139].

Palestinian refugees in host countries have suffered displacement after displacement. For example, during the US-led campaign and occupation of Iraq in 2003, about half of the Palestinian refugees in Iraq were forced to leave to the surrounding deserts. In Lebanon in 2007, 31,000 Palestinian refugees were forced to leave the Nahr al-bared camp without refuge, to nowhere [140].

It is important to note that many of the Palestinian refugees in Syria have been displaced as a result of the current Syrian war. Palestinians who remain in Syria have suffered together with other Syrians as a result of the war.

Health and Social Issues Facing the Palestinian Children and Adolescents

Children and adolescents represent about 40% of the Palestinian population with population growth of over 3% per year, one of the highest rates in the world according to the World Bank; Population Growth Report 2009 [141]. According to UNICEF *State of the World's Children, At a glance: State of Palestine. 2015*, the majority of Palestinian adolescents and children are affected by the displacements, migration, occupation, closure, conflict, and poor environmental conditions [142].

Under-five mortality (UFM) is a key indicator to monitor the health and socioeconomic status of children and is used for international comparisons. In the occupied Palestinian territories, the UFM indicator is over 20 per 1000 (as a comparison, for children in Israel it is 4 per 1000). The causes of child and youth mortality include congenital anomalies, perinatal complications, respiratory infections, accidents and violence, road traffic accidents, missile and firearm injuries, and malignancies. Morbidities include malnutrition and its complications, including iron deficiency anemia. Most of the people in Gaza (56%) and many in the West Bank (25%) experience food insecurity [143].

In Gaza, most water piped to households is unfit for human consumption. This is due to the reliance on a single aquifer in Gaza, which has been contaminated, and the destruction of the single sewage processing plant by Israeli bombing. Since the bombing of the sewage plant, sewage has been largely untreated and dumped into the Mediterranean Sea, which then flushes back to the shore; open untreated sewage runoff and agrichemicals seep into the remaining aquifer. The population is dependent on desalinated water that contains chemical contaminants [144]. These conditions create a very-high-risk situation for the outbreak of endemic disease and public health crises as has taken place in Haiti, Yemen, and Iraq. A report prepared by RAND Corporation [145] based on data collected by the Water Sanitation and Hygiene (WASH) over several years emphasizes the urgency of cooperation between the Palestinian Authority, Israel, and Egypt to pre-empt an epidemic outcome. About 26% of all childhood diseases in Gaza were identified by UNICEF as water-borne [146]. Though typhoid fever, hepatitis A, and viral meningitis have been detected, the fact that there has not been a major epidemic and humanitarian crisis is significant; however, the effort is being undermined by the elimination of funding support from the United States for UNRWA [147].

Mental health problems in the occupied Palestinian territories are of great concern: 93% of adolescents and children feel unsafe, threatened, and fearful. The exposure to violence and trauma is much higher than in other countries: 8 out of 10 adolescents had witnessed a shooting, about 3 out of 10 had witnessed killing, and 1 out of 10 saw a relative or neighbor killed. Almost half of all adolescents were exposed to body searches. The prevalence of post-traumatic stress disorder among children is particularly high ranging from 23% to 70%. Of the Palestinian children who experienced traumatic events during the 2012 Israeli bombing of the Gaza Strip, 30% developed PTSD. According to the World Health Organization "the time spent in detention for children and families represents a period of chronic stress, traumatic experiences including threats to physical integrity that are experienced as overwhelming and are accompanied by intense fear and helplessness, loneliness and loss of faith in adults, possibly even their own parents." The psychological toll of demolitions and forced evictions hits women harder [148].

More than 8000 children were arrested and exposed to maltreatment, torture, or other severely traumatic acts such as beating, kicking, cuffing, yelling, blindfolding, sleep deprivation, denial of access to toilets, lack of showers, exposure to loud noise, excessive heat or cold, and other acts by the soldiers of Israeli army in the period between 2000 and 2017. Consequently, 10% experienced manifestations of depression, 10% had somatic disorders, and about 15% suffered from emotional difficulties [149].

According to *Defense for Children International/Palestine section*, 500–700 children are detained by the Israeli military yearly. The highest figure occurred in 2016, during which 375 children and adolescents per month were imprisoned [150].

The reasons behind this persistently negative health situation are many. They include the occupation by the Israeli forces, lack of resources and aid dependency, lack of international support, the failure of internal governance, difficult socioeconomic situations, healthcare access difficulties, absence of adequate housing and food, deficient electrical supply, and the lack of safe drinking water [151, 152]. Palestinian children and families continue to be negatively affected by occupation-related policies and practices including house demolitions and displacement, denial of access to livelihoods, administrative detention, psychosocial distress, and exposure to explosive remnants of war [152].

With a population of about 2 million and an area of 360 square kilometers, Gaza has the highest population density in the world and a high growth rate. It is a resource-poor region. There are no local well-equipped referral or tertiary health centers for patients, who must be referred to centers outside the borders, which requires them to obtain special security permits from the Israeli authorities through a very complicated process and often ends in denial. During 2014 and 2015, more than 10,000 patients were denied permission to cross borders or checkpoints to reach a referral health center. In February 2017, 40% of the requests to travel from Gaza for medical advice or treatment were refused by Israeli authorities [153]. The International Committee of the Red Cross, among others, has declared this a policy of "collective punishment" and called for Israel to lift its closure. Amnesty International, Human Rights Watch, Physicians for Human Rights Israel, and others have called for an end to the decades-long closure of the Gaza Strip. Israel continues to control all Gaza access, with the exception of the Rafah crossing to Egypt, and all crossing from Gaza to the West Bank and Jordan [154].

North Africa

The majority of asylum-seeking minors from North Africa tend to be Eritreans fleeing religious persecution. Many practice the banned Pentecostal religion in secret and are subject to severe punishment if discovered. Youth can present with wounds from torture and beatings after dangerous journeys through Libya and the Mediterranean. The changing political situation and clan warfare in Somalia and unrest in Sudan have generated large numbers of refugee children and adolescents; in addition, many young males escape from persecution related to their sexual orientation; homosexual practices are punishable by death.

Climate change, drought, and crop failure play an important role in driving displacement and migration, in particular in Somalia, where there were 250,000 new refugees due to drought in 2018 increasing the national total to 850,000 displacements [17].

Armed conflict and ethnic tensions also drive conflict particularly in West and Central Africa, in particular the Democratic Republic of the Congo which has one of the worst humanitarian crises in the world with about 3 million internally displaced persons. The Central African Republic produced about 600,000 refugees and 500,000 internally displaced persons. The Democratic Republic of the Congo and the Central African Republic were both among the top ten origin countries for refugees in the world at the end of 2018 [17].

Refugees from Africa commonly use Libya as a hub for migration to cross the Mediterranean. Libya itself is subject to civil conflict and refugees are exposed to sexual and gender-based violence, forced labor (i.e., slavery), extortion, and other abuses [17].

North Africa is a key route for migration to Europe, with most leaving Libya for Italy in 2016 and 2017 (principally from Tunisia, Eritrea, Sudan, Iraq, and Pakistan, about 15% were unaccompanied children), but in 2018 most took a route from Morocco to Spain [17].

Sexually trafficked young women tend to be brought through Nigeria, Uganda, and other African countries by more direct routes such as air travel, accompanied by "minders" or pimps on false documents that portray the youth as older than they actually are since fewer questions are asked of the traffickers if they are not travelling with minors. The girls are often made up and dressed as older with bras stuffed with cloths. This commonly causes problems for the girls later, when after some months in sexual slavery, they might escape and then be branded as adults by the authorities who insist on going by the date of birth in their forged passports – even when they know they are forged. Hence young traumatized girls end up in adult detention jails.

Many desperate irregular migrants in North Africa face perilous and life-threatening conditions, including being trafficked as slaves. They are faced with few options and seek refuge in Europe through a life-endangering journey across the Mediterranean Sea in poorly equipped vessels. Irregular migrants to Europe frequently enter by crossing the Mediterranean Sea on boat. Casualties related to this crossing are impossible to estimate accurately, given that bodies disappear in the ocean, and there are no written records, but there has been more scrutiny of the number of these deaths since the tragic sinking of two boats off the coast of Italy in 2013 resulting in the deaths of an estimated 368 migrants.

The International Organization of Migration Missing Migrant Project (IOM MMP) now estimates from multiple sources that of 7927 missing migrants in 2016 worldwide (an increase of 26% over 2015) over 60% (5143 in 2016) were among irregular migrants attempting to migrate across the Mediterranean to Europe, adding to 1400 deaths in North Africa due to starvation, violence, sickness, unsafe travel conditions, and a harsh natural environment [155]. In February 2017, the bodies of 74 migrants were recovered near a beach town in western Libya from a shipwrecked inflatable raft found on the shore [156].

Routes to Europe from Africa commonly pass through Libya and then by boat to the Italian island of Lampedusa. In October 2013, 368 migrants died in the sinking of two boats off the coast of Lampedusa. In another event in January 2019, 117 African migrants, including 10 women, two toddlers, and one 2-month-old infant (one of the women was pregnant) died in a tragic sinking of a rickety inflatable dinghy off the Libyan coast [157]; survivors were rescued by the Italian navy and brought to Lampedusa. On the same day, in a separate incident, Sea Watch reported that it had rescued an additional 47 people in the Mediterranean; one of the boats had been stranded at sea for weeks with its passengers after being denied entry to several European ports [157].

The Institute of Migration estimates that at least 17,919 people died attempting to cross the Mediterranean Sea between 2014 and 2018 and that a total of 30,900 women, men, and children lost their lives trying to reach other countries [3].

European practices towards these desperate refugees in life-threatening situations have been varied; in June 2018, Italy's newly elected government turned away a rescue boat with 600 migrants [158]. The Italian Government has now banned the boats from landing which has diverted the problem to Malta and Spain.

The path of irregular migration across the Mediterranean is the most deadly region for irregular migrant transit in the world [7]. Nonetheless, the "Western Mediterranean route" continues to be used by people escaping violence, abuse, sickness, and starvation.

The routes from Afghanistan and the Middle East generally pass through the Middle East to Turkey, across the very dangerous Bosporus narrows where drownings in flimsy boats are common, on to Greece or sweeping further north and then across Europe to France and then the channel.

The above examples are far from complete but illustrate the desperation that refugees face in multiple parts of the world that drive the need to find new homes. The conditions that refugees have faced cannot be separated from the historic effects of colonialism in Africa, the Middle East, and other parts of the world.

Part 4: Meaningful Approaches to Improve the Health of Migrant and Refugee Children and Youth

The Right to Health: A Fundamental Human Right

Migrant and refugee children and adolescents have clear support from multiple international representative bodies to healthcare, nutrition, potable water, education, unification with parents and families, and safety. A number of inclusive agreements have been reached and signed by all, or almost all, nations of the world including the UN Convention on the Rights of the Child and the UN Universal Declaration of Human Rights.

The right to health for refugees and migrants is recognized in the International Framework of Human Rights elaborated by the Member States of the United Nations and is upheld by international human rights law [30]. These rights are further affirmed by the United Nations High Commissioner for Refugees (UNHCR) Convention Relating to the Status of Refugees [31, 32].

The Right to Health is recognized in the inherent dignity of the equal and inalienable rights of all members of the human family by the United Nations Universal Declaration of Human Rights signed in 1948 by all countries which states that:

- "Everyone has the right to a standard of living adequate for the health and well-being of himself and of his family" [28].

The UN Conventions on the Rights of the Child Article 9 assures that:

- "States Parties shall ensure that a child shall not be separated from his or her parents against their will, except when competent authorities subject to judicial review determine, in accordance with applicable law and procedure, that such separation is necessary for the best interests of the child...such as one involving abuse or neglect of the child by the parents, or one where the parents are living separately and a decision must be made as to the child's place of residence" [68].

The World Health Organization Constitution affirms "the highest attainable standard of health is one of the fundamental rights of every human being" [33].

The International Covenant on Economic, Social and Cultural Rights clearly expresses that the right to health obligates governments to ensure that "health facilities, goods and services are accessible to all, especially the most vulnerable or marginalized sections of the population in law and in fact, without discrimination on any of the prohibited grounds" [29].

- Further, the UN Committee on Economic, Social and Cultural Rights in its comments on implementing the International Covenant on Economic, Social and Cultural Rights, affirms the necessity of "being able to receive care which is available, accessible, acceptable and of good quality." Accessibility is described in four dimensions: non-discrimination, physical accessibility, economic accessibility, and information accessibility [35]. The right to health must be interpreted broadly to embrace key socioeconomic factors that promote conditions in which people can lead a healthy life. These include "food and nutrition, housing, access to safe and potable water and adequate sanitation, safe and healthy working conditions, and a healthy environment" [159].

In addition, the World Health Organization is explicit in articulating the basic principles needed to provide healthcare to migrants and refugees [34]:

1. Promoting universal health coverage
2. Reducing mortality and morbidity among refugees and migrants through public health interventions
3. Protecting and improving the health and well-being of women and girls
4. Promoting continuity of care
5. Promoting gender equality and empowering women and girls
6. Improving communication and countering xenophobia
7. Strengthening partnerships, coordination, and collaboration

Coercive practices implemented against parents or youth, such as the use of tear gas, beatings, shackling, involuntary detention, or isolation are highly traumatizing for children and youth, as well as parents, and must not be implemented. Soldiers, police, and others who engage in these practices must be held accountable for their actions.

Stabilization of Migrant Youth in the United States

Today 25% of children in the United States live in an immigrant family, that is, they are an immigrant themselves or one of their parents is an immigrant. The immigration status of children and their parents directly relates to their access to healthcare and is intertwined with other social determinants of health including poverty, food insecurity, housing instability, discrimination, and health literacy [44].

Migrants, in particular children and adolescents, require access to vital acute and preventive healthcare, housing assistance, and nutrition and commonly require access to public benefits. These benefits include accessing Medicaid, the Supplemental Nutrition Assistance Program (SNAP), and the Children's Health Insurance Program (CHIP).

Children covered by Medicaid and CHIP miss fewer school days due to illness or injury, perform better in school, are more likely to graduate and attend college, and may become healthier adults who earn higher wages and pay more in taxes than their uninsured peers. The investment in the health of children and youth, including migrant and refugee children and youth, is an investment in the future of society. Unfortunately, in the United States children and adolescents who are seeking asylum or were brought by parents and do not have legal status are excluded from federally funded programs, including health insurance, by most states [44].

As affirmed by the American Academy of Pediatrics [2, 160], it is essential that utilization of public benefits, in particular healthcare and nutrition benefits, not be used as a barrier to obtaining legal residency or future citizenship as has been proposed as a misguided means to deter migration to the United States. Increased fears about the consequences of using public programs and affecting immigration status have deterred immigrants from accessing programs regardless of eligibility. Immigration enforcement activities that occur near healthcare facilities, schools, places of worship, or other sensitive locations may prevent families from accessing needed medical care [44]. The negative impact of limiting access to public benefits for healthcare and nutrition on the health and well-being of children and youth is massive.

Education for Migrant Children and Young People: A Key Determinant of Health

Education is a key determinant of health and a common point of access for nutrition, health education, healthcare, and counseling for children and youth. Education is integral to the improvement of population health. Refugee and migrant children commonly have challenges in accessing education related to lack of fluency in the language of their new home, prior interruption of education for months or years, and commonly a need to catch up with peers; they may also struggle in school because of post-traumatic repercussions, loss of family members and/or learning disabilities.

All migrants and refugees have the right to education as articulated by the Universal Declaration of Human Rights, the UN Conventions on the Rights of the Child, and multiple other international agreements [45].

For children and youth who have missed out on their education due to circumstances they had no control over, there may be accelerated learning programs available to complete primary education in a shorter period of time providing certification and allowing continuation in formal post primary education.

Education is essential for refugee and migrant children, youth, and adults to fully participate in their new society and can play a signal role in enabling economically and socially marginalized children and adults to leave poverty. In the United States, all children are entitled to free public education and specialized educational services regardless of immigration status [44].

Indigenous people who are refugees and migrants, including children and adolescents, face additional barriers when migrating. They have commonly been traumatized by military persecution prior to leaving, do not speak the dominant language (e.g., indigenous refugees fleeing persecution in Guatemala who arrive in the United States commonly speak neither English nor Spanish), have poor educational background, and face significant barriers to integrating into the host society, including accessing education, housing, and healthcare.

The process of immigration can take months or years. During this period refugee children and youth may languish in refugee camps, not attend school, or live in areas where their native language is not spoken. They may not have opportunities to develop job skills; participate in healthy opportunities of leisure, sports, or recreation and at times be further traumatized. It is essential that in environments where children and youth are held, including refugee camps and temporary shelters, their educational needs be prioritized to prepare them for social integration and employment at the earliest opportunity.

What Can Be Done

Safety in the host country:

- Assure the safety of all children and youth regardless of ethnicity, country, or culture of origin, gender, sexual orientation or identity, or economic status

Access to healthcare:

- In accordance with the recommendations of the UN High Commissioner on Refugees, refugees should be provided with a suitable safety net, such as health insurance, to ensure access to preventive and curative care [39].
- Assure that all children and youth have access to appropriate vaccinations, potable water, stable nutrition, and suitable housing.
- Assure access to primary healthcare for all refugee and migrant children.

Family stability and prompt reunification:

- Strive whenever possible to assure that families stay together and, in particular, that children and youth are not separated from parents and siblings.
- Assure that when parents or responsible adult family members cannot be located that unaccompanied minors have stable placement with a consistent caring adult.
- Children and adolescents who have undergone trauma and significant loss need to know the truth of their family's experience or loss of parents to the extent it is known. It is useful to engage an experienced therapist to guide the conversation and disclosures and support the involved adults and youth.

- Promote factors that increase bonds and connectedness between the schools, families, and children.

Education for all refugee and migrant children and youth:

- Assure that all children and youth are engaged in appropriate education and development of employable skills.
- Direct funding to support the development of small projects for families and youth and promote increasing skills for independence among youth and families.
- Allow children and adolescents to express themselves in the physical, cultural, artistic, writing, and educational fields.
- Promote and educate children and youth about their original history and culture and foster engagement with their families and cultural groups.
- Engage children and youth in a variety of extracurricular activities and encourage them to participate in the learning process and teaching of younger children.
- Encourage reading, writing, painting, and theater and search for and find talented persons in varied fields.
- Find opportunities to teach children and youth in age-appropriate settings to develop skills in utilizing computers and encourage them to be digitally active.
- Establish and support youth clubs for boys and girls with a particular emphasis on sports and creative arts.
- Encourage the development of leadership skills among the youth.

Policy development should include youth involvement in those policies that affect them:

- Governments, policy makers, donors, and nongovernmental organizations can involve adolescents and older children in initiatives concerned with their benefit, including planning, designing, and implementation of support and intervention initiatives.
- Assure that all children and youth have a voice and not be excluded or overwhelmed by dominant individuals or groups.
- Support all aspects of positive support and the feeling of being valued individuals.
- Open and encourage dialogue between the children, teachers, leaders, and families and promote multiple approaches to providing a meaningful voice to youth.
- When the children and adolescents are politically active, they should be given the space and opportunities to express themselves and to engage them in the political dialogues.

Conclusion

The historic numbers of refugee and migrant children youth and families will inevitably continue for the foreseeable future. The factors driving these – war, climate change, ethnic persecution, poverty, and social violence – continue to evolve and in many ways worsen. There are multiple treaties that foster international collaboration to stabilize the lives of these young people and their families including the Universal Declaration on Human Rights in 1948 and the United Nations Conventions on the Rights of the Child which have been ratified by almost all countries of the world that call for providing safe haven for all refugees. Unfortunately, these international agreements are respected more in the breach than in compliance. The future of millions of children and adolescents depends on the permanent, safe, and secure resolution of international conflicts, respectful of the conditions, history, culture, and needs of children, youth, and families.

In areas of conflict, every action must be evaluated in view of its impact on the health and well-being of children and youth. It cannot be ignored that we live in a time that poses serious challenges to respecting the rights of refugees and migrants, and to the fundamental international values and lessons learned that had been arrived at after the disasters of two world wars. These values include human equity, accountability, fairness, justice, and due process. It is largely from the outcomes of the two world wars that the international consensus demonstrated by the Universal Declaration of Human Rights includes the recognition that “Everyone has the right to seek and to enjoy in other countries asylum from persecution.”

The institutions and values that were adopted to foster cooperation are being undermined by the emergence of aggressive nationalism and racism and the rejection of migrant and refugee children and families. The recognition of the rights of migrants and refugees are under threat. In some countries, there has been a kind of weaponization of immigration by demagogic figures to inflame nativism, racism, and xenophobia and undermine democracy. We know from history that this dynamic can escalate to grave attacks on human rights and be targeted against vulnerable groups of people within society because of their perceived characteristics, cultures, or religions; this process has become enhanced through the use of social media to heighten irrational fear, polarize societies, and increase hostility towards migrants, ethnic minorities, sexual minorities, and religious groups. We need to recognize and promote understanding of the great value that immigrants and refugees bring to the societies they join and, notwithstanding the challenges, find a path to welcoming those who join us, most especially the children and youth. The politicization of migration is not new, but we must learn from prior tragic outcomes of xenophobia and racism, recognize the grave threat that they represent to democracy and peace, and strive to provide a safe, healthy, and welcoming environment for those young people and their families who have been forced to leave their homes.

Practices that involve creating unnecessary and gratuitous barriers to migration or obtaining asylum, in particular those barriers that result in separating children and adolescents from their parents and families and/or involve involuntary placement, are inconsistent with international agreements and have been vehemently rejected by leading advocates and experts in child and adolescent health, in particular the American Academy of Pediatrics and the Society for Adolescent Health and Medicine.

Children and adolescents are the most vulnerable of refugees and migrants. They need and deserve to be welcomed and find stability, safety, potable water, food security, sanitation, housing, education, reproductive health, healthcare, and age-appropriate recreational activities. It is essential that children remain together with their families whenever safe and possible and continue to be engaged in their home cultural traditions.

Migrants and their children and families have historically made, and will continue to make, great contributions to the societies that welcome them. The investment that is made in the welfare of children and youth and their families will pay off for all of us in their future contributions.

References

1. World Migration Report 2020, International Organization of Migration, Geneva, Switzerland. Publications.iom.int. Accessed 28 Nov 2019.
2. Cheng I-H, Advocat JR, Vasi S, Enticott J, Willey S, Wahidi S, et al. A rapid review of evidence-based information, best practices and lessons learned in addressing the health needs of refugees and migrants: report to the World Health Organization, Melbourne. 2018. Accessed Nov 2018.
3. World Migration Report 2020, International Organization of Migration, Geneva, Switzerland. Publications.iom.int. Accessed Nov 2019 https://publications.iom.int/system/files/pdf/wmr_2020.pdf.
4. World Vision 2019; https://www.worldvision.org/refugees-news-stories/syrian-refugee-crisis-facts. Accessed 20 Oct 2019.
5. World Vision. From the Field, Syrian refugee crisis: Facts, FAQs, and how to help. https://www.worldvision.org/refugees-news-stories/syrian-refugee-crisis-facts. Accessed 20 Oct 2019.
6. UNHCR 2017 Global Trends Forced Displacement in 2017; https://www.unhcr.org/5b27be547.pdf. Accessed 13 March 2019.
7. Ardittis S, Laczko F. Migration policy practice, Vol VII, Number 2, April–September 2017, measuring irregular migration: innovative data practices publications.iom.int. Accessed 21 Jan 2019.
8. Achilli L, Sanchez G. Migration policy practice, Vol VII, Number 2, April–September 2017, methodological approaches in human smuggling research: documenting irregular migration facilitation in the Americas and the Middle East, publications.iom.int. Accessed 21 Jan 2019.
9. Hannigan A, O'Donnell P, O'Keeffe M, MacFarlane A. How do variations in definitions of "migrant" and their application influence the access of migrants to health care services? Copenhagen: WHO Regional Office for Europe; 2016.
10. De Vito E, Parente P, de Waure C, Posicia A, Ricciardi W. Health evidence network synthesis report No. 53: a review of evidence on equitable delivery, access and utilization of immunization services for migrants and refugees in the WHO European region. Copenhagen: WHO Regional Office for Europe; 2017.
11. WHO.int; Refugee and migrant health. Promoting the right to health. Accessed Nov 2018.
12. World Health Organization January 31, 2017, The Second Declaration on Global Migrant Health, New York Declaration for Refugees and Migrants https://refugeesmigrants.un.org/declaration. Accessed 20 Dec 2019.
13. Guidelines on International Protection No. 9: Claims to Refugee Status based on Sexual Orientation and/or Gender Identity within the context of Article 1A(2) of the 1951 Convention and/or its 1967 Protocol relating to the Status of Refugees; UN High Commissioner for Refugees (UNHCR). https://www.refworld.org/docid/50348afc2.html. Accessed 21 May 2019.
14. http://www.thenewhumanitarian.org/analysis/2013/05/07/plight-lgbti-asylum-seekers-refugees. Accessed 21 May 2019.

15. Climate change and health in the Western Pacific Region : synthesis of evidence, profiles of selected countries and policy direction; https://www.who.int/westernpacific/health-topics/climate-change Accessed 20 Dec 2019.
16. WHO.int; Health of refugees and migrants, Regional situation analysis, practices, experiences, lessons learned and ways forward; WHO Western Pacific Region 2018. Accessed Nov 2018.
17. World Migration Report 2020, International Organization of Migration, Geneva, Switzerland. Publications.iom.int. Accessed 28 Nov 28 2019.
18. New York Times, April 2, 2019. Cholera is spreading in Mozambique, and it's far from the only health threat. DG McNeil.
19. WHO.int; Health of refugees and migrants, Regional situation analysis, practices, experiences, lessons learned and ways forward; WHO Region of Americas 2018; https://www.who.int/migrants/publications/PAHO-report.pdf?ua=1. Accessed 20 Dec 2019.
20. The World Bank, Internal Climate Migration in Latin America; Groundswell, Preparing for Internal Climate Migration, Policy Note No.3. Accessed 20 Dec 2019.
21. Fourth National Climate Assessment, U.S. Global Change Research Program, Department of Commerce, National Oceanic and Atmospheric Administration, 2018 https://www.globalchange.gov/nca4. Accessed 20 Oct 2019.
22. Laczko F, Aghazarm C. Migration, environment and climate change: assessing the evidence. Geneva: international Organisation for Migration. 2009; https://publications.iom.int/system/files/pdf/migration_and_environment.pdf. Accessed 20 Oct 2019.
23. Lancet. The 2018 report of the Lancet Countdown on health and climate change: shaping the health of nations for centuries to come; November 2018; https://www.thelancet.com/journals/lancet/article/PIIS0140–6736(18)32594–7/fulltext. Accessed 20 Oct 2019.
24. Fourth National Climate Assessment, U.S. Global Change Research Program, Department of Commerce, National Oceanic and Atmospheric Administration, 2018; https://nca2018.globalchange.gov/. Accessed 20 Oct 2019.
25. Special Report, Global Warming of 1.5 C; Summary for Policymakers, Intergovernmental Panel on Climate Change (IPCC); https://www.ipcc.ch/sr15/. Accessed 20 Oct 2019.
26. Kennedy S, Kidd MP, McDonald JT, et al. J Int Migr Integr. 2015;16:317. https://doi.org/10.1007/s12134-014-0340-x.
27. Doryniak D, Melo JS, Farrell RM, Ojeda VD, Strathdee SA. Epidemiology of substance use among forced migrants: a global systematic review. PLoS One. 2016; https://doi.org/10.1371/Journal.pone.0159134.
28. Cheng I-H, Advocat JR, Vasi S, Enticott J, Willey S, Wahidi S, et al. A rapid review of evidence-based information, best practices and lessons learned in addressing the health needs of refugees and migrants: report to the World Health Organization, Melbourne. 2018. p. 6. Accessed Nov 2018.
29. Cheng I-H, Advocat JR, Vasi S, Enticott J, Willey S, Wahidi S, et al. A rapid review of evidence-based information, best practices and lessons learned in addressing the health needs of refugees and migrants: report to the World Health Organization. Melbourne. 2018. p.16. Accessed Nov 2018.
30. Cheng I-H, Advocat JR, Vasi S, Enticott J, Willey S, Wahidi S, et al. A rapid review of evidence-based information, best practices and lessons learned in addressing the health needs of refugees and migrants: report to the World Health Organization. Melbourne. 2018. p. 2. Accessed Nov 2018.
31. UNHCR. Convention and protocol relating to the status of refugees: the 1951 convention relating to the status of refugees; the 1967 protocol relating to the status of refugees; and resolution 2198 (XXI). New York: United Nations General Assembly; 2010.
32. OHCHR. Report on principles and practical guidance on the protection of the human rights of migrants in vulnerable situations. Geneva: United Nations. Office of the High Commissioner for Human Rights; 2017.

33. Cheng I-H, Advocat JR, Vasi S, Enticott J, Willey S, Wahidi S, et al. A rapid review of evidence-based information, best practices and lessons learned in addressing the health needs of refugees and migrants: report to the World Health Organization. Melbourne. 2018. p. 3,15. Accessed Nov 2018.
34. Cheng I-H, Advocat JR, Vasi S, Enticott J, Willey S, Wahidi S, et al. A rapid review of evidence-based information, best practices and lessons learned in addressing the health needs of refugees and migrants: report to the World Health Organization. Melbourne. 2018. p. 14. Accessed Nov 2018.
35. Cheng I-H, Advocat JR, Vasi S, Enticott J, Willey S, Wahidi S, et al. A rapid review of evidence-based information, best practices and lessons learned in addressing the health needs of refugees and migrants: report to the World Health Organization. Melbourne. 2018. p.41,42. Accessed Nov 2018.
36. OHCHR. UN Committee on Economic, Social and Cultural Rights, General Comment No. 14: the right to the highest attainable standard of health (Art. 12 of the covenant). Geneva: United Nations, Office of the High Commissioner for Human Rights; 2000. https://www.ohchr.org/Documents/Issues/Women/WRGS/Health/GC14.pdf. Accessed 20 Oct 2019.
37. Cheng I-H, Advocat JR, Vasi S, Enticott J, Willey S, Wahidi S, et al. A rapid review of evidence-based information, best practices and lessons learned in addressing the health needs of refugees and migrants: report to the World Health Organization. Melbourne. p. 26. Accessed Nov 2018.
38. Cheng I-H, Advocat JR, Vasi S, Enticott J, Willey S, Wahidi S, et al. A rapid review of evidence-based information, best practices and lessons learned in addressing the health needs of refugees and migrants: report to the World Health Organization. Melbourne. 2018. p. 120. Accessed Nov 2018.
39. Cheng I-H, Advocat JR, Vasi S, Enticott J, Willey S, Wahidi S, et al. A rapid review of evidence-based information, best practices and lessons learned in addressing the health needs of refugees and migrants: report to the World Health Organization. Melbourne. 2018. p. 27. Accessed Nov 2018.
40. Cheng I-H, Advocat JR, Vasi S, Enticott J, Willey S, Wahidi S, et al. A rapid review of evidence-based information, best practices and lessons learned in addressing the health needs of refugees and migrants: report to the World Health Organization. Melbourne. 2018. p. 26. Accessed Nov 2018.
41. Cheng I-H, Advocat JR, Vasi S, Enticott J, Willey S, Wahidi S, et al. A rapid review of evidence-based information, best practices and lessons learned in addressing the health needs of refugees and migrants: report to the World Health Organization. Melbourne. 2018. p. 19. Accessed Nov 2018.
42. Cheng I-H, Advocat JR, Vasi S, Enticott J, Willey S, Wahidi S, et al. A rapid review of evidence-based information, best practices and lessons learned in addressing the health needs of refugees and migrants: report to the World Health Organization. Melbourne. 2018. p. 55. Accessed Nov 2018.
43. Guinto RLLR, Curran UZ, Suphanchaimat R, Pocock NS. Universal health coverage in 'One ASEAN': are migrants included? Global Health Action; 2015:8(10) https://core.ac.uk/download/pdf/29050489.pdf. Accessed 20 Oct 2019.
44. Linton JM, Green A, AAP Council on Community Pediatrics. Providing care for children in immigrant families. Pediatrics. 2019;144(3):e20192077.
45. Cheng I-H, Advocat JR, Vasi S, Enticott J, Willey S, Wahidi S, et al. A rapid review of evidence-based information, best practices and lessons learned in addressing the health needs of refugees and migrants: report to the World Health Organization. Melbourne. 2018. Accessed Nov 2018 6,19,98,99,100.
46. Cheng I-H, Advocat JR, Vasi S, Enticott J, Willey S, Wahidi S, et al. A rapid review of evidence-based information, best practices and lessons learned in addressing the health needs of refugees and migrants: report to the World Health Organization. Melbourne. 2018. Accessed Nov 2018 134.

47. Cheng I-H, Advocat JR, Vasi S, Enticott J, Willey S, Wahidi S, et al. A rapid review of evidence-based information, best practices and lessons learned in addressing the health needs of refugees and migrants: report to the World Health Organization. Melbourne. 2018. p 29. Accessed Nov 2018.
48. Cheng I-H, Advocat JR, Vasi S, Enticott J, Willey S, Wahidi S, et al. A rapid review of evidence-based information, best practices and lessons learned in addressing the health needs of refugees and migrants: report to the World Health Organization. Melbourne. 2018. Accessed Nov 2018 136.
49. Cheng I-H, Advocat JR, Vasi S, Enticott J, Willey S, Wahidi S, et al. A rapid review of evidence-based information, best practices and lessons learned in addressing the health needs of refugees and migrants: report to the World Health Organization. Melbourne. 2018. Accessed Nov 2018 138,156,157.
50. Cheng I-H, Advocat JR, Vasi S, Enticott J, Willey S, Wahidi S, et al. A rapid review of evidence-based information, best practices and lessons learned in addressing the health needs of refugees and migrants: report to the World Health Organization. Melbourne. 2018. Accessed Nov 2018 155.
51. Cheng I-H, Advocat JR, Vasi S, Enticott J, Willey S, Wahidi S, et al. A rapid review of evidence-based information, best practices and lessons learned in addressing the health needs of refugees and migrants: report to the World Health Organization. Melbourne. 2018. Accessed Nov 2018 163.
52. Cheng I-H, Advocat JR, Vasi S, Enticott J, Willey S, Wahidi S, et al. A rapid review of evidence-based information, best practices and lessons learned in addressing the health needs of refugees and migrants: report to the World Health Organization. Melbourne. 2018. Accessed Nov 2018 161.
53. Cheng I-H, Advocat JR, Vasi S, Enticott J, Willey S, Wahidi S, et al. A rapid review of evidence-based information, best practices and lessons learned in addressing the health needs of refugees and migrants: report to the World Health Organization. Melbourne. 2018. Accessed Nov 2018 141, 142, 10.
54. Cheng I-H, Advocat JR, Vasi S, Enticott J, Willey S, Wahidi S, et al. A rapid review of evidence-based information, best practices and lessons learned in addressing the health needs of refugees and migrants: report to the World Health Organization. Melbourne. 2018. Accessed Nov 2018 227.
55. Cheng I-H, Advocat JR, Vasi S, Enticott J, Willey S, Wahidi S, et al. A rapid review of evidence-based information, best practices and lessons learned in addressing the health needs of refugees and migrants: report to the World Health Organization. Melbourne. 2018. p.12. Accessed Nov 2018.
56. Cheng I-H, Advocat JR, Vasi S, Enticott J, Willey S, Wahidi S, et al. A rapid review of evidence-based information, best practices and lessons learned in addressing the health needs of refugees and migrants: report to the World Health Organization. Melbourne. 2018. Accessed Nov 2018 228.
57. Cheng I-H, Advocat JR, Vasi S, Enticott J, Willey S, Wahidi S, et al. A rapid review of evidence-based information, best practices and lessons learned in addressing the health needs of refugees and migrants: report to the World Health Organization. Melbourne. Accessed Nov 2018 227, 229.
58. Cheng I-H, Advocat JR, Vasi S, Enticott J, Willey S, Wahidi S, et al. A rapid review of evidence-based information, best practices and lessons learned in addressing the health needs of refugees and migrants: report to the World Health Organization. Melbourne. 2018. p.35. Accessed Nov 2018.
59. Cheng I-H, Advocat JR, Vasi S, Enticott J, Willey S, Wahidi S, et al. A rapid review of evidence-based information, best practices and lessons learned in addressing the health needs of refugees and migrants: report to the World Health Organization. Melbourne. 2018. Accessed Nov 2018 190.
60. Cheng I-H, Advocat JR, Vasi S, Enticott J, Willey S, Wahidi S, et al. A rapid review of evidence-based information, best practices and lessons learned in addressing the health needs of refugees and migrants: report to the World Health Organization. Melbourne. 2018. Accessed Nov 2018 197.

61. Cheng I-H, Advocat JR, Vasi S, Enticott J, Willey S, Wahidi S, et al. A rapid review of evidence-based information, best practices and lessons learned in addressing the health needs of refugees and migrants: report to the World Health Organization. Melbourne. 2018. Accessed Nov 2018 198.
62. World Migration Report 2020, International Organization of Migration, Geneva, Switzerland. Publications.iom.int. Accessed November 28 2019.
63. Cheng I-H, Advocat JR, Vasi S, Enticott J, Willey S, Wahidi S, et al. A rapid review of evidence-based information, best practices and lessons learned in addressing the health needs of refugees and migrants: report to the World Health Organization. Melbourne. 2018. p 46, 226,230,231. Accessed Nov 2018.
64. Cheng I-H, Advocat JR, Vasi S, Enticott J, Willey S, Wahidi S, et al. A rapid review of evidence-based information, best practices and lessons learned in addressing the health needs of refugees and migrants: report to the World Health Organization. Melbourne. 2018. Accessed Nov 2018 191.
65. Cheng I-H, Advocat JR, Vasi S, Enticott J, Willey S, Wahidi S, et al. A rapid review of evidence-based information, best practices and lessons learned in addressing the health needs of refugees and migrants: report to the World Health Organization. Melbourne. 2018. p. 37. Accessed Nov 2018.
66. Cheng I-H, Advocat JR, Vasi S, Enticott J, Willey S, Wahidi S, et al. A rapid review of evidence-based information, best practices and lessons learned in addressing the health needs of refugees and migrants: report to the World Health Organization. Melbourne. 2018. p. 37–38; 202. Accessed Nov 2018.
67. Cheng I-H, Advocat JR, Vasi S, Enticott J, Willey S, Wahidi S, et al. A rapid review of evidence-based information, best practices and lessons learned in addressing the health needs of refugees and migrants: report to the World Health Organization. Melbourne. 2018. Accessed Nov 2018 150.
68. UN Conventions on the Rights of the Child, Article 9; https://www.ohchr.org/en/professionalinterest/pages/crc.aspx.
69. SAHM Statement on Forced Family Separation, adolescenthealth.org. Accessed 21 Jan 2019.
70. Cheng I-H, Advocat JR, Vasi S, Enticott J, Willey S, Wahidi S, et al. A rapid review of evidence-based information, best practices and lessons learned in addressing the health needs of refugees and migrants: report to the World Health Organization. Melbourne. 2018. Accessed Nov 2018 151.
71. Cheng I-H, Advocat JR, Vasi S, Enticott J, Willey S, Wahidi S, et al. A rapid review of evidence-based information, best practices and lessons learned in addressing the health needs of refugees and migrants: report to the World Health Organization. Melbourne. 2018. Accessed Nov 2018 191,192,193.
72. New York Times, Family Separation May Have Hit Thousands More Migrant Children Than Reported, M Jordan, January 17, 2019.
73. The New York Review of Books, Lee Gelernt, The Battle to Stop Family Separation; December 19, 2018; www.nybooks.com.
74. New York Times, Inside the Vast Tent City Housing Migrant Children in a Texas Desert. October 12, 2018.
75. NBC News, Trump admin projected it would separate 26,000 migrant kids at border, DHS watchdog says. Nov 27, 2019. https://www.nbcnews.com/politics/immigration/trump-admin-projected-it-would-separate-26-000-migrant-kids-n1092571.
76. NPR "Migrant Youth Go From A Children's Shelter to Adult Detention On Their 18th Birthday, February 22, 2019.; https://www.npr.org/2019/02/22/696834560/migrant-youth-go-from-a-childrens-shelter-to-adult-detention-on-their-18th-birth.
77. Alan Yuhas, New York Times, U.S. Agents Fire Tear Gas Across Mexican Border, 1 Jan 2019.
78. AAP Statement Opposing the Border Security and Immigration Reform Act, Colleen Kraft, President American Academy of Pediatrics, June 15, 2018 available at aap.org. Accessed 21 Jan 2019.
79. Jordan M, Dickerson C. U.S. Continues to Separate Migrant Families Despite Rollback of Policy. New York Times. 9 March 2019.

80. New York Times, Spring brings surge of migrants, stretching border facilities far beyond capacity, M Jordan and S Romero. March 30, 2019.
81. Mobed K, Gold EB, Schenker MB. Occupational health problems among migrant and seasonal farm workers. West J Med. 157(3):367–73.
82. Moyce SC, Schenker M. Migrant workers and their occupational health and safety. Annu Rev Public Health. 2018;39:351–65.
83. WHO.int; Health of refugees and migrants, Regional situation analysis, practices, experiences, lessons learned and ways forward; WHO Region of Americas 2018; https://www.who.int/migrants/publications/PAHO-report.pdf?ua=1. Accessed Nov 2018.
84. World Migration Report 2020, International Organization of Migration, Geneva, Switzerland. Publications.iom.int. Accessed Nov 2019.
85. WHO.int; Health of refugees and migrants, Regional situation analysis, practices, experiences, lessons learned and ways forward; WHO Region of Americas 2018; Accessed Nov 2018.
86. World Migration Report 2018, International Organization of Migration, Geneva, Switzerland. Publications.iom.int. Accessed December 2018.
87. UNHCR Turkey Factsheet - August 2018; https://reliefweb.int/report/turkey/unhcr-turkey-factsheet-august-2018.
88. Report on the health of refugees and migrants in the WHO European Region: no public health without refugee and migrant health (2018). http://www.euro.who.int/en/publications/abstracts/report-on-the-health-ofrefugees-and-migrants-in-the-who-european-region-no-public-health-without-refugee-and-migrant-health-2018.
89. Birch DML; Views from a Practitioner: the Holistic Approach' - in the IGC (Intergovernmental Consultations on Migration, Asylum and Refugees) Workshop on Strategies and Policies for Age Assessment of Unaccompanied Minors Geneva June 2011.
90. Professor Sir Al Aynsley-Green Kt. The assessment of age in undocumented migrants. Professor Emeritus of Child Health, University College London; Children's Commissioner for England; March 2011.
91. Parliamentary Assembly, Council for Europe; 'Child-friendly age assessment for unaccompanied migrant children' Rapporteur: Ms Doris Fiala, Switzerland, ALDE Committee: Doc. 14175, Reference 4257 of 23 January 2017.
92. Birch DML Asylum Seeking Children; Including Adolescent Development and the Assessment of Age. April 2010 ISBN 1 870717 22 8.
93. Birch DML, Iverson E, MacKenzie R. 'Age assessment of young people - preliminary findings of A blind study' – Platform Presentation Atlanta – Society for Adolescent Health and Medicine 2013 and Abstract publication Journal Adolescent Medicine.
94. Birch DML; Challenges to Professionals Involved with Asylum Seeking Adolescents - a special International supplement to the Brazilian journal for adolescent health: REVISTA ADOLESCENCIA & SAUDE (Adolescence and Health) 2012.
95. The Refugee Council Children in the Asylum System November 2018. https://www.refugeecouncil.org.uk/latest/news/5372_minister_announces_children_from_calais_to_be_granted_right_to_remain_in_the_uk/.
96. https://www.bbc.com/news/uk-politics-46738126 Sajid Javid under fire over Channel migrant comments, January 2019.
97. Jack Dutton 'For refugees in Calais, police brutality is a daily occurrence' 10 December 2018 The Independent.
98. Australian Human Rights Commission. The forgotten children: national inquiry into children in immigration detention. Sydney: Australian Human Rights Commission; 2014. ISBN: 978-1-921449-56-7
99. Dudley M, Steel Z, Mares S, Newman L. Children and young people in immigration detention. Curr Opin Psychiatry. 2012;25(4):285–92. https://doi.org/10.1097/YCO.0b013e3283548676.
100. Save the Children (Australia) and UNICEF (Australia). At what cost? The human, economic and strategic cost of Australia's asylum seekers policies and the alternatives. Save

the Children (Australia) and UNICEF, Australia., Melbourne and Sydney; 2016. Available: https://www.unicef.org.au/Upload/UNICEF/Media/Documents/At-What-Cost-Report.pdf.
101. UNHCR. Submission by the United Nations High Commissioner for Refugees on the "Inquiry into serious allegations of abuse, self-harm and neglect of asylum seekers in relation to the Nauru Regional Processing Centre, and any like allegations in relation to the Manus Island Regional Processing Centre'. UNHCR, Switzerland, Geneva; 2016. Available: https://www.refworld.org/pdfid/591597934.pdf
102. Phillips J, Spinks H. Boat arrivals in Australia since 1976. Parliamentary Library. Research Paper. Department of Parliamentary Services, Parliament of Australia, Canberra; 2013. Available: https://www.aph.gov.au/About_Parliament/Parliamentary_Departments/Parliamentary_Library/pubs/BN/2011–2012/BoatArrivals.
103. Phillips J. Boat arrivals and boat 'turnbacks' in Australia since 1976: a quick guide to the statistics. Parliamentary Library. Research Paper Series 2016–2017. Department of Parliamentary Services, Parliament of Australia, Canberra; 2017. Available: https://www.aph.gov.au/About_Parliament/Parliamentary_Departments/Parliamentary_Library/pubs/rp/rp1617/Quick_Guides/BoatTurnbacks.
104. Coddington K, Mountz A. Countering isolation with the use of technology. J Indian Ocean Region. 2014;10(1):97–112. https://doi.org/10.1080/19480881.2014.896104.
105. Human Rights and Equal Opportunity Commission. A last resort? National Inquiry into children in immigration detention. Sydney: HREOC; 2004. ISBN: 0-642-26989-0
106. Drury J, Williams R. Children and young people who are refugees, internally displaced persons or survivors or perpetrators of war, mass violence and terrorism. Curr Opin Psychiatry. 2012;25(4):277–84. https://doi.org/10.1097/YCO.0b013e328353eea6.
107. Mares S. The mental health of children and parents detained on Christmas Island: secondary analysis of an Australian Human Rights Commission data set. Health Human Rights J. 2016;16(2):219–232. PMCID: PMC5395006.
108. Elliott E, Gunasekera H. The health and well-being of children in immigration detention: report of the Australian Human Rights Commission monitoring visit to Wickham Point Detention Centre, Darwin, NT, Australian Human Rights Commission. Australia, Sydney; 2015. Available: https://www.humanrights.gov.au/sites/default/files/document/publication/Health%20and%20well-being%20of%20children%20in%20immigration%20detention%20report.pdf.
109. O'Connor C. Cruelty in our name: children in immigration detention. Precedent 2014; 124:4–9. Available: http://138.25.65.17/au/journals/PrecedentAULA/2014/42.pdf
110. Killendar A, Harris P. Australia's refugee policies and their health impact: a review of the evidence and recommendations for the Australian Government. Aust N Z J Public Health. 2017;41(4):335–7. https://doi.org/10.1111/1753-6405.12663.
111. Refugee Council of Australia and Asylum Seeker Resource Centre. Australia's man-made crisis in Nauru: six years on. RCA and ASRC, Melbourne Australia, Melbourne; 2018. Available: https://www.refugeecouncil.org.au/publications/reports/nauru-full/.
112. Royal Australian College of Physicians. RACP submission: conditions and treatment of asylum seekers and refugees at the regional processing centres in the Republic of Nauru and Papua New Guinea. RACP. Sydney, Australia, Sydney; 2016. Available: https://www.racp.edu.au/docs/default-source/advocacy-library/pa-sl-senator-l-pratt-racp-submission-to-inquiry-into-nauru-and-manus-island.pdf?sfvrsn=d830361a_16.
113. Jesuit Social Services. Submission to the 'Inquiry into serious allegations of abuse, self-harm and neglect of asylum seekers in relation to the Nauru Regional Processing Centre, and any like allegations in relation to the Manus Island Regional Processing Centre'. Jesuit Social Services: Melbourne, Australia, Melbourne; 2016. Available: http://jss.org.au/wp-content/uploads/2016/11/SUB-161020-Senate-Inquiry-into-Manus-Island-and-Nauru-FINAL.pdf.
114. Refugee Council of Australia and Asylum Seeker Resource Centre. Australia's man-made crisis in Nauru: six years on. RCA and ASRC, Melbourne Australia, Melbourne; 2018. page 7 Available: https://www.refugeecouncil.org.au/publications/reports/nauru-full/.

115. Global Trends Forced Displacement in 2018, UN High Commissioner on Refugees, UN Refugee Agency, 2018 in Review, https://www.unhcr.org/5d08d7ee7.pdf. Accessed 5 Nov 2019.
116. World Migration Report 2018, International Organization of Migration, Geneva, Switzerland. https://publications.iom.int/system/files/pdf/wmr_2018_en.pdf p 18; Accessed 18 Oct 2019.
117. WHO.int; Health of refugees and migrants, Regional situation analysis, practices, experiences, lessons learned and ways forward; WHO Region of Americas 2018; https://www.who.int/migrants/publications/PAHO-report.pdf?ua=1 Accessed Nov 2018.
118. An Apology for A Guatemalan Coup, 57 Years Later. E Malkin. New York Times, Oct 20, 2011.
119. America's Role in El Salvador's Deterioration. R Bonner. The Atlantic. Jan 20, 2018.
120. Honduran President Is Ousted in Coup. E Malkin. New York Times. June 28, 2009.
121. Missing Migrants, Tracking Deaths Along Migratory Routes; missingmigrants.iom.int. Accessed 21 Jan 2019.
122. Iraq conflict has killed a million Iraqis: survey, World News January 30, 2008 https://www.reuters.com/article/us-iraq-deaths-survey/iraq-conflict-has-killed-a-million-iraqis-survey-idUSL3048857920080130.
123. Mortality after the 2003 invasion of Iraq: a cross sectional cluster sample survey, G Burnham, R Lafta, S Doocy, L Roberts, The Lancet October 12, 2006. https://www.thelancet.com/journals/lancet/article/PIIS0140-6736(06)69491-9/fulltext.
124. Watson Institute, International and Public Affairs, Brown University, Costs of War; https://watson.brown.edu/costsofwar/costs/human/refugees/iraqi.
125. 2018 Humanitarian Review https://reliefweb.int/report/syrian-arab-republic/unicef-syria-crisis-situation-report-november-2018-humanitarian-results.
126. UNHCR Syria Regional Refugee Response. https://data2.unhcr.org/en/situations/syria. Retrieved 17 April 2018.
127. Yemen Humanitarian Bulletin Issue 30, January 28, 2018; United Nations Office for the Coordination of Humanitarian Affairs. reliefweb.int, retrieved February 9 2019.
128. New York Times, Yemen girl who turned world's eyes to famine is dead; Declan Walsh, November 1, 2018.
129. New York Times Magazine, November 6, 2018; How the war in Yemen became a bloody stalemate - and the worst humanitarian crisis in the world; Robert F. Worth.
130. UN News, Looming famine in Yemen could put two million mothers at risk of death - UN agency. November 1, 2018; https://news.un.org/en/story/2018/11/1024652.
131. "Yemen could be 'worst famine in 100 years'" https://www.bbc.com/news/av/world-middle-east-45857729/yemen-could-be-worst-famine-in-100-years.
132. World Health Organization, Cholera Situation in Yemen. Situation Report SEPTEMBER 2019 ISSUE NO.9 Yemen Conflict. http://applications.emro.who.int/docs/yem/Yem-Sitrep-Sept-2019.pdf?ua=1.
133. UNHCR, UN Refugee Agency; Yemen humanitarian crisis; https://www.unrefugees.org/emergencies/yemen/.
134. Yemen Humanitarian Bulletin Issue 30, January 28, 2018; United Nations Office for the Coordination of Humanitarian Affairs. reliefweb.int, retrieved 9 Feb 2019.
135. Israel Ministry of Foreign Affairs, The Balfour Declaration. https://mfa.gov.il/mfa/foreign-policy/peace/guide/pages/the%20balfour%20declaration.aspx. Accessed 20 Oct 2019.
136. Institute for Palestine Studies. W Glazer; The Palestinian Exodus in 1948. http://www.palestine-studies.org/jps/fulltext/38640. Accessed 20 Oct 2019.
137. UN Refugee Works Agency for Palestine Refugees in the Near East. https://www.unrwa.org/palestine-refugees. Accessed 20 Oct 2019.
138. Badil, Survey of Palestinian Refugees (2008–2009). http://badil.org/en/publication/survey-of-refugees.html. Accessed 20 Oct 2019.
139. Abu Shakrah, Jan, "Palestinian refugees: a discussion paper", American Friends Service Committee's Middle East Program, 2000. https://www.afsc.org/resource/palestinian-refugees-and-right-return.

140. Badil, Research Center for Palestinian residency and refugee rights. Accessed 20 Oct 2019.
141. https://data.worldbank.org/indicator/SP.POP.GROW. Accessed 20 Oct 2019.
142. UNICEF in the State of Palestine; https://www.unicef.org/infobycountry/oPt_statistics.html. Accessed 20 Oct 2019.
143. Tony Waterston, Dina Nasser; Access to healthcare for children in Palestine. BMJ Paediatr Open. 2017;1(1):e000115. https://bmjpaedsopen.bmj.com/content/bmjpo/1/1/e000115.full.pdf. Accessed 20 Oct 2019.
144. UN Office for the Coordination of Humanitarian Affairs. Nov 16.2018; https://www.ocha-opt.org/content/study-warns-water-sanitation-crisis-gaza-may-cause-disease-outbreak-and-possible-epidemic#ftn_ref34. Accessed 20 Oct 20 2019.
145. The public health impact of Gaza's water crisis: analysis and policy options, https://www.rand.org/pubs/research_reports/RR2515.html. Accessed 20 Oct 2019.
146. Israel, Ministry of Justice, Israel's Investigation and Prosecution of Ideologically Motivated Offences Against Palestinians in the West Bank, Oct 2018, p. 1. Accessed 20 Oct 2019.
147. UN Office for the Coordination of Humanitarian Affairs. Nov 16.2018; https://www.ocha-opt.org/content/study-warns-water-sanitation-crisis-gaza-may-cause-disease-outbreak-and-possible-epidemic#ftn_ref34.
148. Manenti A, de Goyet CV, Reinicke C, Macdonald J, Donald J; Report of a field assessment of health conditions in the occupied Palestinian territory. Feb 2016. World Health Organization http://apps.who.int/gb/Statements/Report_Palestinian_territory/Report_Palestinian_territory-en.pdf. Accessed 20 Oct 2019.
149. Giacaman R, Shannon HS, Saab H, Arya N, Boyce W, Eur J. Public Health. 2007;17(4):361–8 Accessed 20 Oct 2019.
150. Palestinian Central Bureau of Statistics; http://www.pcbs.gov.ps/post.aspx?lang=en&ItemID=1801. Accessed 20 Oct 20 2019.
151. R Giacaman, R Khatib, L Shabaneh, A Ramlawi, Belgacem Sabri, G Sabatinelli, et al. Health status and health services in the occupied Palestinian territory. Lancet. 2009;373(9666):784–8. T. March 07, 2009; https://doi.org/10.1016/S0140-6736(09)60107-0.
152. Manenti A, de Goyet CV, Reinicke C, Macdonald J, Donald J. Report of a field assessment of health conditions in the occupied Palestinian territory. Feb 2016. World Health Organization.
153. World Health Organization Special Situation Report Gaza, occupied Palestinian territory May to July 2017; http://www.emro.who.int/images/stories/palestine/WHO-Special-Situation-Report-on-_Gaza_May-June_final_2.pdf.
154. Human Rights Watch; Israel: record-low in Gaza medical permits, February 13, 2018; https://www.hrw.org/news/2018/02/13/israel-record-low-gaza-medical-permits.
155. World Migration Report 2018, International Organization of Migration, Geneva, Switzerland. Publications.iom.int Accessed Dec 2018 and International Organization of Migration, Missing Migrants Project: https://missingmigrants.iom.int/about.
156. World Migration Report 2018, International Organization of Migration, Geneva, Switzerland. Publications.iom.int. Accessed December 2018 and International Organization of Migration, Missing Migrants Project: https://missingmigrants.iom.int/about.
157. New York Times, January 19, 2019, "More Than 100 Migrants Die at Sea in Wreck Off Libya, Survivors Say, G Pianigiani,
158. New York Times, June 11, 2018, "Italy's New Populist Government Turns Away Ship With 600 Migrants Aboard".
159. OHCHR. UN Committee on Economic, Social and Cultural Rights, General Comment No. 14: the right to the highest attainable standard of health (Art. 12 of the covenant). Geneva: United Nations, Office of the High Commissioner for Human Rights; 2000. https://www.ohchr.org/Documents/Issues/Women/WRGS/Health/GC14.pdf Accessed 20 Oct 2019.
160. AAP Opposes Dangerous Public Charge Proposal Sept 19, 2018 https://www.aap.org/en-us/about-the-aap/aap-press-room/Pages/AAP-Opposes-Dangerous-Public-Charge-Proposal.aspx. Accessed 20 Oct 2019.

Chapter 18
Meaningfully Engaging Homeless Youth in Research

Annie Smith, Maya Peled, and Stephanie Martin

Introduction

McCreary Centre Society (McCreary) is a not-for-profit organization in British Columbia (BC), Canada, committed to improving the health of youth through research, evaluation, and community-based projects. Since its inception over forty years ago, McCreary has engaged adolescents in all aspects of its work, including through designated seats on the Board, youth-adult partnership projects, and long-standing youth-led groups such as the Youth Advisory and Action Council (YAC).

The Society is recognized for its engagement of vulnerable populations of young people in community-based research and is also internationally known for its BC Adolescent Health Survey (BC AHS), a population-level questionnaire used to gather information about young people's physical and emotional health and about factors that can influence health during adolescence and in later life. The survey has been conducted in collaboration with the provincial government and public health system, and with the cooperation of BC's school districts since 1992. It is completed by approximately 30,000 Grade 7–12 students every five years. The survey results are used by school districts, community agencies, all levels of government, and young people themselves to identify and help to address current youth health concerns.

A. Smith (✉) · M. Peled · S. Martin
McCreary Centre Society, Vancouver, BC, Canada
e-mail: annie@mcs.bc.ca; maya@mcs.bc.ca; stephanie@mcs.bc.ca

C. Warf, G. Charles (eds.), *Clinical Care for Homeless, Runaway and Refugee Youth*, https://doi.org/10.1007/978-3-030-40675-2_18

However, the survey is limited to students who are attending mainstream public schools, and while a small percentage of homeless youth are included in the survey, it misses many adolescents who are struggling with homelessness. This omission means that decisions about youth health which are based on the survey results are unlikely to be inclusive of the unique health challenges and experiences of homeless youth.

In 2000, McCreary embarked on its first Homeless and Street-Involved Youth Survey (HSIYS) in communities across the province. Unlike the "captive audience" available to researchers in a school setting, homeless youth can be difficult to locate and reluctant to engage in research as participants. It was therefore decided to take a participatory action research approach and to develop a youth-engaged methodology. This approach has proved effective and continues to be used to this day.

Youth Engagement

Youth engagement has been described as the meaningful and sustainable involvement of young people in decision-making that affects them [1, 2]. Meaningful youth engagement allows youth to take action, have their voice heard, and actively participate in their own development [3]. Many benefits of youth engagement have been identified, including improved mental health and reduced health risk behaviors among males and females [3, 4].

Gaining a variety of skills and knowledge is also a benefit of youth engagement, including among marginalized young people [5–7]. For example, youth have been found to develop skills in public speaking, leadership, teamwork, time management, planning and facilitating workshops, and creating written documents. Other benefits might include increased awareness and knowledge of community issues [6].

Youth-serving organizations can benefit from youth engagement, as they develop a better understanding of youth issues, become more responsive to the needs of the youth they serve, and gain a more focused vision [8].

One established model of youth engagement is Hart's "Ladder of Participation" [9]. According to this model, the lower rungs of the ladder (i.e., manipulation, decoration, and tokenism) reflect youth participation that is not genuine. At these lower rungs, youth are not informed or consulted in decision-making processes and instead are involved solely for adults to achieve their own goals. The higher rungs of the ladder are models of genuine participation, where youth are consulted in meaningful and authentic ways or can share decision-making with adults.

However, the highest rungs of the ladder, which reflect youth-led initiatives or genuine youth-adult partnerships, should not be considered as the ideal for all youth in all situations. Different youth might prefer varying degrees of participation and responsibility, depending on their circumstances, abilities, and interests. Their ability to choose their level of engagement is key to genuine youth participation [9].

Youth-Adult Partnerships

Youth-adult partnerships are an essential element of youth engagement and have been described as shared decision-making between youth and adults [10]. These partnerships generally include multiple youth and multiple adults working together in a democratic way over a sustained period of time to positively impact the wider community [11]. These partnerships can also be a way to address the isolation of youth and an opportunity for adults to contribute to their community [11].

There are four core elements that effective youth-adult partnerships incorporate: authentic decision-making (which includes youth at the center), natural mentors (who are non-judgmental, passionate, and well organized), reciprocity (where co-learning occurs), and community connectedness [11]. In addition, for youth-adult partnerships to be successful, organizations must understand the importance of working together to achieve common aims and must put resources into supporting the adults and youth involved [7].

Specific benefits of youth-adult partnerships include an increase in youth's sense of community connectedness and enhanced social networks [2, 9, 10]. Youth-adult partnerships can also increase access to social capital which in turn can improve self-concept and a sense of social acceptance by peers and can reduce risk behaviors [12].

Further, meaningful youth-adult partnerships can have an overall positive impact on the greater community through gaining active citizens who are versed in addressing challenges through collaboration, improved intergenerational understanding, breakdown of stereotypes, and increased social capital [13].

An example of a youth-adult partnership initiative was McCreary's Aboriginal Next Steps II project (2007–2009), which took place in 10 communities across BC. The Next Steps is a workshop series created in 1998 to share the results of the BC AHS with youth who had participated in the survey. The workshops gather youth's feedback and perspectives on the results and support them to design and deliver sustainable projects which address health issues they identify through the survey results. This process has been found to provide young people with a voice and sense of empowerment [14]. The Aboriginal Next Steps is an adapted version of the BC AHS Next Steps, specifically designed for (and with) Indigenous communities.

Through Aboriginal Next Steps II, Indigenous youth aged 13–19, including those with experience of street involvement, substance use challenges, and justice involvement, developed sustainable youth health projects in their communities, which they delivered in partnership with local adult supports (including teachers, youth workers, and parents). The initiative also created meaningful partnerships among community agencies which ensured the youth-led projects were reflective of the unique needs and culture of each community, and increased the likelihood of longer-term project sustainability.

Aboriginal Next Steps II evaluation findings (survey data and qualitative accounts) indicated improvements among youth participants in various areas which they attributed to their involvement in the initiative. Most youth reported reductions in their substance use and criminal behavior (among those who had engaged in these activities), as well as improved mental health, including enhanced self-confidence and hopefulness, and reduced suicidal ideation and self-harm. The majority of participants also reported improved school and community connectedness, and peer and family relationships because of their involvement in a project which they described as personally meaningful [15]. This initiative was awarded the 2009 Solicitor General's Award for Children and Youth Leadership.

Youth Participatory Action Research

Youth participatory action research (YPAR) is an approach to facilitate youth engagement in research, with support and guidance from adults. This type of research attempts to support those who have commonly been the objects or participants of research to become collaborators or coresearchers [16].

A successful YPAR project allows youth to participate and make decisions in areas where young people's voices are commonly omitted. Such projects aim to reduce inequities, place an emphasis on collaboration and on collective knowledge generation, and create an iterative process of research, action, and reflection, which results in personal or collective change for participants [17, 18].

McCreary's Positive Mental Health initiative (2015–2016) focused specifically on engaging vulnerable youth in research and provides an example of a time-limited YPAR project. The aim of this project was to support youth who had experienced mental health challenges to create a report to increase people's awareness and understanding of youth mental health issues, as well as supports and protective factors that can contribute to positive mental health among young people. A total of 28 youth with diverse backgrounds and experiences, including homelessness, attended a Design Lab where they discussed factors that contribute to positive mental health and developed research questions they were interested in answering using data from the 2013 BC Adolescent Health Survey.

Youth then selected one of five roles they were interested in being involved in. These included quantitative analysis (youth learned how to conduct statistical analysis using SPSS and carried out analyses to address their research questions), qualitative analysis (youth categorized open-ended survey responses which related to mental health and documented the themes), report writing (youth integrated and organized the quantitative and qualitative data into a report), dissemination/design (youth worked with a graphic designer to lay out the report and developed promotional material), and facilitation/presentation (youth created an interactive workshop to engage other young people with the key findings from the report and created a slide show for more formal presentations). Participants in each group met regularly over the course of two months to complete these tasks, and all project participants reconvened for a follow-up session to develop the report's key findings and create a dissemination plan.

After launching the report [19] to an audience of policy makers, service providers, and community members, youth participants shared the findings through a number of presentations and workshops across the province, to both youth and adult audiences.

Evaluation findings from the Positive Mental Health initiative highlighted that all participants stayed engaged throughout the project and felt the experience was meaningful to them. The majority reported improvements in their research skills and their confidence carrying out research, as well as their knowledge of youth mental health issues. Further, most reported improvements in their social-emotional functioning, including their sense of well-being, connections to other young people, and connection to their community [20].

Based on the success of the Positive Mental Health project and other youth engagement initiatives, McCreary developed a Youth Research Academy (YRA) for youth aged 16–24 with experience of the government care system. All of these youth have also been homeless or precariously housed and most have experienced associated challenges (e.g., substance use and mental health challenges). The YRA takes one cohort of eight youth each year. Over the course of the year, members of the YRA are trained to conduct research projects that are of interest to youth in and from care and the agencies that serve them. Since its inception in 2016, the YRA have worked on a range of evaluation and research projects, and participants have reported gaining not only research skills but also transferable skills (e.g., communication, teamwork, conflict resolution, work-place etiquette) and improved job prospects [21].

The final project of each cohort of the YRA is to carry out peer-to-peer training with other young people who are interested in learning about community-based research and in participating in a research project. The overall goal is for the YRA to support other at-risk youth to gain skills and interest in community-based research as well as transferable education and employment skills. The first cohort of the YRA (2016–2017) chose to carry out a project on how young people experience and manage stress, to gain a better understanding of how youth can best be supported to manage their stress. The second cohort (2017–2018) was interested in the relation between mental health and nutrition and how youth with mental health challenges can be supported to engage in healthy eating.

The ensuing Youth Research Slam (in March 2017 and March 2018) was a fast-paced project that trained youth in community-based research. It involved six 4-hour sessions which took place over a 2-week period during Spring Break. With support from McCreary staff, youth developed and distributed an online survey, conducted quantitative data analysis, wrote up the results, and disseminated the findings. Evaluation results indicated that the vast majority of participants reported their involvement in the Research Slam helped to improve their skills and interest in research, as well as their skills in other areas such as teamwork and critical thinking. In addition, members of the YRA reported improved leadership skills because of the peer-to-peer training they were involved in through the Research Slam [22].

Homeless and Street-Involved Youth Survey (HSIYS)

While all the youth engagement projects discussed in the previous section included young people with homelessness experience, McCreary's Homeless and Street-Involved Youth Survey (HSIYS) is an example of a youth-adult partnership approach that specifically targets homeless and street-involved youth.

This project embodies the principles, practices, and values of meaningful youth engagement and YPAR. It illustrates a method for engaging street-involved youth throughout the research process, from survey development and delivery to interpretation and dissemination of the findings.

For McCreary, securing funding for a population-level study of homeless youth which engages them throughout the process has proved challenging. This is partly because youth homelessness is less visible than adult homelessness, as young people are often couch surfing and reluctant to access services targeted at homeless adults or at street-entrenched young people. As a result, many municipalities in BC do not provide services for homeless youth or acknowledge that there is a homeless youth population in their city.

In 2000, funding was secured for a more targeted study, which focused on homeless youth in the seven communities considered to have the largest populations of homeless youth in BC. The HSIYS was expanded to nine communities in 2006 and thirteen communities in 2014.

Methodology Overview

The HSIYS was designed to include many of the same questions as the BC Adolescent Health Survey as well as additional questions which provide information about risk and protective factors among BC youth who are homeless, precariously housed, or involved in a street lifestyle. The content of each wave of the survey is determined by an advisory committee made up of young people with experience of homelessness, and youth homelessness experts from Indigenous and non-Indigenous youth-serving agencies in each of the communities participating in the survey.

In addition to updating the content of the survey to capture new and emerging issues and ensure items remain relevant, members of the advisory committee also guide data analysis, take responsibility for the recruitment and support of community coresearchers hired to administer the survey (one youth worker and one or more youth with experience of homelessness in each participating community), and oversee dissemination of findings in their community.

Engaging Youth as Coresearchers

The HSIYS is administered by an experiential youth in partnership with a frontline youth worker. Steering committee members recruit the youth and frontline worker, and both are paid for the hours they work on the project. Youth researchers are selected based on their experience and knowledge of youth homelessness in the community, as well as availability. The position requires flexible work hours and is best suited to a young person who has recently exited homelessness or who is looking to make changes away from a street lifestyle.

Before data collection begins, the community coresearchers attend a comprehensive two-day training session where they learn about community-engaged research and are trained to administer the survey. They work together to develop a strategy to survey typically hard-to-reach homeless youth to participate in the study, as well as to create a list of local services they could approach where youth can be accessed. They also determine procedures for safe storage of blank and completed surveys and honoraria, engage in role playing to practice the necessary steps for obtaining informed consent (e.g., reading the consent form aloud and answering frequently asked questions from participants), and divide up the administrative tasks between them as appropriate.

Upon completion of data collection, a debrief session with all the community coresearchers is held to guide the analyses, and then a final session brings together the advisory committee members and coresearchers to review a draft of the results and to identify key findings and messages.

Dissemination of Findings

After each wave of the survey is completed, the community coresearchers and youth and adult members of the steering committee work together to select key findings for dissemination and to determine the format the dissemination will take. After each survey, a series of Next Steps workshops takes place to share the results with youth. These workshops are designed to provide homeless youth with an opportunity to discuss the results of the survey, to make recommendations for change, and to plan (and sometimes deliver) projects for improving the health of homeless youth in their community and across the province. The interactive workshops are held in spaces which are welcoming to homeless youth, including youth drop-in centers, Aboriginal friendship centers, youth resource centers, and youth shelters.

Following the 2014 HSIYS, youth coresearchers produced three stop-motion films of their key findings to share the results with youth during the workshops. Developing a trivia game based on the survey findings has been another approach youth researchers have used to disseminate the results and engage participants in a dialogue of key findings. Workshop participants respond to trivia questions, share why they chose a particular answer, and discuss how results reflect what they see in their own community.

By using the results of the survey to spark a dialogue, youth who may have participated in the survey have the opportunity to see how their answers compare to those of homeless youth in other parts of the province and to observe and comment on trends and patterns in the data. They are also asked for their suggestions on how the health picture of homeless youth which emerges from the data can be improved. The community coresearchers' participation in these dissemination activities ensures that youth's recommendations are incorporated into the final Homeless and Street-Involved Youth report and can be further disseminated.

Impacts

Coresearchers on the HSIY project have reported gaining skills and knowledge through their involvement, including skills in survey design and implementation, as well as workshop facilitation and public speaking. Many have also felt the experience improved their job prospects and helped them find their career path.

Further, coresearchers have expressed appreciation for the opportunity to make a difference in their community and to improve the lives of homeless youth. Youth researchers who participated in the 2014 HSIYS noted that creating a report which they could take to policy makers locally and provincially was one of the most meaningful and impactful parts of the project. It inspired a sense of pride in their accomplishments, as well as a desire to continue to disseminate the results widely and to address issues in their community and for homeless youth.

The coresearchers also reported making new contacts with workers and agencies in their community they had been previously unaware of, which helped to improve their sense of connection to the community and their access to needed services.

> I have learned quite a lot while working on the HSIY project, from learning computer skills to learning how to connect with youth of all ages, and how to facilitate an effective workshop. I had a lot of fun conversing with people and learning new skills each day. The most enjoyable thing was knowing that I was doing something to help the younger generation of youth that are going through the same challenges as I previously had. – Youth coresearcher

> The HSIY project was a great experience and being part of it helped me learn facilitating skills and public speaking skills which are both things that have/will help me in my future career. I really enjoyed having the opportunity to go out in the community and do the presentations. Overall it was an awesome experience for me. My favourite part was being able to see all the work we put into it come out during our presentations. – Youth coresearcher

> The youth researcher got to be the expert. She now wants to be a youth worker because of this experience. – Adult coresearcher

Beyond benefits to the youth coresearchers, over the years there has been consistent feedback from youth survey respondents and Next Steps workshop participants that they appreciated the joint leadership role of the youth in the project. Many have stated that having youth as coresearchers motivated them to complete the survey which they otherwise would not have felt comfortable or interested in completing. Also, youth workshop participants have expressed appreciation for the opportunity to hear the results of the survey, reflect on the findings, and offer their suggestions to improve the lives of homeless youth in their community.

> I like that the survey goes directly to the youth and you get all the information first hand, from youth themselves. – Youth participant

> Youth felt safe doing the survey because youth researchers were handing it out. – Adult coresearcher

> I loved that the youth wanted to do the survey because they wanted to give back and to make this a success. – Youth coresearcher

The youth-adult partnership approach has also been welcomed by local service providers who have seen legitimacy in the recommendations that came from each report and Next Steps workshop. For example, one service provider added provisions for pets when they learned from the survey results how many youth were not accessing services because they had nowhere to leave their pet, and another added gym equipment to their housing program after learning about the lack of opportunities for homeless youth to engage in physical activity in the winter. The information and feedback youth have shared in the workshops have provided important directions for community-based action and further research.

Challenges and Benefits of Engaging Homeless Youth in Research

There are a number of challenges to engaging homeless youth in youth-adult partnerships in general and in a YPAR project such as the HSIYS in particular. Not least is the need for significant time, energy, staff, and financial commitments to make the project a success, and to increase the likelihood of success, it is essential to anticipate these challenges and the resources that will be required.

Adults are often unfamiliar with working in partnership with homeless youth, and it may be necessary to work through their concerns about homeless youth's abilities or conversely the tendency of some adults to give all control and too much responsibility to the youth.

When selecting youth coresearchers, it is important that the youth are at a place where they are able to be objective and fulfill the role of neutral researcher when collecting data. Young people who are too close to their own homelessness experience or who wish to act as counsellor or confidante to the research participants may need significant training to ensure they can fulfill the researcher role appropriately and safely.

Young people with homelessness experience who become coresearchers have often experienced additional challenges beyond homelessness, including a history of trauma, mental health challenges, or substance use, which, although extremely helpful for guiding the project, may interfere with their ability to fully commit to the entirety of the project for its duration. A contingency plan should be in place should the youth need additional support or to withdraw from the project on a temporary or permanent basis.

Many youth who become homeless have been let down by the adults in their lives, and it may be difficult for them to develop trust in the partnership process. It is therefore vital that youth are consistently kept informed of all elements of the project and are given the time and opportunity to develop trusting relationships with the adults involved.

Our experience with the HSIYS has shown that the challenges are outweighed by the benefits of engaging homeless youth throughout the process. Their involvement in survey design can help to identify new and emerging relevant issues to be included and can support the accessibility and readability of the survey layout for young people. Their involvement in data collection can ensure "hard-to-reach" youth are located and can increase the likelihood of these youth agreeing to participate.

Young people's role in guiding the data analysis can help to identify issues that adults might miss. For example, the most recent HSIYS included analyses on the role that having pets can play in missing out on needed health care and on feeling safe at night – analyses the youth had proposed and which had not been considered by any adult expert involved in the project, and which yielded significant findings.

Having youth engaged in selecting the key findings for dissemination and playing a role in that dissemination ensures youth who participated in the research see themselves reflected in the data and highlights the issues of importance to young people.

In addition, partnerships with community agencies can be enhanced when they see the value of engaging young people as coresearchers. Community agencies may become less hesitant about facilitating connections between the youth they serve and research agencies if they know the research embodies a participatory action approach and that the youth may benefit from their involvement.

Adopting youth engagement practices across various projects within an agency, rather than only for a specific time-limited project, can also build greater capacity within the agency to sustain meaningful youth engagement.

Lessons Learned for Engaging Homeless Youth in Research

Authentic youth-adult partnerships take time to develop, especially with youth who have reason to distrust adults. Additionally, building the capacities of diverse adults and youth to work in partnership requires skilled staff support and an understanding and commitment to the process.

A project such as the HSIYS can take up to 18 months from beginning to end, and it is important that the commitment required is fully understood and that the costs of youth and staff involvement in terms of workload, time, and resources are fully understood and covered.

Also, statutory agencies and bodies such as ethics boards which may be involved may require a lengthy approval process and additional submissions and assurances before agreeing to a survey using a YPAR methodology. These time considerations should be factored into the project timeline.

It is important that homeless youth become engaged at the outset of the project so they can be involved in meaningful planning, decision-making opportunities, and implementation processes alongside adults throughout the project. It is also important to clearly identify and articulate the roles and responsibilities of adults and youth and to regularly – formally and informally – recognize young people's contributions.

Piloting the survey is vital to ensure it is understandable to youth and is of an appropriate length. It also allows youth researchers to understand what questions may come up during survey administration and to prepare an answer to those questions.

When surveying homeless youth, it is important to factor in the weather and time of year. For example, many homeless young people travel to BC for the summer before returning to their home provinces in the fall, meaning survey results may differ at different times of the year. Additionally, in communities which experience severe weather, it may be difficult to find young people to survey during the winter months.

It is important to take a strengths-based approach where each youth is encouraged to work in a way that draws on their strengths and skills. Also, giving youth the opportunity to be creative within the delivery and design of data collection or dissemination workshops increases their sense of ownership and enjoyment.

Creating spaces which are physically and emotionally safe and welcoming for youth is important for fostering their meaningful participation. For example, the timing and location of steering committee meetings should be carefully planned to be youth friendly and easily accessible.

Ensuring the physical and emotional safety of youth conducting research activities in the community is also important. This includes implementing a buddy system to ensure youth researchers do not administer surveys alone and providing regular opportunities to debrief youth's experiences and address any challenges that may have arisen.

Finally, acknowledging that youth who will engage in a project such as this one may be homeless or have recently transitioned out of homelessness, it is necessary to ensure their needs are met so they can fully participate. This can include providing youth with food; transportation to get to meetings, workshops, and other project-related activities; honoraria to acknowledge their time and contributions; and access to the Internet (to coordinate research activities, to communicate with project partners, and to connect to resources to meet their basic needs).

Conclusion

Meaningfully engaging homeless youth and other vulnerable young people in research that affects them can be challenging. These youth often have histories of trauma, mental health challenges, and substance abuse and can struggle to meet their basic needs, which can create barriers to their engagement and to supporting their sustained involvement.

It is therefore important to ensure youth's basic needs are met and to be aware of other challenges they may be experiencing, to ensure they can be supported to fully participate and fulfill their roles on the project. It is also important to create safe youth-friendly spaces and to allow time for youth to develop trusting relationships with the adults involved.

Young people should be involved in the research project from the outset, and there should be clear and transparent communication about roles, responsibilities, and progress throughout the project. Taking a strengths-based approach is also important, whereby youth are encouraged to work in a way that draws on and further develops their strengths and skills.

Meaningfully engaging homeless young people in research can benefit not only these youth (e.g., skill development, improved education and employment prospects, and increased connections) but also other marginalized young people who might otherwise not be reached and have their voice included. YPAR and youth-adult partnerships can also be beneficial to the wider community by supporting the development of engaged and skilled young people who are motivated to contribute to positive change and are hopeful for their future.

References

1. Checkoway B. What is youth participation? Child Youth Serv Rev. 2011;33:340–5.
2. Smith A, Peled M, Hoogeveen C, Cotman S, McCreary Centre Society. A seat at the table: a review of youth Engagement in Vancouver. Vancouver: McCreary Centre Society; 2009.
3. BC Healthy Communities. Provincial youth engagement scan. 2011. http://bchealthycommunities.ca/res/download.php?id=961. Accessed 23 Aug 2018.
4. Paglia A, Room R. Preventing substance use problems among youth: a literature review & recommendations. J Prim Prev. 1998;20(1):3–50.
5. Libby M, Rosen M, Sedonaen M. Building youth-adult partnerships for community change: lessons from the youth leadership institute. J Community Psychol. 2005;33(1):111–20.
6. Ramey H, Rose-Krasnor L. The new mentality: youth-adult partnerships in community mental health promotion. Child Youth Serv Rev. 2015;50:28–37.
7. Zeldin S, Petrokubi J, McCart S, Khanna N, Collura J, Christens B. Strategies for sustaining quality youth-adult partnerships in organizational decision making: multiple perspectives. Prev Res. 2011;18(Suppl):7–11.
8. Ramey HL. Organizational outcomes of youth involvement in organizational decision making: a synthesis of qualitative research. J Community Psychol. 2013;41(4):488–504.
9. Hart RA. Children's participation: from tokenism to citizenship. 1992. http://www.unicef-irc.org/publications/pdf/childrens_participation.pdf. Accessed 1 Aug 2018.
10. Zeldin S, Camino L, Mook C. The adoption of innovation in youth organizations: creating the conditions for youth-adult partnerships. J Community Psychol. 2005;33(1):121–35.
11. Zeldin S, Christens BD, Powers JL. The psychology and practice of youth-adult partnership: bridging generations for youth development and community change. Am J Community Psychol. 2013;51:385–97.
12. Thomason JD, Kuperminc G. Cool girls, inc. and self-concept: the role of social capital. J Early Adolesc. 2014;34(6):816–36.

13. Ministry of Children and Family Development. *Youth engagement toolkit: resource guide*. 2013. https://www2.gov.bc.ca/assets/gov/family-and-social-supports/data-monitoring-quality-assurance/information-for-service-providers/youth_engagement_toolkit_resource_guide.pdf. Accessed 2 Aug 2018.
14. Morsillo J, Prilleltensky I. Social action with youth: interventions, evaluation, and psychopolitical validity. J Community Psychol. 2007;35(6):725–40.
15. Peled M. Aboriginal next steps II: final evaluation report. 2010. http://www.mcs.bc.ca/pdf/ANS_Final_Evaluation.pdf. Accessed 5 Jun 2018.
16. Brown L, Strega S. Research as resistance: critical, indigenous, and anti-oppressive approaches. Ontario: Canadian Scholars' Press/Women's Press; 2005.
17. Kindon SL, Pain R, Kesby M. Participatory action research approaches and methods: connecting people, participation and place. London: Routledge; 2007.
18. London JK, Zimmerman K, Erbstein N. Youth-led research and evaluation: tools for youth, organizational, and community development. New Dir Eval. 2003;98:33–45.
19. McCreary Centre Society. Unspoken thoughts & hidden facts: a snapshot of BC youth's mental health. 2016. http://www.mcs.bc.ca/pdf/Unspoken_thoughts_hidden_facts.pdf. Accessed 1 Aug 2018.
20. Peled M, Smith A, Martin S. Engaging experiential youth in a youth-led positive mental health research initiative. Paper presented at the 6th Conference of the International Society for Child Indicators (ISCI), Montreal, Canada, Jun 2017.
21. Peled M, Martin S, Smith A. Youth research academy: a model for engaging youth from government care in community-based research. Paper accepted for presentation at the European Scientific Association on Residential & Family Care for Children and Adolescents (EUSARF), Porto, Portugal, Sept 2018.
22. Peled M, Smith A, Martin S. Research slam: creating a model of meaningfully-engaged youth research in an urban setting. Paper presented at the 14th International Conference on Urban Health (ICUH), Coimbra, Portugal, Sept 2017.

Chapter 19
Conclusion: Next Steps for Investigation and Research

Grant Charles, Curren Warf, and Gary Tennant

Over the last several decades, there has been significant progress in research development concerning the homelessness of adolescents in the United States and in Canada. Many of the key points evolving from contemporary research and practice have been described in the chapters contained in this book. The suggestions below are not meant to supplant the current agendas which are under development, but to augment current trajectories based on contemporary review and gaps identified.

Introduction

The population of homeless youth changes and evolves over the years as does our appreciation of the various influences that shape and characterize the young people making up this population. Our sensitivity to (or neglect of) specific groups including LGBTQ2S (lesbian, gay, transgender, questioning, two-spirited) youth, specific ethnic or racialized minorities (in particular, African American and Indigenous youth), youth with disabilities (including young people with less visible disabilities such as cognitive deficits, childhood attachment disorder, and post-traumatic stress disorder), and migrant youth have been highlighted by several authors in this book.

This concluding chapter will identify a number of key areas that need to be better understood to effectively support the young people we are serving, identify their needs, and prevent homelessness before it begins or intervene as early as possible

G. Charles
School of Social Work, University of British Columbia, Vancouver, BC, Canada

C. Warf (✉)
Department of Pediatrics (Retired), Division of Adolescent Health and Medicine, British Columbia Children's Hospital, University of British Columbia, Vancouver, BC, Canada

G. Tennant
Faculty of Child, Family and Community Studies, Douglas College, Vancouver, BC, Canada

C. Warf, G. Charles (eds.), *Clinical Care for Homeless, Runaway and Refugee Youth*, https://doi.org/10.1007/978-3-030-40675-2_19

before youth are acculturated to the streets. This will require a concerted cross system effort.

Understanding the Early Childhood and Family Precedents to Youth Homelessness and Developing Strategies to Reduce Vulnerability

Youth homelessness is best understood as a series of systemic failures that begin long before a young person experiences homelessness. These systemic failures can begin prenatally with parents struggling with the intergenerational legacy of marginalization, poverty, discrimination, alcoholism, and other substance use and who are provided inadequately funded, developed, and targeted services.

Many adolescent and adult women of childbearing age still confront the lack of ready access to non-stigmatizing full-spectrum contraceptive services, inclusive of medical and surgical termination. Access to full spectrum reproductive health services is essential to enable women to have full control over their reproductive lives, enable conscious decision making, and plan productive lives of their choosing.

Public health education informing potential mothers of the harm to brain development from prenatal alcohol and other drug exposure may reduce exposure and negative influences on the developing fetus. Public health initiatives that put the highest priority on ensuring safe drinking water, in particular a water supply free of lead contamination, can make a significant contribution to the future neurological development of children and youth.

The family context in which children grow is critical to healthy emotional development and development of characteristics of resiliency. Providing all parents with support from family, community, and professional resources to assure stable, loving, and consistent environment for every child is a critical social goal. The child's experience can also be shaped by parental misuse of alcohol and drugs, childhood experiences of emotional neglect or maltreatment, and the impact of exposure intense conflict between parents and caregivers or to intimate partner violence.

Poverty interferes with housing stability and healthy family and child nutrition; systemic approaches to assure that every person and every family has adequate stable housing regardless of income, with continued support as needed, can set up new families for success. Poverty interferes with every parent's ability to provide the loving and stable environment that their children need and that parents strive to provide. The need for assuring stability of housing and food security for families with children is particularly critical in an era characterized by structural barriers including escalating housing prices, incomes of even fully employed people that are far below the cost of living, widespread unemployment, and insecure employment.

Other significant influences shaping early childhood development and family stability include timely availability and funding of preschool and other early childhood services, parental education in early childhood development, and early access to formal child developmental assessments. Inaccessibility or delay of these childhood supports and pediatric screening services result in delayed detection of early developmental issues and lack of support to optimize development.

Improvement in access to universal high-quality childcare, preschool, and primary and secondary education will support the development of children and youth. Caring connections between school personnel and youth can provide a safe haven for children and young people struggling with unstable housing or homelessness.

All of these factors influence eventual life outcomes, including adolescent homelessness, and can be improved by targeted public health initiatives. In fact, there have been many broad policy initiatives in the United States over the years that have made successful contributions such as Project HeadStart, Medicaid, Supplemental Nutrition Assistance Program, Child Health Insurance Program and others. It is essential that the data on outreach, engagement, efficacy, and outcomes be documented regularly so that there are strong arguments to expand and sustain services during periods of budget shortfalls and cutbacks.

Family Poverty Contributing to Adolescent Vulnerability to Homelessness

The problems manifested during adolescence and leading to homelessness may be grounded in challenges that parents face such as lack of secure employment and living wage jobs. These problems are bound to escalate as the gap between family income and cost of living continues to widen. Youth who have been homeless commonly enter the job market with poor educational background and lack of job skills and are at a disadvantage that becomes increasingly significant with the increased role of technological jobs; their futures will disproportionately be shaped by poverty, unstable housing and severe challenges in providing support for their own families. The disparity between the preparation of youth experiencing homelessness and the accessible economic opportunities is a compelling argument for prevention and early intervention of homelessness, continuing education and accessible job skill development. There may be no realistic response to this tragic situation without some kind of guaranteed minimum income, universal health care, rent subsidies, realistic program for food security, and other major, even unprecedented, policy changes in the United States. At a minimum, research documenting the adverse effects of family economic insecurity on child and youth development and health, including relevance to adolescent homelessness, can play an influential role in shaping public policy to address the challenges that families face.

Support for Families Struggling with Insufficient Resources

Supporting families through emergency financial aid, low barrier food programs, public transportation support and increased rent supplements can reduce significant stressors on parents and reduce the incentives for youth to leave home prematurely.

However, growing income disparities and unaffordability of housing for many families has led to increased visibility of homelessness among adults and children in both urban and rural environments. This phenomenon is increasingly apparent with the growth of "tent cities" in many US urban centers. Significant initiatives are called for to provide stable housing for families with children, employment with realistic income to meet the costs of living, including housing, and employment preparation and opportunities accessible to both parents and youth.

Child Neglect, Maltreatment, and Abuse

Risk of child maltreatment and adolescent homelessness is decreased among children growing up in safe and violence-free homes and neighborhoods, among families with adequate housing, secure food sources, and safe drinking water. The absence of any of these protective and resiliency factors increases the risk for eventual homelessness; these are all factors that can occur prior to a young person reaching school age.

The drivers for childhood neglect, maltreatment, and abuse need to be more clearly understood to improve approaches to prevention and intervention and reduce the frequency of removal of children and youth from families. Many factors have been identified including parents' own experience of maltreatment as children; parental anxiety and fear that their children will come to the attention of police or other authorities; parental alcoholism and other substance abuse; parental mental illness; long-term incarceration of parents; lack of social and financial support for children in the event of parental death or serious illness; high levels of economic pressure and insecurity on families; and other factors. Though there has been significant attention in research focused on childhood trauma and maltreatment, the drivers of child maltreatment are less well studied and could provide tools for effective approaches to prevention.

Systemic Threats Faced by Parents in Providing a Stable Home

In the United States, many parents face long-term incarceration in dehumanizing conditions that, in addition to removing them from the care of their children and families, leaves them after release with a record that continues to haunt their prospects for employment. This practice of long-term incarceration disproportionately affects African American men and has had a grave impact on their health and health and well-being of their children, removing parents, largely fathers, from involvement with their children. How can youth be expected to believe in equality before the law and the promise of a just future in the face of the reality of their family experiences? Continued review and documentation of these effects with a new openness to significant policy changes and criminal justice reforms is urgently needed.

Similarly, the criminalization of undocumented immigrant status in the United States has led to the arrest without warning, incarceration, and deportation of thousands of parents in many urban centers. This process leaves their children, including adolescent children who are commonly citizens of the United States, highly traumatized and left without supervision, without warning; thousands of immigrant children and adolescents who do not have documentation are held in indefinite detention. These practices have ripple effects of driving other immigrant families away from accessing necessary public services for their children including health care, nutrition and even school.

Research focused on the consequences for children and youth of disproportionate incarceration and deportation of parents without warning, as well as the consequences of involuntary detention of immigrant children and youth separated from parents, is urgently needed to provide the strongest possible arguments for rational humane social policies. Similarly, research on the benefits for child and family development of social inclusion of immigrants and refugees, family stabilization and safety from deportation, and access to public education and to universal health care can provide objective evidence for an alternative path to deportations and xenophobia.

What can we do to improve support for parents and families to reduce the chances that young people will experience neglect or maltreatment? This involves developing a better understanding of what factors interact with experiences of abuse and violence to increase vulnerability to homelessness. We know that, by far, not all young people who have experienced abuse and violence become homeless, so what other dynamics are at play?

Environment for Children After Removal from Family of Origin

Though it is at times necessary for children or youth to be removed from parental custody, the environment in which they are placed and the relationships that are fostered need to provide a higher level of love, hope, resources, and security from the environment from which they were taken. That is, the challenge of providing a loving, secure, stable, and consistent environment for children after removal from their family of origin must be successfully met, beyond an institutional setting. In addition, removal of children from parental custody requires that the child protective services take responsibility through adolescence and young adulthood to provide for their housing, education, preparation for employment, and transition to self-sufficiency following emancipation. It is also important that there be universal access for youth in care to continued tuition and other needed financial supports for young adults to attend trade school or college, and additional support when youth confront housing and social instability or “failure to fly.” There has been an increased recognition of the obligations of child protective services under these circumstances, and some of the larger programs have invested resources in providing necessary supports, but there remain many challenges that need to be evaluated with the development of, and funding for, effective intervention and transition strategies.

Instability of housing for children and youth is exacerbated in the context of parental mental health problems, alcoholism or other substance abuse, unemployment, and poverty. Notwithstanding these family and parental concerns, attachment of children and adolescents to parents commonly remains quite strong and early intervention with supportive resources may be effective in encouraging sustained engagement of parents with their adolescent children and prevent adolescent homelessness.

Public Schools as a Core Resource for Adolescent Stability and Development

While a well-resourced school system may meaningfully, if insufficiently, compensate for deficiencies in family support and help address risk factors for youth, under-resourced schools where students are unsafe or exposed to interpersonal violence may inadvertently increase the likelihood of future homelessness and undermine schools' capacity to make connections with young people through sports, arts, and other activities. For many unstably housed or homeless youth, schools remain a major source of stability and of contact and relationships with supportive adults. However, schools do not exist in a vacuum and confront many of the same challenges as their surrounding communities.

The broader society's cultural acceptance of, or rejection of, racism, sexism, homophobia, xenophobia, and other forms of discrimination play a critical role in shaping the cultural climate in schools, so that it may be unsafe for youth to be seen as different if diversity is not celebrated, in particular for LGBTQ2S and migrant youth. Schools that are not provided the resources to support children with disabilities and special needs, especially cognitive disabilities, or cannot provide access to appropriate health and mental health services for students, may also be unable to protect these most vulnerable of children. All of these factors contribute significantly to eventual youth homelessness.

Social Biases, School Environment and Youth Homelessness

There has been solid work conducted that both broadens and deepens our understanding of the relationship between specific risk factors and youth homelessness. While we are becoming better at appreciating the relationship between youth homelessness and certain forms of discrimination such as racism, xenophobia, or homophobia, we have only a beginning understanding of other issues that are seen as setting some young people apart from their peers. In some regions there are growing and ominous problems with xenophobia, Islamophobia, or discrimination against migrant or foreign-born youth. All of these forms of bias against children, youth, and their families threaten their emotional and material stability, create a sense of exclusion and marginalization and are important factors in contributing to their inability to access needed resources.

Youth in schools and other settings are commonly subjected to "implicit bias" or social presumptions of their generalized and "intrinsic" characteristics based on appearance or racialization or immigration status. Though these implicit biases are pervasive in society, they play out more commonly with immigrant and ethnic minority youth, in particular African American and Indigenous youth. In fact, the National Academy of Medicine released their 2017 report "Perspectives on Health Equity and Social Determinants of Health" with a sobering but apt section titled "The Character Assassination of Black Males: Some Consequences for Research in Public Health."[1] How can adolescents' experience of stigma be reduced and eliminated? How can the adults who interact with adolescents become more self-aware so that implicit biases are not communicated to or modeled for young people? How can we strengthen the capacity for every individual adult to play a stabilizing, caring, and supportive role in the lives of youth?

Other characteristics that may influence social exclusion include speech or language issues or even factors such as clumsiness or perceived differences in appearance such as being overweight or having a visible disability or difference. Any one of these can contribute to peer exclusion of certain youth, driving "othering" and disconnection.

The same holds true for mental health issues. We can see the connection between mental illness and homelessness, but we do not have as much knowledge about which mental health conditions make a young person more vulnerable to exclusion in school settings. We also need to better understand how early childhood trauma contributes to vulnerability in adolescence in ways that push beyond just the acknowledgement of the connection, and what factors foster resiliency among children and adolescents who have experienced significant trauma and/or loss.

How can the educational system be further utilized to connect young people with responsible adults, secure food access, provide specific learning supports, access sports and arts programs, and what potential does school connectedness have to promoting reunification with parents, extended family, or foster care? An empathetic and supportive relationship with even one adult in the school system for a youth who is isolated or whose family faces instability and exclusion can make the difference whether a youth stays in school or leaves for the streets. How can we systematically assure that every youth at high risk has a genuine opportunity to develop an authentic and supportive relationship with a teacher, librarian,

[1] National Academy of Medicine 2017, Perspectives on health equity and social determinants of health, Alford Young PhD; Section 3, p. 47–61: The character assassination of black males: some consequences for research in public health 2017.

counselor, nurse, youth worker, or other adult in the school setting? How can we foster connections and acceptance for young people who have been marginalized due to racialization, ethnicity, migration status, disability, gender identity, or sexual orientation?

Youth who are highly stressed or who have been subjected to bullying or social exclusion may have difficulty expressing their sense of isolation and exclusion in constructive or clear ways and consequently may face undue disciplinary actions by school personnel or be further excluded by peers. How can we assure that these difficult periods are used as opportunities to create understanding and connections?

Given the recent era in the United States of the mass shootings that have taken place in school settings, with armed guards present and visible on school grounds, and students experiencing repeated frightening rehearsals of what to do, how can young people experience a safe learning environment at school? What will be the long-term impact on youth of encountering these experiences?

Improving the Transition for Adolescents from State Care to Independent Living

A critical area that needs better understanding is the connection between being in state care, including foster care, group homes, and youth justice, and youth homelessness. Given that the US data shows that up to 19% of youth leaving foster care experience homelessness within two years, it is essential that we better understand what factors enable youth to avoid homelessness to guide efforts to better support youth during transition and prepare youth for independence.

While it is clear there is a strong relationship to being in state care and experiencing homelessness, we need to better understand the dynamics at play. For example, is it the experience of neglect or maltreatment, or of disrupted relationships with parents or primary care givers, or of being in care itself that makes young people more vulnerable? Is it the inadequate preparation for transition? Does transition take place too early? Are there too few resources available to support recovery when youth stumble and cannot manage finances or sustain engagement in employment? Is the vulnerability to homelessness a consequence of trauma experienced prior to coming into care, being separated from their family of origin, or are there multiple factors at work?

Clearly, not all young people who have been in care become homeless, so there are the questions of if and how those who become homeless differ from those who do not and what additional barriers they confront. Is it a matter of accessing the right supports at the right time that decreases vulnerability or are there other factors involved? Part of this examination would be an evaluation of how supports, such as post-care counselling, free post-secondary tuition, increased financial support for housing, or continued support and monitoring into young adulthood contribute to decreasing vulnerability to homelessness.

While examining transition and youth homelessness, it is essential that we gain a better understanding about how to improve outcomes for youth who graduate from state care or foster care, or who are released from the youth justice system.

Related to this is the need to better understand the systemic barriers that decrease the likelihood that young people who transition from child protection, youth justice, mental health, and substance misuse systems will engage with available supports. What is needed to better engage with them to avoid homelessness or recover from homelessness once experienced? How can we facilitate youth employment, affordable housing, and social supports? How do we match needed and effective services and supports for specific young people? We need to examine how to reduce the vulnerability of youth in care: promote safe family reconnections, successful placement in foster care, and successful transition out of care to employment preparation, steady employment, or college.

Significantly, American and Canadian parents with sufficient income and stability now support their children into their twenties as the young people navigate the twenty-first-century challenges of short-term contract employment, barely affordable housing, the costs of post-secondary education, student loans, new relationships, and broken hearts. Who supports the homeless youth? How can young people experiencing homelessness, without family support to rely on, gain stability of housing and assurance that their experience of homelessness will be brief and not a predictor for their future?

Reducing Stigma of Lesbian, Gay, Bisexual, Transgender, and Other Sexual Minority Youth

LGBTQ2S youth make up from 20 to 40% of the homeless youth population, far in excess of their prevalence in society. The factors behind this, including social and family exclusion and stigma, need to be closely studied with the goal of increasing family and social acceptance and normalization. LGBTQ2S youth's family environments need to be evaluated to promote acceptance and strengthen connections with parents, siblings, and extended family as well as school. This is an area that needs new initiatives for research and evidence-informed approaches to decreasing social stigma and increasing social and family acceptance.

Reducing the Disproportionate Representation of Ethnic Minority Youth Among the Homeless Population

We also need to more fully understand systemic factors that contribute to the overrepresentation of specific groups of young people within the homeless population. This should include the evaluation of interventions that reduce the multiple inequalities that create disproportionate vulnerability to homelessness among, for example, racialized, Indigenous, immigrant and refugee youth. Factors that play significant roles include intergenerational trauma, historic exclusion and poverty, disproportionate incarceration of parents, the threat of deportation of immigrant parents and loved ones, differing rates of alcohol and other drug misuse, and widespread and historic social and institutional bias that seeps into health-care settings, shapes the attitudes of many in law enforcement, governs housing patterns and quality of community primary and secondary schools, and restricts access to employment. All of these factors, and more, promote a sense of exclusion and reduce educational and employment opportunities for children and youth. There is a great need to view these issues as pressing public health challenges and develop research with evidence-informed interventions to assure that all children are provided equal and meaningful opportunities and do not have their life options restricted by historic inequities.

Reducing Overrepresentation of Youth with Disabilities Among the Homeless Population

We also need to fill in the gaps in our knowledge about specific populations of homeless young people who continue to be largely hidden. This includes young people with cognitive challenges, fetal alcohol effects, and other forms of disabilities. We need to better understand what specific ways these young people differ from their peers among the broader population of homeless youth and what they need that is not currently available to them.

Understanding and Reducing Homelessness Among Other Vulnerable Adolescent Populations

Homelessness among adolescents in rural areas is a poorly studied subject. Little is known about prevalence, resources, drivers, and approaches to addressing this problem. Indigenous (or Native American) youth seem to experience homelessness disproportionately and carry an historic intergenerational legacy of displacement, maltreatment and family disruption, including coerced childhood placement in residential schools, which continues to shape the development of and access to ostensibly supportive resources.

Adolescent mothers who are homeless or at high risk for homelessness have critical additional needs. How can they be rapidly brought into more stable environments? How can their parents be constructively involved and under what circumstances is it realistic? How can their partners or fathers of their children be engaged effectively? What do they and their children need that may be different from other young people who are homeless?

Inclusion of Migrant and Refugee Children and Youth in Stabilization, Housing, Health-Care Access, and Education

Both Canada and the United States have historically welcomed and included migrants, including children and youth, from around the world. The rights of migrants, in particular children, are well recognized through the Universal Declaration of Human Rights and the United Nations Convention on the Rights of the Child. The forces driving migration are far beyond the abilities of individual parents or youth to challenge and include war, ethnic persecution, sex trafficking, threats by gangs, experiences with intimate partner violence, displacement due to climate change, drought, starvation, and more. There are powerful and threatening political and social forces that have emerged, strengthened by racism and xenophobia that promote wholesale deportation of migrants and the refusal of asylum. As care providers for children and youth, we have professional and ethical responsibilities to uphold their fundamental human rights and protect the safety of all children and youth regardless of nationality, ethnicity, religious background or racialization. This includes assuring the safety, housing, education, nutrition, access to health care, stability of families, and granting of asylum without undue barriers.

The World Health Organization holds that universal health coverage is a key aspect of the right to health:

> Ensuring that all people have access to needed promotive, preventive, curative, and rehabilitative health services, of sufficient quality to be effective, while also ensuring that people do not suffer financial hardship when paying for these services.[2]

Inclusion of migrants and refugees in universal health care is a human rights imperative because they may be vulnerable to discrimination and exploitation and their access to health care may be hampered by political, legal, economic, cultural, and practical barriers.[3]

Monitoring and assessing access to health care as advocated by the World Health Organization is essential to assuring that the needs of migrants, in particular migrant children and youth, are able to participate fully in civic life. The definitive statements of the World Health Organization and the United Nations in this regard reflect international consensus on the importance and urgency of including all migrants in existing health-care systems.

These areas cry out for interdisciplinary research, public advocacy, political independence, and professional courage to assure that the rights of all children and youth are respected and protected. In this regard, the American Academy of Pediatrics and the Society for Adolescent Health and Medicine serve as outstanding examples.

---

[2] WHO.int; WHO; A rapid review of evidence-based information, best practices and lessons learned in addressing the health needs of refugees and migrants-report to the World Health Organization April 2018, Cheng, I-Hao et al. Accessed November 2018, p. 120

[3] WHO.int; WHO; A rapid review of evidence-based information, best practices and lessons learned in addressing the health needs of refugees and migrants-report to the World Health Organization April 2018, Cheng, I-Hao et al. Accessed November 2018, p. 26

Improving Engagement and Reducing Homelessness of Youth with Opioid and Other Serious Substance Use Disorders and Mental Health Disorders

While there has been a great deal of work done in recent years about how to engage youth who are experiencing homelessness with existing services, we still need to better understand the dynamics and processes underlying successful and unsuccessful engagement strategies. This holds particularly true for youth who have significant mental health issues and who are involved in serious substance misuse, particularly with opioids. Opioid overdose related to both pharmaceutical opioids and to illicit opioids including fentanyl and heroin has emerged as the leading cause of death for all adults under age 55 in both the United States and Canada; opioid overdose is increasingly found to be the cause of death for adolescents. Opioid misuse commonly starts during adolescence; many of the adolescents who are brought to the emergency department in overdose are homeless, though many retain some contact with parents. Due to the urgency of this situation, new models of care for the management of opioid overdose by adolescents are developing, including certification (or involuntary hospitalization) of adolescents for medical stabilization and engagement in treatment services up to, and including, longer-term certified secure care usually with engagement of parents or other caregivers. We need to document the efficacy of more assertive services such as secure care for young people who abuse opioids and are at high risk for death from overdose. These assertive approaches should be seen as part of a developmentally appropriate approach to care that includes for adults and youth more entrenched in opiate addiction, harm reduction approaches such as access to clean needles, safe injection sites and access to pharmaceuticals as indicated. There is an urgent need to better understand which programs and interventions enable youth to discontinue use and why, or to reduce risk of potentially lethal overdose or HIV infection and translate this research to practice.

Assuring That All Youth, Inclusive of Homeless Youth, Have Access to Health Care, in Particular Contraception and Other Sexual Health Care; HIV Screening, Prevention, and Management; and Protection from Sex Trafficking

All adolescents, and especially adolescents experiencing homelessness, need timely, confidential, full-spectrum access to contraception including free access to condoms, oral contraception, post-coital contraception, injectable contraception, implants, and timely medical or surgical termination. They also need access to PEP and PrEP. Homeless youth, given the common lack of contact with conventional health education, the instability of sexual relationships, and vulnerability to participation in "survival sex" and vulnerability to sexual assault have relatively increased risk of exposure to sexually transmitted infections. These infections, if left untreated, may have long-term effect on fertility among females and can cause a wide spectrum of serious complications. Evaluation and presumptive treatment, including partner treatment, needs to be readily available.

Advances in medical science have made HIV, if not curable, a preventable and treatable chronic infection. This is among the historic advances of medicine of the twentieth and twenty-first centuries. It is essential that all adolescents at risk receive free and confidential access to HIV screening, prevention education, medical prevention, and management. For those youth who use injection drugs, it is essential that they have access to clean needles and syringes and are engaged in other harm reduction approaches and treatment on demand. Ongoing monitoring with early diagnosis and treatment of complications needs to be conducted.

In addition, homelessness for adolescents is a condition that brings with it a very high risk for being victimized by sexual assault or driven into "survival sex" or marketed in sex trafficking. Every young person needs the highest level of sensitivity, patience, understanding, and protection possible to assure their stability and safety. Victims of sex trafficking are commonly highly stigmatized and marginalized youth, including migrants and sexual minority youth. Perpetrators of sexual assault, or individuals engaged in sex trafficking, need to be held accountable by the law to the fullest extent possible. Guidelines for sexual assault evaluation are included in this text; examinations should take place by clinicians trained and experienced in forensic examinations and evidence collection.

These are areas that requires ongoing vigilance and new research initiatives of the consequences and more importantly, of effective strategies to intervene, interrupt, and prevent these traumatic experiences of young people.

Evaluation of Incremental Steps Toward Building Connections with Homeless Youth

There are a number of other areas that would benefit from further research. The first would be an examination of micro interventions that promote a sense of mattering to the young people within our individual services. This principle of showing young people that they matter in life is a powerful instrument of change.

Coordination of Systems to Effectively Engage Youth and Reduce Homelessness

We see an increase in communication between the health care, youth serving community agencies, social service departments, mental health, police, addictions, and education sectors. In Vancouver, BC, for example, youth-serving practitioners in one district have organized a lunchtime roundtable that meets twice a month to share information on programs and to provide updates on specific homeless youth and youth at risk. Practitioners who attend this meeting include street youth workers, health-care providers, addictions workers, community youth workers, police, social work, and school youth workers. Similar interdisciplinary meetings have been organized in other districts in the city to coordinate information on youth at risk. These roundtables provide opportunities for practitioners to learn about programs and build contacts that will help current and future homeless youth. Interdisciplinary collaboration holds the promise to build professional skills, effectively support transition and stabilization of youth experiencing homelessness, build sustainable services and meaningfully engage community partners.

Short-Term and Long-Term Interventions and Strategies

The needs of homeless youth are complex and multifaceted and require short- and long-term interventions sustained over time. Determining what specifically works can be a costly approach, although in the long run it can contribute to creating interventions that are more effective and efficient, saving both time and money. There is little evidence to suggest that complex, systemic issues can actually be solved by a single type of intervention. Integrated service networks are successful in health and human service areas. It would be beneficial to document and more closely examine how principles of an integrated service network address the issue of adolescent and young adult homelessness. These principles could then be used to identify what services should be included in a full service network and how various networks link with each other. This process would need to include the difficult task of sustaining funding for effective and responsive organizational leadership and effective networks of services, while eliminating funding and organizational ownership of ineffective services, to be able to build truly responsive networks.

Professional Openness to Self-Examination and Evaluation

Collectively, we continue to be good at identifying other professionals, organizational and system practices, shortcomings, and policies that contribute to youth homelessness. However, in our experience and observations, we are collectively not so willing to examine how we ourselves may contribute to the problem. Practitioners, organizations, or systems need to take the time to critically examine how and what we do may unwittingly contribute to youth homelessness or unintentionally create barriers to stabilization.

The place to start a significant change process may be in our own backyard. One simple example is about connection. We know that there is a relationship between feelings of disconnection and youth homelessness and that there is an equally strong relationship between feeling connected to others and moving out of homelessness. We may ask ourselves what in our practice, both as individual health practitioners and as members of our professions, contributes to connection and what contributes to disconnection. This may mean evaluating our tone of voice when we are talking to young people, the time we have available to talk with youth or questioning our assumptions about and attitudes towards homeless people or people who misuse substances. It may mean looking through the eyes of a young person at our office space, the attitudes of staff, or design of waiting areas. This would include questioning our practices, policies, and procedures by asking a simple question: Is what we are doing helping or hurting? Once we have answered this question on an individual basis, we should next ask the same question on organizational and systemic levels.

Conclusion

Though the prevalence of homelessness among adolescents remains alarming, we have come a long way in the identification of homeless youth, in developing professional collaboratives, in monitoring and identifying high-risk populations, and in identifying the risks to long-term youth development. Some communities and governments have developed housing and longer-term housing and education supports for homeless youth. Given that we are building on the substantive research that has already been conducted, we can approach the challenging work of helping stabilize this very-high-risk population of young people and contribute to their promising future despite the many challenges that have been placed in their path.

Excellent resources on contemporary research on adolescent homelessness include:

U.S. Resources on Youth Homelessness

- US Interagency Council on Homelessness; Preventing and Ending Youth Homelessness, A Coordinated Community Response
  - https://www.usich.gov/resources/uploads/asset_library/Youth_Homelessness_Coordinated_Response.pdf
- National Academy of Medicine 2017, Perspectives on Health Equity and Social Determinants of Health
  - https://nam.edu/perspectives-on-health-equity-and-social-determinants-of-health/
- US Interagency Council on Homelessness; Criteria and Benchmarks for Achieving the Goal of Ending Youth Homelessness
  - https://www.usich.gov/resources/uploads/asset_library/Youth-Criteria-and-Benchmarks-revised-Feb-2018.pdf;

- Ending Youth Homelessness, Guidebook Series: Promising Program Models; US Department of Housing and Urban Development's Office of Community Planning and Development
  - https://files.hudexchange.info/resources/documents/Ending-Youth-Homelessness-Promising-Program-Models.pdf
- LP Pope, Housing for Homeless Youth, National Alliance to End Homelessness
  - www.endhomelessness.org

Canadian Resources on Adolescent Homelessness

- The Homeless Hub:
  - https://www.homelesshub.ca/

Canadian Observatory on Homelessness

At a national level the Canadian Observatory on Homelessness (COH) out of York University has developed a "non-partisan research and policy partnership between academics, policy and decision makers, service providers and people with lived experience of homelessness". The COH completed the first pan Canadian survey of homeless youth in 2016 and provided a series of federal, provincial and community recommendations:

- https://www.homelesshub.ca/about-homelessness/population-specific/youth.
- https://www.homelesshub.ca/resource/what-works-and-whom-framework-promising-practices

Additional findings and the recommendations can be reviewed in the Executive Summary of the report:

- https://www.homelesshub.ca/sites/default/files/attachments/WithoutAHome-execsummary.pdf

Systems Planning Collective with Four Part Learning Modules

The Systems Planning Collective is led by *A Way Home Canada*, *Canadian Observatory on Homelessness* and *Turner Strategies* and is dedicated to helping communities and governments to prevent and end all forms of homelessness in Canada by supporting evidence-based systems planning, capacity building and technical assistance and has released a four-part learning module series developed to help communities across Canada take actionable steps towards systems planning for prevention and sustained exits from homelessness.

- https://www.homelesshub.ca/hub-solution/systems-planning-collective

Index

C. Warf, G. Charles (eds.), *Clinical Care for Homeless, Runaway and Refugee Youth*, https://doi.org/10.1007/978-3-030-40675-2

Z